Review of NEUROSCIENCE

REVIEW OF
NEUROSCIENCE

Duane E. Haines, Ph.D.

Professor and Chairman
Department of Anatomy
and Professor of Neurosurgery
The University of Mississippi Medical Center
Jackson, Mississippi

John A. Lancon, M.D.

Assistant Professor of Neurosurgery
Department of Neurosurgery
The University of Mississippi Medical Center
Jackson, Mississippi

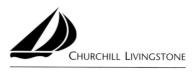

CHURCHILL LIVINGSTONE

An Imprint of Elsevier Science
New York Edinburgh London Philadelphia

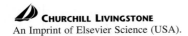
An Imprint of Elsevier Science (USA).

The Curtis Center
Independence Square West
Philadelphia, Pennsylvania 19106

Notice

Neuroscience is an ever-changing field. Standard safety precautions must be followed, but as new research and clinical experience broaden our knowledge, changes in treatment and drug therapy may become necessary or appropriate. Readers are advised to check the most current product information provided by the manufacturer of each drug to be administered to verify the recommended dose, the method and duration of administration, and contraindications. It is the responsibility of the treating physician, relying on experience and knowledge of the patient, to determine dosages and the best treatment for each individual patient. Neither the Publisher nor the editor assumes any liability for any injury and/or damage to persons or property arising from this publication.

The Publisher

Library of Congress Cataloging-in-Publication Data

Haines, Duane, E.
Review of neuroscience / Duane E. Haines, John A. Lancon.–1st ed.
  p. ; cm.
    ISBN 0-443-06625-6
  1. Neurophysiology.   I. Lancon, John A.   II. Title.
    [DNLM: 1. Central Nervous System–physiology.   2. Central Nervous System–anatomy
  & histology.   3. Nervous System Physiology.   WL 300   H153r2003]
  QP355.2 .H35 2003
  612.8–dc21

                                                           2002031449

Acquisitions Editor: Jason Malloy
Developmental Editor: Kevin Kochanski
Production Manager: Norman Stellander

BS

Printed in the China.

Last digit is the print number: 9   8   7   6   5   4   3   2   1

PREFACE

Neuroscience, as taught to medical, dental, and a variety of other students entering the medical profession (as broadly defined), is somewhat different from other basic sciences in three respects. First, most neurobiology courses start by stressing fundamental concepts and then building on these throughout the course. There is a particular emphasis on correlating the basic science concepts with the reality of their clinical application. Second, during their clinical years, students will revisit a very high percentage of what they learned in their first neuroscience course. In other words, a great deal of what they learn is directly transferable to, and applicable in, the clinical setting. Third, neurologic deficits resulting from rather small lesions may have a profound impact on the quality of life, or even on life itself. For example, a lesion of the cervical spinal cord, a structure no greater in diameter than one's little finger, can result in complete paralysis of movement or even in the inability to breathe! The formation of microscopic plaques, and the related loss of neurons, can completely alter the personality of a patient.

The questions in *Review of Neuroscience* are designed to provide a comprehensive review of neuroscience, with a particular emphasis on its applicability to clinical issues. While based primarily on *Fundamental Neuroscience*, second edition (FN2e), some questions draw on the broad knowledge base that the student should have acquired by the end of the first year or the beginning of the second year. Although following the general organization of *Fundamental Neuroscience*, the vast majority of the questions cover topics that are basic to neuroscience as a subject in general. In this respect, the questions and answers in this review include concepts, topics, and clinical examples covered in many neuroscience courses regardless of the primary textbook(s) used in a particular course. These questions should be useful to students in their initial learning experience, in preparation for course examinations, as well as in preparation for standardized examinations.

A unique innovation in this review regards the illustrations and how they are presented. First, illustrations are used liberally and include MRI and CT scans, photographs, and line drawings that show representative structures and lesions. Second, all illustrations showing structures, pathways, and lesions are presented in a format/orientation that correctly reflects how that particular part of the central nervous system (brain or spinal cord) is viewed on MRI or CT images in the clinical environment. For example, on an axial MRI scan of the medulla oblongata, the pyramids, representing the anterior (ventral) medullary surface and containing corticospinal fibers, are "up" in the image, and the fourth ventricle representing the posterior (dorsal) aspect of the medulla is "down" in the image. Recognizing the reality of how brain structures are viewed on MRI and CT scans in the clinical setting, the drawings of the brain and especially those of the brainstem in this review are oriented to match the MRI/CT view. This allows the user to review structures, vascular patterns, pathways, and deficits resulting from trauma and/or lesions in the orientation in which these same parts of the central nervous system are seen in the clinical setting. This represents the direct translation of important basic science information to the clinical setting without intervening, and potentially confusing, steps.

The questions in *Review of Neuroscience* are formulated in the general style used by the USMLE. The most frequently used style is the *single one best answer* question. Single one best answer questions consist of a statement or question followed by a series of choices, usually lettered A, B, C, D, E. Although some choices may be *partially correct*, there is only one best answer. These questions may briefly describe a clinical situation (patient vignette version or application of knowledge version) or may require the recall of an important fact (isolated fact version or non-vignette version) as related to a general clinical example or a point of general knowledge of the basic sciences as applied to a clinical issue.

The other style of question used in this review is the sample item set. This consists of a brief description of a patient, including deficits, laterality of these deficits, and other related information followed by a series of questions (usually 2 to 4) specifically related to this patient. In general, the questions in this sample item set follow the single one best answer approach. This style of question allows a diagnosis of the patient's condition by presenting a series of deficits followed by questions that, through a series of logical steps, lead to an appropriate conclusion.

The correct answer to each question is given at the end of the chapter along with a concise description of why that particular response is correct. In most cases the correct answer is referenced to *Fundamental Neuroscience*, second edition, by the specific page number(s). The exceptions are those questions that rely on a general knowledge base. In some cases the answer is referenced to page numbers that are in chapters other than the one from which the question is generated. For the large part, illustrations are taken from *Fundamental Neuroscience*, second edition. Recognizing that the physician encounters a slight variation on a general theme every time he or she looks at an MRI or CT scan of a new patient, however, some additional representative images are included.

The questions in this review are purposefully challenging. While some are to the point and the single best answer is clear, other questions are more three dimensional and require analysis, integration, and interpretation to arrive at the correct response. This seems to be an appropriate approach since the physician must analyze, integrate, and interpret information to arrive at the correct diagnosis of the neurologically compromised patient. This review does not replace a textbook. Rather, it can be used to assess general progress at any point during a course, to practice/review before examinations

in a course, and to practice/review prior to taking standardized examinations.

A review experience should also be a learning experience. Consequently, all the questions and answers in this review cover basic neuroscience facts and especially how this information applies to a clinical situation or example. Some questions are specifically designed to broaden the user's knowledge base by requiring the integration of information from prior educational experiences and/or by providing new but related information in the answer.

Recognizing that education is a dynamic, ongoing, and ever-changing endeavor, we welcome suggestions, comments, and corrections from users of this review.

D.E. Haines, Ph.D.

J.A. Lancon, M.D.

ACKNOWLEDGMENTS

We wish to express our sincere appreciation to those individuals who have been essential to the completion of this project. Churchill Livingstone, the publisher of *Fundamental Neuroscience*, second edition (2002), has generously allowed us to borrow images, and obviously a lot of text information, as we developed these review questions and answers.

We are appreciative of the time and effort of Drs. J. David Dickman, S.G. Pat Hardy, Craig K. Henkel, James B. Hutchins, James C. Lynch, Paul J. May, Gregory A. Mihailoff, John P. Naftel, and Robin W. Rockhold in the construction of some questions for this project. Photographs of new MRI and CT images were made by Mr. G. William (Bill) Armstrong (Director of Biomedical Photography at The University of Mississippi Medical Center), Mr. Chuck Runyan, Mr. Robert Gray, and Mr. William (Bill) A. Buhner II (Director of Computer Graphics at The University of Mississippi Medical Center). Ms. Jean Henderson created the visual fields used in Chapter 20. We also express our appreciation to Lippincott Williams & Wilkins for permission to use two MRI images (Figs. 2–37A and 4–17, upper left) from their publication *Neuroanatomy, An Atlas of Structures Section and Systems*, fifth edition (2000) in this review. We are indebted to Ms. Amanda Ellis for tracking down new MRI and CT images and to Ms. Lisa Boyd for her timely work correcting the text in a number of chapters. Ms. Katherine Squires typed all chapters and the prefatory material. We greatly appreciate her cooperation and patience as we attempted to complete this project in a timely manner.

We also wish to express our appreciation to Mr. Jason Malley, our editor at Elsevier Science (USA), for his encouragement and numerous helpful hints; to Mr. Kevin Kochanski (Mr. Malley's assistant) for his help in getting everything into the pipeline; to Ms. Susan Kelly for reviewing drafts of our questions/answers and for her helpful suggestions; to Mr. Norman Stellander, Production Manager, Elsevier Science (USA), and his staff for putting the text and images into a production format, and to Churchill Livingstone and Elsevier Health Science for support and confidence in this project. Last, but certainly not least, we express our sincere appreciation to Dr. Gretchen C. Haines for her skilled proofreading of the chapters. Her attention to details revealed inconsistencies (spelling, punctuation, and otherwise) that had escaped us.

As the authors we are responsible for any oversights that may be discovered in this work. We welcome comments, suggestions, and corrections from our colleagues and from students.

REMEMBER, THINK CLINICAL

One unique innovation in *Review of Neuroscience* is the presentation of all images in clinical orientation, that is, a presentation of basic science information images (of tracts, nuclei, blood supply, lesions, and so on) in an orientation that directly correlates with how the corresponding areas of the brain are seen in the clinical environment.

The vast majority of users of this review will be embarking on a medically related career (as a practitioner or instructor/faculty member) or may already be in advanced standing (resident, fellow). Therefore, it seems only logical and appropriate to present images in a format that correctly reflects how these brain areas are viewed on MRI or CT images. This is especially important when describing a patient vignette in which *laterality of lesion versus deficit in an essential issue*. When reviewing basic science information in preparation for a clinical experience or examination, the basic science information should be presented in a format that flows seamlessly into its clinical application.

When viewing an MRI or CT image in the axial plane, the forebrain is cut parallel to the long axis of the hemisphere (the frontal-occipital axis) and perpendicular to the coronal plane. The image is viewed as if the patient were lying on his or her back and the physician is standing at the patient's feet looking toward the patient's head. Consequently, the physician's right side is the left side of the image (and of the patient) and the physician's left is the right side of the image (and of the patient). When the axial plane is extended through the brainstem, this part of the central nervous system is cut, more or less, in cross-section. The anterior (ventral) aspect of the brainstem is "up" in the image and the posterior (dorsal) aspect of the

brainstem is "down" in the image. This same orientation extends into the spinal cord; the anterior horn is "up" and the posterior horn is "down."

When viewing an MRI or CT image in the coronal plane, the forebrain is cut in a plane parallel to the coronal suture and perpendicular to the long axis of the hemisphere (a line passing through the frontal-occipital axis). The image is viewed as if the physician were looking at the face of the patient; the physician's right is the left side of the image and the left side of the patient. The physician's left is the patient's right. While the forebrain is viewed in coronal images, the brainstem is cut in an oblique plane. This is due to the fact that there is a sharp bend in the long axis of the nervous system at the midbrain-diencephalon junction. The coronal plane through the forebrain extends obliquely through the brainstem. This requires skill in interpreting coronal images that extend into and through the brainstem.

When viewing an MRI or CT of the brain in the sagittal plane, the frontal lobe is to the left in the image and the occipital lobe is to the right. The cerebellum is inferior to the occipital lobe and, along with the brainstem, caudal to the diencephalon.

The approach of emphasizing basic science information in a clinical orientation yields two important benefits. First, the right/left orientation within images is constantly reviewed and reinforced. This includes the essentials of understanding the laterality of the lesion as correlated with the deficits resulting therefrom. Second, basic science information presented and reviewed in this way can be directly applied to a clinical question without the confusing intervening steps of going from an "anatomical orientation" to a "clinical orientation".

ILLUSTRATION CREDITS

Figures 1–1, 1–2, 3–1, 3–2, 5–1, 6–1, 6–2, 6–3, 6–4, 7–3, 7–4, 7–5, 7–6, 8–1, 8–2, 8–3, 8–4, 8–5, 9–1, 9–2, 9–3, 9–4, 9–5, 10–2, 10–3, 10–5, 10–6, 10–8, 10–9, 12–2, 12–4, 12–5, 12–6, 12–7, 13–2, 13–3, 13–4, 13–5, 13–8, 14–1, 14–2, 14–4, 14–5, 15–1, 15–2, 15–3, 15–4, 15–6, 16–1, 16–2, 16–3, 16–4, 16–6, 16–7, 17–1, 17–2, 17–4, 17–5, 17–6, 19–1, 21–1, 21–2, 21–4, 24–2, 24–3, 24–5, 24–6, 24–8, 24–9, 24–10, 24–11, 26–1, 30–1, 30–2, 30–3, 32–2, 32–5, 32–6, 33–1, 33–2, 33–3, and 33–4 are from Haines DE: Review of Neuroscience. Philadelphia, Churchill Livingstone, 2002.

Figures 7–1 and 7–2 are from Haines DE: On the question of a subdural space. Anatomical Record 230:3–21, 1991.

Figures 10–1, 15–5, 15–8, 16–5, 16–8, 17–3, 17–9, and 24–12 are from Haines DE: Neuroanatomy: An Atlas of Structures, Sections, and Systems, 5th ed. Philadelphia, Lippincott Williams & Wilkins, 2000.

Figure 13–1 is from Haines: Neuroanatomy: An Atlas of Structures, Sections, and Systems, 5th ed. Philadelphia, Lippincott Williams & Wilkins, 2000. Modified from the original.

Figures 14–3, 14–5, 14–6, and 14–7 are modified from Parent A: Carpenter's Human Neuroanatomy, 9th ed. Philadelphia, Lippincott Williams & Wilkins, 1995.

Figures 15–7 and 15–10 are adapted from Haymaker W, Anderson E, Nauta WJH: The Hypothalamus. Springfield, Ill, Charles C Thomas, 1969.

Figure 15–9 is modified from Haines DE: Neuroanatomy: An Atlas of Structures, Sections, and Systems, 5th ed. Philadelphia, Lippincott Williams & Wilkins, 2000.

Figures 17–7, 17–8, 17–10, 24–1, 24–4, and 24–7 are adapted from Penfield W, Rasmussen T: The Cerebral Cortex of Man: A Clinical Study of Localization of Function. New York, Hafner Publishing, 1968.

CONTENTS

Essential Concepts

CHAPTER 1

Orientation to the Structure and Imaging of the Central Nervous System

1. A 66-year-old man presents with paralysis of the upper and lower extremities on the right and paralysis of most movement of the left eye. Which of the following represents the best "localizing sign" in this patient?

- ○ (A) Paralysis of the right upper extremity
- ○ (B) Paralysis of the right lower extremity
- ○ (C) Paralysis of upper and lower extremities
- ○ (D) Paralysis of most eye movements on the left
- ○ (E) Sensory deficits on the right side

2. A patient presents to the emergency department with a sensory deficit involving the same side of the face and body. This would most likely suggest a lesion in which of the following structures?

- ○ (A) Cerebral hemisphere
- ○ (B) Brainstem
- ○ (C) Cervical spinal cord
- ○ (D) Lumbosacral spinal cord
- ○ (E) Peripheral nerve roots

3. During a routine physical examination the physician discovers a lemon-sized tumor in the small intestine of a 42-year-old man. This portion of the gut is composed predominately of which of the following?

- ○ (A) Smooth muscle only
- ○ (B) Smooth muscle and cardiac muscle
- ○ (C) Smooth muscle and glandular epithelium
- ○ (D) Smooth muscle and striated muscle

- ○ (E) Smooth muscle, cardiac muscle, and glandular epithelium

4. A 69-year-old woman is brought to the emergency department after being found unresponsive. On examination she is unconscious and has abnormalities of eye movement. An MRI reveals a lesion in the midbrain. Which of the following cranial nerves would most likely be directly involved in this lesion?

- ○ (A) CNs II, III, and IV
- ○ (B) CN III only
- ○ (C) CNs III and IV
- ○ (D) CNs IV and V
- ○ (E) CNs III, IV, and VI

5. Which of the following represents the most likely location of neurons of the visceromotor (autonomic) nervous system?

- ○ (A) Central nervous system only
- ○ (B) Peripheral nervous system only
- ○ (C) Peripheral ganglia
- ○ (D) Intramural ganglia in the gut only
- ○ (E) Central and peripheral nervous systems

6. A 57-year-old woman presents with symptoms that have progressed slowly over several years. The MRI of this patient, shown below, indicates that the tumor causing this deficit is located in which of the following?

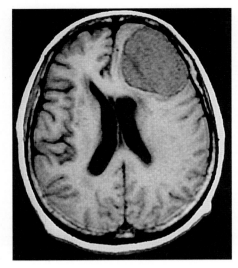

Figure 1–1

○ (A) Right cerebral hemisphere
○ (B) Left cerebral hemisphere
○ (C) Right side of the patient's brainstem
○ (D) Left side of the patient's brainstem

7.   A 12-year-old girl presents with a decreased level of consciousness and range of motor and sensory deficits. After a series of tests, the examining physician concludes that this patient has a tumor infiltrating the "brainstem." Which of the following represents the most likely location of this lesion?

○ (A) Medulla oblongata
○ (B) Medulla and pons
○ (C) Medulla, pons, and cerebellum
○ (D) Medulla, pons, and midbrain
○ (E) Medulla, pons, cerebellum, and midbrain

8.   A 62-year-old man presents with difficulty in speaking and swallowing. His voice is hoarse and gravelly. The physician concludes that this lesion involves the nuclei of cranial nerves IX, X, and XII. This lesion is located in which of the following parts of the nervous system?

○ (A) Spinal cord
○ (B) Medulla
○ (C) Pons
○ (D) Midbrain
○ (E) Thalamus

9.   A 19-year-old man presents with motor deficits on one side of the body and sensory deficits on the other side of the body after an automobile collision. It is most likely that the lesion causing these deficits is located in which of the following parts of the nervous system?

○ (A) Spinal cord
○ (B) Medulla
○ (C) Pons
○ (D) Midbrain
○ (E) Telencephalon

10.   A 38-year-old woman presents with neurological symptoms that wax and wane. The physician orders an image that shows blood vessels, brain structures in detail and white (hyperintense) cerebrospinal fluid. Which of the following most correctly describes this image?

○ (A) CT
○ (B) CT bone window
○ (C) MRI, T_1-weighted
○ (D) MRI, T_2-weighted
○ (E) PET

11.   A 78-year-old man presents with weakness of the muscles of mastication and of facial expression, both on the same side of the face. The examining physician concludes that the lesion involves the nuclei of cranial nerves V and VII. Which of the following parts of the nervous system is the most likely site of this lesion?

○ (A) Medulla
○ (B) Pons
○ (C) Midbrain
○ (D) Thalamus
○ (E) Telencephalon

12.   A 23-year-old woman presents with progressive weakness of muscles that move the eyes followed by weakness of the extremities. The attending physician concludes that this patient has a neurotransmitter disease. Which of the following structures is most likely the specific site of the dysfunction leading to these deficits?

○ (A) Neuron cell body
○ (B) Dendrites
○ (C) Axon
○ (D) Sensory receptor
○ (E) Synapse

13.   An elderly patient presents with weakness of the upper and lower extremities combined with a loss of most eye movement. The deficits seen in this patient represent injury to a functional system plus a brain region. This lesion most likely includes which of the following?

○ (A) Corticospinal tract and hypoglossal nerve
○ (B) Monosynaptic reflex arc
○ (C) Corticospinal tract and oculomotor nerve
○ (D) Spinal cord only
○ (E) Corticospinal tract and facial nerve

14.   A 67-year-old man presents with a motor deficit that, based on an MRI, the attending physician concludes is located in the basal nuclei (basal ganglia). This indicates that the lesion is most likely located in which of the following parts of the brain?

○ (A) Medulla
○ (B) Pons
○ (C) Midbrain
○ (D) Thalamus
○ (E) Telencephalon

15.   A physician taps the patellar tendon of a 22-year-old woman and notes that the resulting reflex (knee jerk)

is less active than normal. Which of the following most accurately describes this reflex?

- ○ (A) Areflexia
- ○ (B) Hyporeflexia
- ○ (C) Hyperreflexia
- ○ (D) Crossed deficit
- ○ (E) Localizing sign

16. A 71-year-old man presents to the emergency department with a severe headache, nausea, and a decreased level of consciousness. The emergency department physician suspects an acute subarachnoid hemorrhage. Which of the following provides the best diagnostic evidence in this case?

- ○ (A) X-ray
- ○ (B) CT
- ○ (C) MRI, T1-weighted image
- ○ (D) MRI, T2-weighted image
- ○ (E) PET scan

17. A 62-year-old farmer was found unresponsive in his barn when he failed to show up for the evening meal. The emergency department physician suspects a subacute (4 + hours old) vascular lesion. Which of the following most likely provides the best diagnostic evidence to support the physician's suspicions?

- ○ (A) X-ray
- ○ (B) CT
- ○ (C) MRI, T1-weighted image
- ○ (D) MRI, T2-weighted image

18. A 31-year-old man is brought to the emergency department after an automobile collision. Following his examination the emergency department physician writes "crossed deficits" on the patient's chart. This indicates a lesion in, or to, which of the following?

- ○ (A) Spinal cord
- ○ (B) Cerebral cortex
- ○ (C) Brainstem
- ○ (D) Peripheral nerves
- ○ (E) Roots of cranial nerves

19. A 16-year-old boy is examined in the emergency department within 45 minutes of a motorcycle collision. The attending physician suspects a potential skull fracture and intracranial hemorrhage. Which of the following would the physician most likely order?

- ○ (A) MRI, T1-weighted image
- ○ (B) MRI, T2-weighted image
- ○ (C) X-ray
- ○ (D) CT
- ○ (E) Brain biopsy

20. A 39-year-old man presents to the neurosurgeon's office with a variety of ill-defined signs and symptoms that have progressed slowly over several months. Suspecting a brain tumor, which of the following would the physician most likely order?

- ○ (A) CT
- ○ (B) MRI, T2-weighted image
- ○ (C) X-ray
- ○ (D) MRI enhanced with a gadolinium
- ○ (E) MRI, T1-weighted image

21. A 67-year-old woman is diagnosed with a brain tumor. During the ensuing neurologic examination the physician discovers that all of her deep tendon reflexes are more active than normal. Which of the following most accurately describes this reflex?

- ○ (A) Hyperreflexia
- ○ (B) Localizing sign
- ○ (C) Areflexia
- ○ (D) Alternating hemiplegia
- ○ (E) Hyporeflexia

22. A 21-year-old woman presents with a small tumor (confirmed by MRI) that has resulted in a change in her eating habits and sexual behavior. She now eats excessively and has become promiscuous. Which of the following represents the most likely location of this lesion?

- ○ (A) Telencephalon
- ○ (B) Hypothalamus
- ○ (C) Midbrain
- ○ (D) Pons
- ○ (E) Medulla

23. A 1-year-old child is brought to the pediatric neurologist. Examination of this infant reveals a somnolent patient with an apparent mass in the parietal-occipital area of the skull. The neurologist orders the MRI shown here. Which of the following most accurately describes this image?

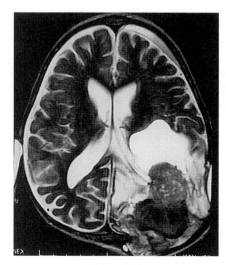

Figure 1–2

- ○ (A) X-ray
- ○ (B) CT
- ○ (C) CT, bone window
- ○ (D) MRI, T1-weighted image
- ○ (E) MRI, T2-weighted image

24. A 19-year-old man is brought to the emergency department after an automobile collision. He has face and head injuries and is semicomatose and when his patellar tendon is tapped there is no response. Which of the following most accurately describes the state of his patellar tendon reflexes?

- ○ (A) Hyperreflexia
- ○ (B) Hyporeflexia
- ○ (C) Areflexia
- ○ (D) Alternating hemiparesis
- ○ (E) Crossed deficit

ANSWERS

1.   **(D)** Long tract signs, such as motor and sensory losses of the extremities, could indicate a lesion at many different levels of the neuraxis. However, these tracts pass through the midbrain. Significant deficits of eye movement in this patient indicate a lesion of the oculomotor nerve, the nucleus of which is located in the midbrain and the root of which exits the midbrain. In fact, the corticospinal tract is quite close to the root of the oculomotor nerve in anteromedial areas of the mesencephalon.
FN2e 8–9

2.   **(A)** In general, sensory and/or motor deficits located on the same side of the face and body signify damage to a cerebral hemisphere. Lesions of the brainstem usually result in alternating deficits or crossed deficits (face/head one side, body opposite side) whereas damage to the spinal cord will result in deficits of the body below the lesion with sparing of the head and/or face.
FN2e 8–9

3.   **(C)** Visceral organs, when considered collectively, are composed of smooth muscle, cardiac muscle, or glandular epithelium or a combination of these tissues. In the case of the small intestines, smooth muscle and glandular epithelium are present but cardiac muscle is not.
FN2e 4

4.   **(C)** The cranial nerve nuclei of the midbrain are the oculomotor (III), trochlear (IV), and the mesencephalic nucleus of the trigeminal nerve (V). Deficits would be seen that would potentially relate to cranial nerves III and IV.
FN2e 7

5.   **(E)** Visceromotor neurons are found in both central (preganglionic) and peripheral (postganglionic) nervous systems. Whereas some peripheral ganglia are made up of visceromotor cell bodies, other peripheral ganglia are sensory in function.
FN2e 4–5

6.   **(B)** This is an axial view of the cerebral hemisphere. When viewing the axial MRI, the physician is looking at the image as if the patient is lying on his or her back and the physician is looking from the feet toward the head.

Consequently, the physician's right is always the patient's left.
FN2e 12–14

7.   **(D)** The brainstem is the medulla, pons, and midbrain; the cerebellum is considered a suprasegmental structure.
FN2e 7

8.   **(B)** The nuclei of cranial nerves IX (glossopharyngeal), X (vagus), and XII (hypoglossal) are located in the medulla. The difficulty in speaking and the gravelly voice reflect damage to the nucleus ambiguus, which innervates muscles served by the glossopharyngeal and vagus nerves, and to the hypoglossal nucleus. These nerves innervate pharyngeal and laryngeal muscles and muscles of the tongue.
FN2e 7

9.   **(A)** A lesion in the spinal cord results in deficits of the body only (no cranial nerve deficits) and may result in a motor deficit on one side of the body and a sensory deficit (pain and temperature loss) on the opposite side of the body.
FN2e 9

10.   **(D)** In a T1-weighted image of the brain, cerebrospinal fluid is white (hyperintense), bone is very dark, gray matter (neuron cell bodies) is light gray (isointense), white matter (axons) is black (hypointense), and muscle is dark gray to black. In a T2-weighted image, cerebrospinal fluid is hyperintense, gray matter is dark gray, and white matter is light gray.
FN2e 10–12

11.   **(B)** The motor nucleus of the trigeminal nerve (mastication) and the motor nucleus of the facial nerve (facial expression) are located in the pons, with the facial nucleus at caudal levels and the trigeminal nucleus at midpontine levels. Both of these nuclei innervate muscles on the ipsilateral side of the face.
FN2e 7

12.   **(E)** A neurotransmitter disease is one that disrupts the activity of the synapse. This may be reflected in a decrease in the amount of neurotransmitter extruded into the synaptic cleft or a decrease in the number of receptors on the postsynaptic membrane available to the neurotransmitter. This result is a decrease in the efficiency of the synapse.
FN2e 5

13.   **(C)** Corticospinal fibers originate in the cerebral cortex and course through all segments of the brain to end in the spinal cord; this is an important long tract, representing one important part of the motor system. As these fibers pass through the midbrain (an important region), they pass in close association with the exiting fibers of the oculomotor nerve.
FN2e 8–9

14.   **(E)** The basal nuclei (ganglia) are located within the cerebral hemisphere, which is part of the telencephalon. Lesions of the basal nuclei result in motor deficits. One commonly known disease of the basal ganglia is Parkinson disease.
FN2e 7

15. **(B)** When a reflex is depressed or less active than normal, it is hyporeflexia. Areflexia refers to a completely absent reflex, and hyperreflexia refers to an excessively active reflex.
FN2e 6

16. **(B)** With CT, acute blood (generally less than 3 hours after a hemorrhage) appears white relative to the gray color of the brain and the black color of normal cerebrospinal fluid.
FN2e 11–12; 119

17. **(D)** This patient had a stroke several hours before being examined by the physician. Ischemia/infarction appears as light gray to white (hyperintense) in T2-weighted MRI images.
FN2e 11–12

18. **(C)** The term *crossed deficits* refers to deficits on one side of the body and the opposite side of the face. Such signs and symptoms usually indicate a lesion in the brainstem. Sometimes these are called alternating (or alternate) deficits.
FN2e 8–9

19. **(D)** CT is especially useful in visualizing bone (it appears very white) and blood in an acute time frame (it also appears white to very white). Because CT of the brain only takes a few minutes to complete, it is particularly useful in evaluating traumatic brain injuries and allows rapid visualization of hematomas, contusions, and fractures.
FN2e 10–12

20. **(D)** Most tumors will show clearly on MRI when enhanced with gadolinium. Without enhancement, the tumor may, or may not, be especially obvious. The tumor enhances because the blood vessels invading the growing tumor do not have a blood-brain barrier and the gadolinium enters the extracellular space. Because of the greater resolution of MRI compared with CT, MRI provides more useful information regarding involvement of specific structures and blood vessels to assist the neurosurgeon in planning resection.
FN2e 12

21. **(A)** When a reflex is excessively brisk or exaggerated, it is hyperreflexia. A reflex that is diminished is hyporeflexia, and a reflex that is absent is areflexia.
FN2e 6

22. **(B)** The hypothalamus is a comparatively small part of the thalamus that is especially concerned with autonomic (visceromotor) functions. (The thalamus is also commonly called the diencephalon.) These functions are very important and include sexual functions, feeding behavior, regulation of body temperature, hormone production, and influence of many visceral centers in the brainstem and spinal cord.
FN2e 7

23. **(E)** In the T2-weighted image, bone is very dark, white matter and gray matter of the brain are shades of gray, cerebrospinal fluid is white, and fat is light gray.
FN2e 10–12

24. **(C)** The complete lack of reflexes is areflexia. Hyporeflexia refers to deep tendon reflexes that are depressed, whereas hyperreflexia refers to reflexes that are excessively brisk.
FN2e 6

CHAPTER 2

The Cell Biology of Neurons and Glia

1. A 31-year-old woman presents with weakness of the extraocular muscles and muscles of the extremities. The attending physician concludes that the patient's own immune system is producing antibodies that attack the ligand-gated synaptic channels in the neuromuscular junction. This patient is most likely suffering from which of the following?

   ○ (A) Multiple sclerosis
   ○ (B) Myasthenia gravis
   ○ (C) Lambert-Eaton syndrome
   ○ (D) Dementia
   ○ (E) Huntington disease

2. Which of the following structures is not typically found in normal healthy axons?

   ○ (A) Synaptic vesicles
   ○ (B) Ribosomes
   ○ (C) Neurofilaments
   ○ (D) Mitochondria
   ○ (E) Microtubules

3. A 37-year-old woman presents with a tumor in the white matter of the brain that has originated from the myelin-forming cells of the CNS. Which of the following represents this cell type?

   ○ (A) Fibrous astrocyte
   ○ (B) Microglia cell
   ○ (C) Oligodendrocyte
   ○ (D) Macrophage
   ○ (E) Protoplasmic astrocyte

4. A 21-year-old woman presents with neurologic deficits that wax and wane over time. After a series of tests, her physician concludes that she has a breakdown/degeneration of myelin sheaths in the CNS resulting in an interruption of the propagation of action potentials on the axon and a likely invasion of the site by the processes of reactive astrocytes. This patient is most likely suffering from which of the following?

   ○ (A) Wallerian degeneration
   ○ (B) Myasthenia gravis
   ○ (C) Oligodendroglioma
   ○ (D) Muscular dystrophy
   ○ (E) Multiple sclerosis

5. A neuropathologist examines the biopsy specimen of a brain tumor from a 48-year-old man and discovers, within the periphery of the lesion, the most common neuronal cell type in the adult CNS. Which of the following most accurately specifies this cell type?

   ○ (A) Unipolar cell
   ○ (B) Apolar neuroblast
   ○ (C) Bipolar cell
   ○ (D) Multipolar cell
   ○ (E) Pseudounipolar cell

6. Which of the following represent the thin type III collagen fibrils and occasional fibroblasts found around individual myelinated axons?

   ○ (A) Epineurium
   ○ (B) Perineurium
   ○ (C) Endoneurium
   ○ (D) Tendon
   ○ (E) Aponeurosis

7. A 7-year-old child is bitten by a rabid squirrel. The virus replicates in the muscle at the site of the bite and then moves toward the cell bodies of the affected neurons by which of the following?

   ○ (A) Anterograde transport
   ○ (B) Retrograde transport
   ○ (C) Transsynaptic transport
   ○ (D) Pinocytosis
   ○ (E) Exocytosis

8. A neuropathologist examines a biopsy specimen from a 22-year-old woman. At the periphery of the section there are neurons with round cell bodies, concentrically located nuclei, and a surrounding layer of satellite cells.

This would suggest that the specimen includes which of the following?

- ○ (A) Anterior horn of the spinal cord
- ○ (B) Visceromotor (autonomic) ganglia
- ○ (C) Basal nuclei (basal ganglia)
- ○ (D) Posterior root ganglia
- ○ (E) Neocortex

9.   During development of the human nervous system, some cells are seen in the adult that do not originate from the neural plate. These cells appear only after blood vessels invade the nervous system during development and may become phagocytic under certain conditions. Which of the following most likely represents this cell population?

- ○ (A) Oligodendroglial cells
- ○ (B) Protoplasmic astrocytes
- ○ (C) Bipolar neuroblasts
- ○ (D) Fibrous astrocytes
- ○ (E) Microglial cells

10.   Which of the following ions is in highest concentration in the intracellular fluid of a resting neuron?

- ○ (A) Sodium (Na^+)
- ○ (B) Potassium (K^+)
- ○ (C) Chloride (Cl^-)
- ○ (D) Nitrogen

11.   A 16-year-old boy, who is a good athlete, presents with a tumor of the sciatic nerve. A histologic analysis reveals that this tumor is composed of the myelin-forming cell of the peripheral nervous system. Which of the following represents this particular cell type?

- ○ (A) Oligodendroglial cell
- ○ (B) Satellite cell
- ○ (C) Schwann cell
- ○ (D) Microglial cell
- ○ (E) Endoneurium

12.   A 36-year-old male construction worker is brought to the emergency department after a serious traumatic injury to his forearm. Injury to the axons innervating the muscles of the hand may result in swelling of the cell body and dispersion of the granular endoplasmic reticulum, and the nucleus of the cell may assume an eccentric position within the cell body. Which of the following most correctly describes this reaction?

- ○ (A) Anterograde degeneration
- ○ (B) Necrosis
- ○ (C) Chromatolysis
- ○ (D) Apoptosis
- ○ (E) Necrosis

13.   A 62-year-old woman presents to the emergency department after a sudden severe headache suggesting a stroke. Which of the following cells within the brain of this patient secrete cytokines, maintain their ability to proliferate in the mature brain, and participate in the formation of a "scar" after brain injury?

- ○ (A) Microglia
- ○ (B) Astrocytes
- ○ (C) Oligodendroglia
- ○ (D) Fibroblasts
- ○ (E) Macrophages

14.   Which of the following most correctly describes the movement of proteins and mitochondria from the neuronal cell body distally down the axon toward its terminals?

- ○ (A) Retrograde transport
- ○ (B) Pinocytosis
- ○ (C) Fast anterograde transport
- ○ (D) Slow anterograde transport
- ○ (E) Transsynaptic transport

15.   An 11-year-old girl presents with a tumor that, when examined histologically, contains neurons with round cell bodies and with single large processes emanating from each side of the cell body. Based on these observations, which of the following would most likely represent the location of this tumor?

- ○ (A) Posterior root ganglia
- ○ (B) Visceromotor (autonomic) ganglia
- ○ (C) Cerebellar cortex
- ○ (D) Retina or olfactory epithelium
- ○ (E) Hippocampus

16.   A 37-year-old man is diagnosed with a brain tumor. Tests reveal that the tumor enhances, indicating a lack of the blood-brain barrier within the tumor. Which of the following contribute most directly to formation of the blood-brain barrier as well as to the glia limitans (glial limiting membrane)?

- ○ (A) Oligodendroglia
- ○ (B) Astrocytes
- ○ (C) Microglia
- ○ (D) Pia mater
- ○ (E) Fibroblasts

17.   Which of the following structures in dendrites helps them to maintain their branched shape?

- ○ (A) Mitochondria and synaptic vesicles
- ○ (B) Mitochondria
- ○ (C) Granular endoplasmic reticulum
- ○ (D) Neurofilaments and microtubules/neurotubules
- ○ (E) Pinocytotic vesicles

18.   A healthy 14-year-old boy grips a baseball bat tightly enough to hold the bat and to make a successful swing. Which of the following represents the process of turning a physical stimulus (grip) into an electrical impulse that can be propagated along an axon?

- ○ (A) Translocation
- ○ (B) Transduction
- ○ (C) Transcription
- ○ (D) Transferrin
- ○ (E) Transfusion

19. A 27-year-old woman presents with a disease that compromises the most common type of synapse found within the mammalian CNS. Which of the following represents this type of synapse?

- ○ (A) Chemical
- ○ (B) Electrical
- ○ (C) Electrotonic
- ○ (D) Dopaminergic
- ○ (E) Cholinergic

20. A neuropathologist examines a small tumor removed from a 15-year-old girl during a surgical procedure for intractable epilepsy. Neurons with pyramid-shaped somata are found in the periphery of this tumor. Based on this information, which of the following represents the most likely source of this tumor?

- ○ (A) Cerebellar cortex
- ○ (B) Posterior root ganglia
- ○ (C) Anterior horn of spinal cord
- ○ (D) Cerebral cortex
- ○ (E) Retina and vestibular ganglia

21. A 27-year-old woman is diagnosed with a disease that results in a decreased function of chemical synapses. Which of the following is characteristic of this type of synapse?

- ○ (A) The synaptic cleft is 200 to 500 nm wide.
- ○ (B) Synaptic vesicles fuse with the presynaptic membrane in response to calcium (Ca^{2+}) influx.
- ○ (C) Neurotransmitter substances are contained in mitochondria.
- ○ (D) Synaptic vesicles cluster near active zones on the postsynaptic membrane.
- ○ (E) Information is transmitted in both directions across the synaptic cleft.

22. Which of the following ion(s) is in highest concentration outside the neuron cell membrane in a resting state?

- ○ (A) Chloride (Cl^-) and potassium (K^+)
- ○ (B) Potassium (K^+) only
- ○ (C) Magnesium (Mg^{2+})
- ○ (D) Chloride (Cl^-) and sodium (Na^+)
- ○ (E) Nitric oxide (NO)

23. A 46-year-old man presents to the emergency department with a severe injury to his left lower extremity resulting in a crushing and tearing injury to the peripheral nerves. The attending physician concludes that the trophic (metabolic) center of the affected neurons will likely disappear. Which of the following is the trophic center of the neuron?

- ○ (A) Nucleus
- ○ (B) Nucleolus
- ○ (C) Axon and axon terminals
- ○ (D) Dendrites and dendritic spines
- ○ (E) Cell body (perikaryon)

24. Which of the following corresponds to the Nissl bodies (or Nissl substances) of the neuron?

- ○ (A) Smooth endoplasmic reticulum
- ○ (B) Rough (granular) endoplasmic reticulum
- ○ (C) Lysosomes
- ○ (D) Mitochondria
- ○ (E) Neurofilaments

25. A neurotransmitter may be described as "excitatory" (leads to depolarization) or "inhibitory" (no change or hyperpolarization). Which of the following determines the action of the neurotransmitter?

- ○ (A) The type of charges (+ or −) on the neurotransmitter
- ○ (B) The type of pores in the presynaptic membrane
- ○ (C) The width of the synaptic cleft
- ○ (D) The receptors on the postsynaptic membrane
- ○ (E) The active zones in the postsynaptic membrane

26. A 58-year-old man has a large tumor in the anterior cranial vault. The neuropathologist examines sections of the tumor and suspects that it is of astrocytic origin. Positive immunostaining for which of the following intermediate filament proteins would be most consistent with an astrocytic origin of this tumor?

- ○ (A) Vimentin
- ○ (B) Keratin
- ○ (C) Desmin
- ○ (D) Neurofilament (heavy chain)
- ○ (E) Glial fibrillary acidic protein

27. A 28-year-old woman, who has been diagnosed as HIV positive, exhibits disturbances of sensation and voluntary movements. These neurologic abnormalities could arise as a result of HIV infection of which type of CNS cell?

- ○ (A) Pyramidal cells of the cerebral cortex
- ○ (B) Multipolar neurons of nucleus ventralis posterolateralis
- ○ (C) Fibrous astrocytes
- ○ (D) Oligodendrocytes
- ○ (E) Microglial cells

28. An autopsy examination of sections of a spinal cord at the C8 level reveals that the cell bodies of many alpha motor neurons appear swollen, have eccentrically located nuclei, and have uniformly dispersed basophilic staining of the cytoplasm. These findings suggest that, before the death of the patient, there had been a recent injury to what?

- ○ (A) A peripheral nerve
- ○ (B) A posterior root ganglion
- ○ (C) A descending tract above the C8 level
- ○ (D) An ascending tract below the C8 level
- ○ (E) A peripheral motor ganglion

29. Peripheral nerves contain both unmyelinated and myelinated axons. Which of the following is a characteristic shared by both of these fibers?

- ○ (A) Fast conduction velocities
- ○ (B) Axon diameters less than 1 μm

○ (C) Schmidt-Lanterman clefts
○ (D) Nodes of Ranvier
○ (E) Coverings derived from Schwann cells

30. An 8-year-old girl has suffered a crush injury that severed the axons of the median nerve at the wrist. If regeneration of the sensory nerve fibers proceeds optimally, what is the approximate minimum possible time for a return of sensation to the tip of the index finger?

○ (A) One day
○ (B) One week
○ (C) One month
○ (D) Four months
○ (E) Four years

31. The structural basis of the blood-nerve barrier is what?

○ (A) The epineurium
○ (B) The perineurium
○ (C) The endoneurium
○ (D) The endothelium of capillaries

32. A 49-year-old man presents to his family physician with headache and lethargy. A gadolinium-enhanced MRI image reveals a tumor in the parietal lobe. The fact that the tumor enhanced suggests that the blood-brain barrier is compromised. Which of the following represents the structural basis of the blood-brain barrier?

○ (A) Endoneurium
○ (B) Pia mater
○ (C) Covering of blood vessels by astrocyte foot processes
○ (D) Endothelium of capillaries
○ (E) Epineurium

33. A neuropathologist wishes to determine whether an electron micrograph of nervous tissue originated from central or peripheral nervous tissue. Inspection of myelinated nerve fibers could provide one basis for a conclusion because, although myelinating Schwann cells and oligodendrocytes share many features, only Schwann cells have which of the following characteristics?

○ (A) Form myelin segments that are not interrupted by nodes of Ranvier
○ (B) Have basal laminae
○ (C) Provide myelin sheaths for multiple axons
○ (D) Myelinate large-caliber axons only
○ (E) Contribute their plasmalemmas to the formation of multiple myelin sheaths

34. Cytoplasm containing extensive rough endoplasmic reticulum (rER) is characteristic of cells that are either actively growing, dividing, or synthesizing proteins for secretion. Although a mature projection neuron is engaged in none of these activities, its cell body contains abundant rER. Which of the following best explains the need for extensive rER in such a neuron?

○ (A) The rER of neurons functions to generate adenosine triphosphate required for active pumping of ions.

○ (B) The cell body produces the proteins needed to maintain the axon.
○ (C) The cell body exports a continuous supply of rER to terminal boutons.
○ (D) The cell body undergoes apoptosis.
○ (E) The cell body needs energy to undergo necrosis.

ANSWERS

1. **(B)** Patients with myasthenia gravis have elevated serum antibodies to nicotinic acetylcholine receptors. The subjunctional folds of the neuromuscular junction are destroyed, and the efficiency of the junction is compromised. The typical symptoms are (a) weakness that may fluctuate over minutes, hours, or days; (b) an initial (about 40%) or ultimate (about 85%) involvement of ocular muscles; and (c) a positive response to the administration of certain cholinergic drugs such as pyridostigmine bromide or neostigmine.
FN2e 25–27

2. **(B)** Ribosomes are present in dendrites and in the soma of the cell's body but are absent in the axon hillock and in the axon.
FN2e 21

3. **(C)** Oligodendroglia are the myelin-forming cells of the CNS, and Schwann cells perform this function in the peripheral nervous system. The membranes from a single oligodendroglial cell may provide myelin sheaths for many (perhaps up to 40) axons.
FN2e 30–32

4. **(E)** In multiple sclerosis, the myelin segments surrounding groups of axons degenerate with a resulting interruption in the transmission of action potentials. The cause of this disease is unknown; it appears in the age range of 20 to 40 years and may involve any part of the CNS. The general progression is inflammation, demyelination, potential damage to or loss of axons, and sclerosis/scarring. The symptoms seen in these patients reflect the regions/structures of the CNS involved.
FN2e 32

5. **(D)** Multipolar neurons are, by far, the most numerous type of neuron in the adult CNS. Multipolar neurons may take shapes that are characteristic of certain areas of the CNS, such as granule cells of the cerebellar cortex, pyramidal cells of the cerebral cortex, or large motor neurons of the anterior horn of the spinal cord.
FN2e 16, 20

6. **(C)** Endoneurium is found around the individual myelinated axons in peripheral nerves and is composed primarily of type III collagen and sparse numbers of fibroblasts.
FN2e 35

7. **(B)** The movement of any substance from an axon terminal to the cell body is retrograde transport. In addition to being an important mechanism in a variety of clinical situations, retrograde transport is used as an

experimental technique to map interconnections between populations of neurons.
FN2e 21

8.   **(D)** Unipolar cell bodies with concentric nuclei and an envelope of satellite cells are found in posterior root ganglia, in sensory ganglia of cranial nerves, and in the mesencephalic nucleus of the trigeminal nerve, although the satellite cells are lacking in this nucleus. Unipolar cells are regarded as sensory neurons.
FN2e 18–20

9.   **(E)** Microglia cells presumably originate from a monocyte-macrophage cell line and do not appear in the CNS until after the developing brain and spinal cord are invaded by blood vessels (and developing blood cells). When stimulated by an injury (traumatic or spontaneous, such as a stroke), microglial cells proliferate and become phagocytic.
(FN2e 32)

10.   **(B)** Whereas potassium (K^+) is in high concentrations in intracellular fluids (in a resting state), sodium (Na^+) and chloride (Cl^-) are in high concentrations in the extracellular fluid.
FN2e 23–24

11.   **(C)** Schwann cells form the internodal myelin segments (the myelin between two nodes of Ranvier) in the peripheral nervous system; one Schwann cell forms the myelin for one internodal segment. Oligodendroglia are the myelin-forming cells of the CNS.
FN2e 29

12.   **(C)** Chromatolysis refers to the color changes seen in degenerating neuron cell bodies resultant to the dispersion of the Nissl substance. Depending on a number of variables (e.g., distance from injury to axon and cell body, type of injury [cut vs. tear]) the chromatolytic cell body may eventually die or may recover and, with time, appear normal. However, the recovered cell, if located in the CNS, may not establish functional synaptic contacts with other CNS neurons.
FN2e 22, 35–36

13.   **(B)** Cytokines secreted by the astrocyte may help regulate immune cells within the CNS. The ability of astrocytes to differentiate/proliferate in the adult brain is reflected in the fact that this cell gives rise to a variety of brain tumors (astrocytomas, anaplastic astrocytomas, glioblastoma multiforme—WHO classification). The astrocytic scar also arises from this cell.
FN2e 28–30

14.   **(C)** Fast anterograde transport may move up to 400 mm/day, use a protein called kinesin, and move vesicles containing large-molecular-weight molecules as well as mitochondria.
FN2e 21

15.   **(D)** Bipolar cells are located in special sensory epithelia (retina, olfactory structures, auditory and vestibular ganglia) and are classified as special somatic afferent. Bipolar neuroblasts are also seen during development between apolar and/or unipolar neuroblasts and multipolar neuroblasts.
FN2e 20

16.   **(B)** Processes of astrocytes form the glial limiting membrane on the surface of the brain and spinal cord. A basal lamina is located on the external surface of the glia limitans. External to the glial limiting membrane there may be a small subpial space containing collagen and then the fibroblasts forming the pia mater.
FN2e 28–30

17.   **(D)** Neurotubules and neurofilaments are filamentous proteins that are found in organized patterns in dendrites and axons. The neurotubule is larger (20 to 25 nm in diameter) than the neurofilament (which is about 10 nm in diameter). In high-resolution electron microscopic micrographs, the neurofilament also appears to have a tubular structure.
FN2e 16

18.   **(B)** In general, transduction is the act of turning one form of energy into another. Within the nervous system, transduction is seen in many areas, for example, in the retina, in receptors in the skin, and even when one strikes his or her "funny bone" (actually the ulnar nerve passing around the medial epicondyle of the humerus) on the edge of a table.
FN2e 25

19.   **(A)** Chemical synapses consist, in general, of a presynaptic element, a postsynaptic element, and an intervening space in the range of 20 to 50 nm wide. Synaptic vesicles in the presynaptic element release a transmitter into the cleft that triggers a change in the postsynaptic membrane. Electronic synapses are rare, are present in the primate nervous system (retina, cerebral cortex, hippocampus), and are made up of a presynaptic and postsynaptic membrane separated by a 2- to 4-nm space containing a connexon.
FN2e 25–36

20.   **(D)** Pyramid-shaped cells may be present in a variety of regions of the CNS. However, cells of this shape are particularly characteristic of the cerebral cortex, where they are found in all layers except lamina I. They range from small pyramidal cells to the giant pyramidal cells (of Betz) found in lamina V of the primary motor cortex.
FN2e 20

21.   **(B)** Depolarization of the presynaptic membrane (resultant to the arrival of an action potential) opens Ca^{2+} channels. The influx of Ca^{2+} causes the synaptic vesicles to fuse with the presynaptic membrane and to release their contents into the synaptic cleft.
FN2e 25–27

22.   **(D)** In the resting state, the extracellular fluid of the neuron has a high concentration of sodium (Na^+) and chloride (Cl^-) and a low concentration of potassium (K^+) whereas the intracellular fluid has a high concentration of potassium (K^+) and a low concentration of sodium (Na^+) and chloride (Cl^-).
FN2e 23–24

23.   **(E)** The cell body (soma or perikaryon) manufactures all the cellular components needed for maintaining the life of the neuron. Injury to the axon may, or may not (based on a number of variables), result in the death of

the cell body. However, injury to the cell body will result in the death of all the processes of the injured soma and in the death of the soma itself.
FN2e 16–18

24. **(B)** Stacked layers of endoplasmic reticulum that are covered by ribosomal RNA comprise the basophilic staining substance commonly called the Nissl substance.
FN2e 17

25. **(D)** Receptors on the postsynaptic membrane determine if a neurotransmitter will move the resting membrane potential from −60 mV to threshold and result in an action potential (excitation) or move the resting membrane from, for example, −60 mV to −80 mV and result in hyperpolarization (inhibition) of the membrane.
FN2e 26

26. **(E)** Intermediate filaments contribute to the cytoskeleton of many neural and non-neural cells types, but specific families of the constituent proteins are characteristic of specific cell types and classes, and this can be useful in determining the origins of tumors. The intermediate filament protein that is characteristic of astrocytes is glial fibrillary acidic protein, whereas neurons express various forms of neurofilaments.
FN2e 21, 28

27. **(E)** Microglia are the CNS representatives of the immune system, and these are the CNS cells that are susceptible to HIV infection. By unknown mechanisms, this can lead to abnormal function of neurons and resultant neurologic deficits.
FN2e 33

28. **(A)** Axotomy results in chromatolysis, that is, swollen perikarya with eccentric nuclei and dispersed rough endoplasmic reticulum (Nissl substance), which would be seen in sections as a uniform distribution of staining by basic dyes. Axotomy of alpha motor neurons results from peripheral nerve injury but not from damage to posterior root ganglia or descending or ascending tracts of the spinal cord.
FN2e 17, 22

29. **(E)** Both myelinated and unmyelinated peripheral nerve fibers have sheaths of Schwann cell cytoplasm. Only myelinated axons have nodes of Ranvier, Schmidt-Lanterman clefts, and fast conduction velocities. The smallest axons (diameter less than 1 μm) are not myelinated but lie within a trough of the Schwann cell plasmalemma.
FN2e 34–35

30. **(D)** Although crush injuries of peripheral nerves sever axons, conduits that guide regenerating axons to their original peripheral targets are likely to be preserved. The growth rate of regenerating axons is approximately 1 mm/day, so about 4 months will be required to extend the roughly 120 mm distance from the wrist to the fingertip of a 10-year-old child.
FN2e 36

31. **(B)** The perineurium is composed of an epithelium-like layer of cells that are interconnected by tight (occluding) junctions. Thus, the perineurium has the structural features necessary to limit and control movement of substances from the surrounding interstitial fluid into a fascicle of peripheral nerve fibers.
FN2e 35

32. **(D)** Capillaries in the CNS are characterized by endothelial cells that are interconnected by extensive tight junctions so that any plasma solutes must traverse the cytoplasm of the endothelial cells to enter the CNS tissue compartment. CNS capillaries also show much less transport of endocytotic vesicles than ordinary tissue capillaries. Astrocytes have an indirect role in establishment of the blood-brain barrier, in that endothelial cells are induced to assume their specialized features as a result of contact by astrocyte end feet.
FN2e 30

33. **(B)** Schwann cells, but not oligodendrocytes, have basal laminae that are important structures in guiding regenerating axons after peripheral nerve injury. Only oligodendrocytes contribute myelin sheaths to multiple axons.
FN2e 35

34. **(B)** The cell body (perikaryon) contains synthetic machinery that must provide proteins for the axon as well as the cell body. In a neuron with a long axon (e.g., a posterior root ganglion neuron) the requirement for protein synthesis is extremely high because the cell body has less than 1% of the volume and surface area of the axon.
FN2e 16–17, 21

CHAPTER 3

The Electrochemical Basis of Neuronal Integration

1. A 7-year-old boy is treated in the emergency department for severe diarrhea of 3 days' duration. The physician suspects that the boy will suffer from excessive loss of extracellular fluid volume and possibly become severely hyponatremic. In general, what effect would this serum electrolyte imbalance most likely have on neuronal membrane excitability?

○ (A) No substantial effect
○ (B) Increased excitability, which might lead to restlessness and seizures.
○ (C) Decreased excitability, which might result in symptoms such as lethargy, hypotonia, and hyporeflexia.
○ (D) Some neurons might be more excitable and others less excitable.
○ (E) The electrolyte imbalance could be treated by restricting water intake.

2. A 54-year-old man in the intensive care unit is diagnosed with acute renal failure caused by renal tubule necrosis. The patient is severely hyperkalemic. In general, what effect would this serum electrolyte imbalance most likely have on neuronal excitability?

○ (A) No substantial effect
○ (B) Increased excitability, which might lead to hyper-reflexia, spastic paralysis, and seizures
○ (C) Decreased excitability, as evidenced by confusion, stupor, hyporeflexia, and flaccid paralysis
○ (D) Some neurons might be more excitable and others less excitable.
○ (E) The electrolyte imbalance could be treated by restricting water intake.

3. A 47-year-old woman is diagnosed with an adenoma of the parathyroid gland. This results in excessive production of parathyroid hormone, which disrupts the normally well-controlled calcium balance and leads to a change in blood calcium levels. As a result of this endocrine disorder, which of the following effects on neuronal function would most likely be observed in this patient?

○ (A) An increased serum calcium level would result in greatly diminished neuronal excitability.
○ (B) A decreased serum calcium level would result in greatly diminished neuronal excitability.
○ (C) An increased serum calcium level would result in greatly enhanced neuronal excitability.
○ (D) A decreased serum calcium level would result in greatly enhanced neuronal excitability.
○ (E) An increased serum calcium level would result in a more electrically stable membrane and only slightly reduced neuronal excitability.

4. Over a period of 6 hours the blood pH level of a 27-year-old woman increases from 7.4 to 7.7. Which of the following statements is most likely correct in regard to neuronal activity?

○ (A) The change in pH signals a severe acidosis that will lead to increased neuronal excitability.
○ (B) The change in pH signals a severe alkalosis that will lead to increased neuronal excitability.
○ (C) The change in pH signals a severe acidosis that will lead to decreased neuronal excitability.
○ (D) The change in pH signals a severe alkalosis that will lead to decreased neuronal excitability.
○ (E) The change in pH will have little or no effect on neuronal excitability.

5. Threshold depolarization is defined as the level of depolarization that results in an action potential

○ (A) 0.5% of the time
○ (B) 25% of the time
○ (C) 50% of the time
○ (D) 75% of the time
○ (E) 100% of the time

6. At the peak of the action potential, the inward sodium current is

○ (A) Equal to the outward potassium current
○ (B) Greater than the outward potassium current
○ (C) Less than the outward potassium current
○ (D) Twice the outward potassium current
○ (E) One third of the outward potassium current

7. During the rising phase of the action potential, additional inward current cannot influence the amplitude of the action potential. Which of the following most specifically describes this period of time in the excitability cycle?

○ (A) Null refractory period
○ (B) Relative refractory period
○ (C) Local response
○ (D) Absolute refractory period
○ (E) Time constant

8. The electrophysiologic evaluation of a 19-year-old man with suspected peripheral neuropathy reveals a decrease of action potential propagation in several classes of fibers. Which one of the following most correctly describes the propagation of the action potential?

○ (A) Depolarization of the inactive membrane occurs as a result of net outward current.
○ (B) Current flows into the membrane segment that is undergoing repolarization.
○ (C) The ratio of the amount of current flowing into the inactive membrane to that needed to exceed threshold is called the safety factor.
○ (D) The action potential moves along the axon by passive electrotonic spread.
○ (E) The action potential conduction velocity is greater in unmyelinated axons than in myelinated axons.

9. Action potential velocity in myelinated axons is enhanced by which of the following?

○ (A) Saltatory conduction
○ (B) Passive electrotonic spread
○ (C) Decreasing the length of internodal segments
○ (D) Decreasing axonal diameter
○ (E) Decreasing thickness of the myelin sheath

10. Under normal physiologic conditions, action potentials are propagated orthodromically; that is, from the soma toward the synaptic terminals. Which of the following most specifically accounts for this phenomenon?

○ (A) An action potential can only be propagated in the orthodromic direction.
○ (B) The membrane proximal to the active region is undergoing repolarization.
○ (C) Sodium and potassium channels are not found in the region of the node of Ranvier.
○ (D) The time constant progressively decreases in the distal (orthodromic) direction.
○ (E) The safety factor progressively decreases in the distal (orthodromic) direction.

11. Before suturing a skin laceration in a 12-year-old boy in the emergency department the physician infiltrates the skin around the wound site with a local anesthetic. The reduction in pain sensation from the wound site is most likely the result of which of the following?

○ (A) Increased frequency of action potentials in the sensory nerves leading from the wound site
○ (B) Opening of the voltage-gated sodium channels
○ (C) Dilation of cutaneous blood vessels around the wound site
○ (D) Decreased action potential propagation in sensory nerves supplying the wound site
○ (E) Blockage of synaptic transmission in the spinal cord dorsal horn where the sensory fibers from the wound site will eventually terminate

Match the correct word(s) listed below with the statements in items 12, 13, and 14:

(A) Transduction
(B) Fiber code
(C) Place code
(D) Modality
(E) Adaptation

12. An action potential firing pattern that describes the specific location of a stimulus in a sensory receptive field (   )

13. The type or category of sensation that stimulates a particular class of receptors (   )

14. When a stimulus is continuously applied to a receptor, the receptor might first respond vigorously but then gradually decrease its firing even though the stimulus intensity is maintained at its initial value (   )

15. Which of the following mechanisms makes it possible to encode and discriminate stimulus amplitude over a range larger than the dynamic range of a single sensory fiber?

○ (A) Frequency coding
○ (B) Place coding
○ (C) Saturation
○ (D) Recruitment
○ (E) Adaptation

16. Compound action potentials are recorded from the median nerve of a 17-year-old boy after a compression injury to the nerve at the wrist 6 months previously. The objective is to see if each of the various populations of motor and sensory fibers in this mixed nerve have recovered and are present in the correct proportions. The histogram shown here illustrates the data recorded from this

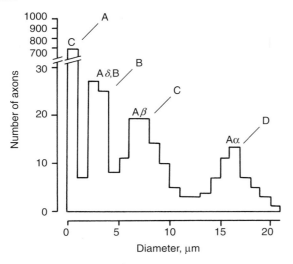

Figure 3–1

patient. Of the four peaks labeled above, which indicates the population of axons with the most rapid conduction velocity? (   )

17.   A 27-year-old woman presents with ocular dysmetria and muscle weakness that waxes and wanes over time. This finding suggests a possible disruption of the effectiveness of the synapse. The time required to release a neurotransmitter agent, allow it to diffuse across the synaptic cleft, and bind to its postsynaptic receptor is called what?

○ (A) Presynaptic inhibition
○ (B) Synaptic delay
○ (C) Reuptake
○ (D) Time constant
○ (E) Postsynaptic inhibition

18.   Which of the following is the most characteristic and distinguishing feature of a second-messenger type synapse?

○ (A) The presence of synaptic vesicles
○ (B) The presence of a presynaptic element or profile
○ (C) A transmitter-receptor complex is directly coupled to an ion channel
○ (D) Produces only excitatory postsynaptic potentials (EPSPs)
○ (E) Involves a guanosine nucleotide-binding protein (G protein)

19.   Which of the following substances functions as a so-called second messenger?

○ (A) Diacylglycerol (DAG)
○ (B) Phosphatidylinositol
○ (C) Adenylyl cyclase
○ (D) G protein
○ (E) Phospholipase A

20.   A key concept in analyzing how neurons process information is the observation that there is typically one area of membrane that has the lowest threshold for action potential initiation (most excitable region), the so-called trigger zone. For most neurons this site is located at the axon hillock. Which of the following best describes why this membrane segment has the lowest threshold for activation of action potentials?

○ (A) It has the smallest concentration of voltage-gated potassium channels.
○ (B) The excitatory presynaptic terminals are typically clustered in this region.
○ (C) It has the largest concentration of voltage-gated sodium channels.
○ (D) The cell membrane is thinnest at this location.
○ (E) The inhibitory presynaptic terminals are typically clustered at this location.

21.   Synaptic potentials differ from action potentials in that synaptic potentials are

○ (A) Typically of the same amplitude regardless of the intensity of stimulation
○ (B) Spread along the membrane by active propagation
○ (C) Typically produced in a presynaptic terminal
○ (D) Graded in amplitude and most are directly proportional to the intensity of stimulation
○ (E) Nearly always depolarizing

22.   Listed below are five events that typically occur in conventional chemical synapses:

○ (A) On depolarization of the presynaptic terminal, voltage-modulated Ca^{2+} channels open, allowing Ca^{2+} into the synaptic terminal.
○ (B) A neurotransmitter is released into the synaptic cleft, diffuses across the cleft, and binds to postsynaptic receptor elements.
○ (C) Synaptic vesicles accumulate in the presynaptic terminal.
○ (D) An action potential depolarizes the presynaptic terminal.
○ (E) The increase in intracellular Ca^{2+} promotes docking of synaptic vesicles to release sites in the presynaptic membrane.

Which of the following represents the proper sequence of these events at a chemical synapse?

○ (A) 4, 1, 3, 5, 2
○ (B) 2, 1, 5, 3, 4
○ (C) 4, 1, 3, 5, 2
○ (D) 3, 4, 1, 5, 2
○ (E) 4, 3, 1, 5, 2

23.   In the figure below, the upper trace illustrates low (1) and high (2) frequency action potential depolarization of an axon terminal and generation of small and large excitatory postsynaptic potentials (EPSPs), respectively, in a postsynaptic target neuron.

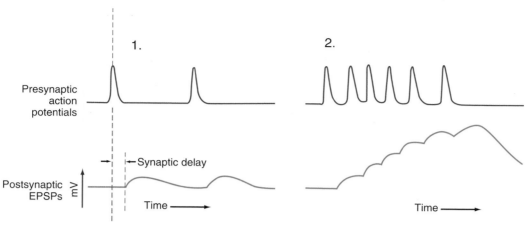

1.

2.

Presynaptic
action
potentials

Synaptic delay

Postsynaptic
EPSPs   mV

Time ⟶

Time ⟶

Figure 3–2

The larger EPSP generated by the high-frequency stimulation (at 2) is an example of

○ (A) Presynaptic inhibition
○ (B) Adaptation
○ (C) A shunt pathway
○ (D) Spatial summation
○ (E) Temporal summation

24. Which of the following most specifically describes voltage-gated sodium channels?

○ (A) The potassium channel has both an activation gate and an inactivation gate.
○ (B) Both the sodium and the potassium channels have an activation gate.
○ (C) An inactivation gate responds to depolarization by opening.
○ (D) An activation gate responds to depolarization by closing.
○ (E) When its channel is in the activated state, sodium flows down its concentration gradient out of the cell.

ANSWERS

1. **(C)** The decreased availability of extracellular sodium ions has a hyperpolarizing effect on the neuronal membrane. This would move the neuronal membrane potential to a more negative value and thus make the neuron less excitable.
FN2e 39–40

2. **(B)** An increase in extracellular potassium would result in decreased movement of potassium ions out of the cell and would have a depolarizing influence on the cell. Consequently, the neuron would become more excitable and cause hyperactive states, such as increased reflex activity, spasticity, and increased seizure activity.
FN2e 39–40

3. **(A)** The presence of additional parathyroid hormone would lead to an increase in extracellular calcium levels. The accumulation of additional calcium in the extracellular space has a stabilizing effect on the neuronal membrane, and thus the neuron would become slightly less excitable.
FN2e 26

4. **(B)** The increase in pH from 7.4 to 7.7 results in alkalosis. In this environment, the neuronal membrane becomes less stable and neuronal excitability is enhanced. Acidosis results in just the opposite response; neuronal excitability is diminished.
FN2e 25

5. **(C)** When the level of depolarization in a neuron reaches its threshold value an action potential is generated 50% of the time.
FN2e 42

6. **(A)** The inward movement of sodium is equal to the outward movement of potassium at the peak of the action potential.
FN2e 43

7. **(D)** The absolute refractory period is the time during the rising phase and the early part of the falling phase in the excitability cycle when inward current cannot influence the amplitude of the action potential. During the relative refractory period, a larger stimulus can initiate an action potential, but this action potential will be of smaller magnitude.
FN2e 44

8. **(C)** The amount of current flowing into the active membrane in excess of that needed to exceed threshold is a measure of that axons safety factor. Depolarization of the membrane is a result of inward current movement, whereas repolarization is accomplished by the outward flow of current. Action potentials are moved along the membrane by active propagation and not passive spread. Action potential velocity is greatest in myelinated axons.
FN2e 45

9. **(A)** The velocity of an action potential is enhanced by the property of saltatory conduction. That is, the action potential is said to "jump" from one node of Ranvier to the next. This mechanism is referred to as active propagation not passive spread. The speed with which this process occurs is directly proportional to the length of the internodal segment, the diameter of the axon, and the thickness of the myelin sheath.
FN2e 45–46

10. **(B)** If the axon is stimulated at some point along its course, an action potential can be propagated in both the orthodromic and antidromic directions. However, under typical physiologic conditions, it originates from the axon hillock and the action potential moves only in the orthodromic direction. This is because the trailing (proximal) edge of the active zone begins to undergo repolarization and cannot support another action potential during this time. The time constant and safety factors have no direct bearing on action potential initiation nor does the presence or absence of ion channels at the node of Ranvier.
FN2e 46

11. **(D)** When infiltrated into the skin, a local anesthetic agent interferes with the normal activity of voltage-gated sodium channels in the axonal membrane and this leads to a reduction in, or blockage of, action potential propagation in the sensory nerves supplying the wound site. Dilation of cutaneous blood vessels and synaptic transmission in the dorsal horn are not relevant.
FN2e 46

12. **(C)** The cochlea contains a receptor sheet distributed over the frequency-tuned basilar membrane. The location of a receptor along the basilar membrane determines the auditory frequency to which it will respond best. This process is called place coding.
FN2e 47

13. **(D)** The type of sensation that stimulates a particular class of receptors is called its modality.
FN2e 47

14. **(E)** A receptor that first responds vigorously to a maintained level of stimulation and then begins to decrease its firing level while the level of stimulation is maintained is said to exhibit adaptation.
FN2e 47

15. **(C)** Sensory axons that might be carrying the same type (modality) of information will have differing thresholds and differing dynamic ranges. Therefore, increasing stimulus intensity will often cause (recruit) more axons to discharge and, thus, signal or encode stimulus amplitudes greater than the dynamic range of any one individual fiber. Place coding and frequency coding are functions of individual axons, whereas saturation and adaptation represent mechanisms whereby responses to a given level of stimulation are damped or limited.
FN2e 47–48

16. **(D)** The peak indicated by the letter D represents the axons with the greatest diameter (x-axis) and, therefore, the fastest conduction velocity. However, as indicated on the y-axis, the most rapidly conducting axons are among the fewest. The largest number of fibers fall within the slowest conducting group. This distribution of conduction velocities and numbers of fibers within each population is typical for a normal mixed nerve such as the median nerve.
FN2e 48–49

17. **(B)** The time required to release a neurotransmitter and allow it to travel to, and bind to, its postsynaptic receptor determines the synaptic delay of the synapse. Reuptake refers to a mechanism whereby the neurotransmitter can be returned to the presynaptic terminal. The time constant is an inherent property of the neuronal membrane and has no relationship to synaptic mechanisms.
FN2e 50

18. **(E)** Activation of a G protein is a characteristic feature of the so-called second messenger synapse. Both single-messenger and second-messenger synapses contain synaptic vesicles, and both types include a presynaptic and a postsynaptic element. In single-messenger synapse the postsynaptic receptor is directly linked to an ion channel, whereas in a second-messenger synapse the postsynaptic receptor can only be indirectly linked to an ion channel via its specific G protein.
FN2e 51–52

19. **(A)** DAG is formed from phosphatidylinositol-4,5-biphosphate and serves as a second messenger. Each of the other items (except for G protein) is an enzyme involved in the formation of a second messenger.
FN2e 52

20. **(C)** The presence of the highest concentration of sodium channels in the membrane of the axon hillock makes this the trigger zone for action potential initiation. Excitatory synaptic input is not necessarily concentrated in this region of the neuron, although it could be. The thickness of the cell membrane at the axon hillock has no relation to its excitability nor does the density of potassium channels in this region.
FN2e 52

21. **(D)** A characteristic feature of synaptic potentials is that they are graded in amplitude and directly proportional to stimulation intensity. This is in contrast to action potentials that are "all or none" in amplitude regardless of stimulus intensity. Synaptic potentials can be either depolarizing or hyperpolarizing, whereas action potentials are only depolarizing. Synaptic potentials spread passively along the membrane and are not actively propagated as are action potentials.
FN2e 52–53

22. **(D)** The sequence of events in a conventional chemical synapse begins with the accumulation of synaptic vesicles in the presynaptic axon terminal. When that terminal is depolarized by the arrival of an action potential, voltage-modulated calcium terminals are opened and calcium enters the synaptic terminal. The entry of calcium promotes docking of synaptic vesicles at specific sites in the presynaptic membrane where the vesicles exocytose their neurotransmitter agent into the synaptic cleft. The neurotransmitter then binds to receptors in the postsynaptic membrane, which typically results in the

activation of ion channels and leads to the development of a postsynaptic potential. If the ion channel activation leads to depolarization of the postsynaptic membrane, an EPSP is generated. Conversely, if the ion channel activation leads to hyperpolarization of the postsynaptic membrane, an inhibitory postsynaptic potential (IPSP) is generated.
FN2e 49–50

23.   **(E)** When action potentials arrive in axon terminals at low frequency, they generate EPSPs in the postsynaptic element that do not overlap in time and thus cannot summate. However, when action potentials arrive at an axon terminal at relatively high frequency, they can generate postsynaptic potentials that overlap in time and these can summate to produce a larger EPSP.
FN2e 54

24.   **(B)** Both the sodium and potassium channels have an activation gate, whereas the sodium channel (but not the potassium channel) also has an inactivation gate. The activation gate responds to depolarization by opening, whereas the inactivation gate responds to depolarization by closing. When the sodium channel is in the activated state, sodium is free to flow into the cell.
FN2e 42–43

CHAPTER 4

The Chemical Basis for Neuronal Communication

1. The syndrome of orthostatic hypotension is often characterized by reduced norepinephrine release from nerve terminals that possess normally functioning autoregulatory presynaptic receptors. Which of the following drugs is most likely to be effective in elevating norepinephrine release and thereby improving blood pressure in a patient with orthostatic hypotension?

- ○ (A) Reserpine
- ○ (B) Propranolol
- ○ (C) Yohimbine
- ○ (D) Guanethidine
- ○ (E) α-Methyltyrosine

2. Twenty-four-hour urine collection in a 27-year-old man shows lower than normal levels of dopamine, norepinephrine, and epinephrine. However, tissue biopsy yields clearly elevated levels of the norepinephrine precursor dopa. A congenital deficiency of which enzyme is most likely to produce such a pattern?

- ○ (A) Tyrosine hydroxylase
- ○ (B) L-Amino acid decarboxylase
- ○ (C) Dopamine β-hydroxylase
- ○ (D) Monoamine oxidase
- ○ (E) Adenylyl cyclase

3. A 35-year-old white man presents with hypertension that is characterized by tachycardia and elevated cardiac contractility, symptoms consistent with increased numbers and/or responsiveness of β-adrenoceptors. Of the following, which agent most specifically addresses the hemodynamic problems of this patient?

- ○ (A) Yohimbine
- ○ (B) Reserpine
- ○ (C) Guanethidine
- ○ (D) Cocaine
- ○ (E) Propranolol

4. Electrical stimulation of nerve fibers innervating the forearm of a 27-year-old woman does not elicit any change, even at supramaximal voltages, until the stimulation frequency exceeds 10 Hz. Above 10 Hz, even very low voltages elicit vasodilation and flushing. The examining physician tentatively concludes what?

- ○ (A) Frequencies of stimulation above 10 Hz elicit effects unrelated to neurotransmitter release
- ○ (B) No neurotransmitters can be released by stimulation frequencies less than 10 Hz
- ○ (C) High-frequency (= 10 Hz) stimulation selectively releases neuropeptides that cause vasodilation and flushing
- ○ (D) High-frequency (= 10 Hz) stimulation selectively releases small molecule neurotransmitters that cause vasodilation and flushing

5. Ingestion of a wild mushroom, identified as *Amanita muscaria*, causes vomiting, abdominal cramping, and diarrhea in an 18-year-old woman. These responses are the result of what process?

- ○ (A) Inhibition of nicotinic cholinergic receptors
- ○ (B) Inhibition of muscarinic cholinergic receptor
- ○ (C) Stimulation of nicotinic cholinergic receptors
- ○ (D) Stimulation of muscarinic cholinergic receptors
- ○ (E) Stimulation of α-adrenoceptors

6. A 24-year-old woman suffering from a severe allergic reaction improves markedly after a subcutaneous injection of epinephrine. Transduction of this epinephrine chemical signal involves which of the following?

- ○ (A) Binding of epinephrine to membrane-bound β-adrenoceptors
- ○ (B) Dissociation of the α subunit from the β-, γ-heterodimer of the G-protein complex
- ○ (C) Binding of the G-protein α subunit to adenylyl cyclase
- ○ (D) Stimulation of adenylyl cyclase to increase intracellular cyclic adenosine monophosphate levels
- ○ (E) All of these steps

7. A 47-year-old man to whom the emergency department physician has just administered an intravenous

injection of epinephrine shows tachycardia (an excitatory effect) and vasodilation of blood vessels in skeletal muscle (an inhibitory effect). Which of the following most specifically describes these apparently divergent postsynaptic responses to the same chemical messenger?

- (A) The responses are mediated by different epinephrine receptors (adrenoceptors).
- (B) Only excitatory responses can be elicited by a single chemical messenger.
- (C) Only inhibitory responses can be elicited by a single chemical messenger.
- (D) The excitatory responses result from membrane hyperpolarization in the target tissue.
- (E) The inhibitory responses result from membrane depolarization in the target tissue.

8. Treatment of a patient with a monoamine oxidase inhibitor will cause a dramatic exaggeration of the effects of which agent?

- (A) Glutamate
- (B) Acetylcholine
- (C) Substance P
- (D) Nitric oxide
- (E) Norepinephrine

9. Ingestion of MPTP (1-methyl-4-phenyl-1,2,3,6-tetrahydropyridine) causes tremor, muscle rigidity, and virtually complete paralysis, a syndrome similar to Parkinson disease, in a 25-year-old man These responses to MPTP require which of the following?

- (A) Destruction of dopamine by the monoamine oxidase isoform MAO-B in brain neurons
- (B) Formation of dopamine by the monoamine oxidase isoform MAO-B in brain neurons
- (C) Activation of MPTP by the monoamine oxidase isoform MAO-B in brain glia
- (D) Destruction of MPTP by the monoamine oxidase isoform MAO-B in brain glia
- (E) Activation of MPTP by the monoamine oxidase isoform MAO-A in the liver

10. Pedigree analysis of a family reveals the presence of a recessive mutation that inactivates transporter proteins for glutamate in neurons and glia. Individuals who are homozygous for the mutation (i.e., who express the mutation fully) will show which of the following?

- (A) More prolonged and more intense responses to glutamate
- (B) Shorter and reduced responses to glutamate
- (C) Enhanced synthesis of glutamate in neurons
- (D) Enhanced release of glutamate from neurons
- (E) Enhanced removal (uptake) of synaptic glutamate by glia

11. A 19-year-old man presents to the emergency department in an agitated state, with hypertension and tachycardia. Plasma and urinary levels of norepinephrine are significantly elevated. Ingestion of which of the following is most likely to be the cause of these symptoms?

- (A) α-Methyldopa
- (B) Propranolol
- (C) Reserpine
- (D) Guanethidine
- (E) Cocaine

12. A 16-year-old woman presents with a diagnosis of pheochromocytoma, a tumor of adrenal chromaffin cells in which excess norepinephrine is synthesized and released, causing multiple symptoms. Of the following agents, which will most specifically reduce norepinephrine synthesis and alleviate her symptoms?

- (A) α-Methyltyrosine
- (B) Cocaine
- (C) Tyramine
- (D) Pargyline
- (E) Corticosterone

13. Chronic hypertension, with symptoms of sympathetic overactivity including tachycardia and elevated cardiac output, has been diagnosed in a 21-year-old white man. Which of the following would be most suitable to manage this patient?

- (A) Corticosterone
- (B) Cocaine
- (C) Tyramine
- (D) Propranolol
- (E) Pargyline

14. Administration of reserpine has mitigated symptoms of sympathetic overactivity (hypertension, muscle tremors, sweating, and tachycardia) in a 47-year-old woman. The beneficial effects of reserpine result from what action?

- (A) Depletion of neuronal norepinephrine after inhibition of the vesicular H^+-monoamine pump
- (B) Interference with coupling of nerve terminal excitation and norepinephrine release
- (C) Blockade of postsynaptic norepinephrine uptake 2
- (D) Inhibition of tyrosine hydroxylase and reduced norepinephrine synthesis
- (E) Inhibition of presynaptic α_2-adrenoceptors

15. A 17-year-old boy who presents with a congenital mutation that causes impaired function of the G_S G protein would most likely show which of the following?

- (A) Reduced activity of monoamine oxidase
- (B) Reduced responses to stimulation of β_2-adrenoceptors by epinephrine
- (C) Increased responses to stimulation of β_2-adrenoceptors by epinephrine
- (D) Increased synthesis of cyclic adenosine monophosphate after administration of epinephrine
- (E) Increased enzymatic activity of adenylyl cyclase by epinephrine

16. Muscle weakness is found to result from a reduction in the amount of acetylcholine released at neuromuscular junctions in a 29-year-old woman. This is most likely to be the result of reduced activity/content of which of the following enzymes?

- ○ (A) Dopamine β-hydroxylase
- ○ (B) Catechol *O*-methyltransferase
- ○ (C) Monoamine oxidase
- ○ (D) Adenylyl cyclase
- ○ (E) Choline acetyltransferase

17. Which of the following receptors is a fundamental component of a ligand-gated ion channel?

- ○ (A) The nicotinic cholinergic receptor
- ○ (B) The β_2-adrenoceptor
- ○ (C) The α_2-adrenoceptor
- ○ (D) The intracellular testosterone receptor
- ○ (E) All of these receptors

18. The endoplasmic reticulum gives rise to peptides that enter the *cis* face of the Golgi complex. The neuropeptides that issue from the *trans* face of the Golgi complex are classically

- ○ (A) Found in large, dense-cored neuronal vesicles
- ○ (B) Found in small synaptic vesicles
- ○ (C) Associated only with synapses showing fast chemical neurotransmission
- ○ (D) Associated only with excitatory postsynaptic potentials (EPSPs)
- ○ (E) Associated only with inhibitory postsynaptic potentials (IPSPs)

19. Amino acid neurotransmitters may increase the activity of postsynaptic neurons (via excitation) or decrease the activity of postsynaptic neurons (via inhibition). Which of the following is an excitatory amino acid neurotransmitter?

- ○ (A) Acetylcholine
- ○ (B) Norepinephrine
- ○ (C) Glutamate
- ○ (D) γ-Aminobutyrate (GABA)
- ○ (E) Serotonin

20. Which of the following is true concerning G protein–coupled receptors?

- ○ (A) Only very few chemical messengers transmit information through such receptors
- ○ (B) G proteins form transmembrane loops in ligand-gated ion channels
- ○ (C) Dissociation of the α subunit from the α-, β-, γ-heterotrimer is essential for signal transfer
- ○ (D) Extracellular G proteins transduce neurotransmitter signals
- ○ (E) G protein–coupled receptors transduce nicotinic cholinergic signals

ANSWERS

1. **(C)** On the presynaptic norepinephrine nerve terminal, stimulation of autoinhibitory α_2-adrenoceptors by an agonist, such as norepinephrine, normally reduces subsequent norepinephrine release from that terminal. Blockade of the α_2-adrenoceptors by yohimbine eliminates that inhibitory influence and yields enhanced norepinephrine release. Yohimbine has been shown to improve blood pressure in patients with orthostatic hypotension.
FN2e 68–70

2. **(B)** The laboratory data should be interpreted to indicate that the synthetic pathway leading to the catecholamines dopamine, norepinephrine, and epinephrine is blocked at the step leading from dopa to dopamine. The enzyme that catalyzes the reaction of dopa to dopamine is L-amino acid decarboxylase.
FN2e 68–70

3. **(E)** Stimulation of β- (β_1-) adrenoceptors in the heart causes tachycardia and increased myocardial contractility. The presence of increased numbers and/or responsiveness of such receptors to normal chemical messengers (norepinephrine, epinephrine) would cause a resultant increase in cardiac output. Such a pattern has been documented to contribute to increased blood pressure (hypertension) in patients such as the individual described here.
FN2e 68–70

4. **(C)** Neuropeptide neurotransmitters are typically *not* released from neuronal large, dense-cored vesicles until stimulation frequencies of 10 Hz or higher are applied to a nerve. In contrast, small molecule neurotransmitters are commonly released by lower frequencies of stimulation. The scenario in this question is consistent with the presence of a neuropeptidergic nerve to the forearm that, when stimulated at high (=10 Hz) frequency, releases a neuropeptide that causes vasodilation and flushing of the forearm.
FN2e 63

5. **(D)** The mushroom *Amanita muscaria* contains muscarine, the prototypical agonist at muscarinic cholinergic receptors and the agent for which the receptors are named. Stimulation of muscarinic cholinergic receptors will elicit symptoms including nausea and vomiting, as well as increased gastrointestinal motility leading to abdominal cramping and diarrhea.
FN2e 63

6. **(E)** Subcutaneous injection of epinephrine (0.3 to 0.5 mL of a 1:1000 epinephrine solution) is a standard therapeutic intervention in a severe allergic reaction, which may present as bronchospasm, mucous membrane congestion and swelling, angioedema, and cardiovascular collapse. Epinephrine binds to highly specific G protein–coupled membrane receptors (in particular, the β-adrenoceptors), and triggers the expected cascade of intracellular events leading to increased levels of cyclic adenosine monophosphate.
FN2e 65–66

7. **(A)** Both excitatory and inhibitory responses can be produced by the same neurotransmitter in different tissues. The important criterion is the presence of either excitatory or inhibitory receptors for that neurotransmitter.
FN2e 67

8. **(E)** Monoamine oxidase is responsible for degradation of norepinephrine after its uptake into the presynaptic nerve terminal by uptake 1. Inhibition of monoamine oxidase reduces that degradation, limiting reuptake and resulting in higher concentrations of norepinephrine in the synaptic space. The effects of norepinephrine (either released from a nerve or exogenously injected) would thus be significantly exaggerated. None of the other chemical messengers is affected by this enzyme.
FN2e 68–70

9. **(C)** MPTP was originally synthesized inadvertently in an illegal effort to produce meperidine, a morphine-like narcotic analgesic. When ingested for recreational purposes, the MPTP caused profound, very rapidly developing and irreversible symptoms similar to those seen in advanced Parkinson disease. MPTP itself is inactive and must be metabolized to the active compound, N-methyl-4-phenylpyridinium (MPP+), following active uptake of MPTP into brain glial cells.
FN2e 68

10. **(A)** Glutamate is the predominant excitatory amino acid neurotransmitter in the mammalian brain. Its actions are terminated almost exclusively through the action of three highly specific glutamate transporters. One of these is localized to neurons, and the other two are found in glia cells. Faulty glutamate transporter proteins would result in less transport out of the synapse into neurons and glia and would result in more prolonged and more intense postsynaptic responses to neuronally released glutamate.
FN2e 68

11. **(E)** The symptoms described are those classically associated with an adverse reaction to/overdosage with cocaine. Cocaine inhibits neuronal uptake 1 of norepinephrine and results in spillover (overflow) of synaptic norepinephrine into blood and urine. All of the other choices are antihypertensive drugs that either reduce the release of norepinephrine or block norepinephrine (β-adrenoceptor) receptors in cardiovascular tissue (e.g., propranolol).
FN2e 68–70

12. **(A)** The agent α-methyltyrosine is a competitive inhibitor of tyrosine hydroxylase, which is the first enzymatic reaction in the cascade leading to norepinephrine synthesis. It has been used to treat the symptoms of pheochromocytoma. All the remaining agents would exaggerate responses to norepinephrine, either by inhibiting uptake 1 (cocaine), monoamine oxidase (pargyline), or uptake 2 (corticosterone) or by stimulating presynaptic release of norepinephrine (tyramine). They would worsen the symptoms of this patient.
FN2e 68–70

13. **(D)** In some patients, particularly younger whites, a so-called hyperdynamic state can exist in the cardiovascular system. This is characterized by increased sympathetic nerve activity, particularly including tachycardia and elevated cardiac output, which contribute to or cause elevated blood pressure. Administration of a β-adrenoceptor antagonist, such as propranolol, is often quite effective in blocking such responses and has often been used in the treatment of hypertension in this group of patients.
FN2e 68–70

14. **(A)** Reserpine is an irreversible inhibitor of the vesicular H^+-monoamine pump that concentrates monoamine neurotransmitters (including dopamine and norepinephrine) in synaptic vesicles. This inhibition blocks storage of monoamines and eventually results in depletion of monoamine neurotransmitters from the tissue.
FN2e 68–70

15. **(B)** The G protein G_S is associated with the β_2-adrenoceptor stimulated by epinephrine. A congenital impairment of G_S would reduce or eliminate the responses to epinephrine and all other β_2-adrenoceptor agonists.
FN2e 65–66, 68–70

16. **(E)** The mammalian neuromuscular junction depends on neuronal release of acetylcholine and subsequent stimulation of nicotinic cholinergic receptors on skeletal muscle. Choline acetyltransferase is the rate-limiting enzyme determining the formation of neuronal acetylcholine. Impairment of this enzyme would reduce the amount of acetylcholine available for release at the neuromuscular junction.
FN2e 61

17. **(A)** Only the nicotinic cholinergic receptor is associated with a membrane-bound ligand-gated ion channel. The adrenoceptors are G protein–coupled receptors, and the testosterone receptor is a protein found intracellularly that acts as a regulator of gene transcription.
FN2e 64–65

18. **(A)** Neuropeptides are most commonly associated with large, dense-cored vesicles. They are released, often at nonsynaptic sites along a neuron, following high frequencies of nerve stimulation. They can be associated with either EPSPs or IPSPs but are more commonly involved in mediation of slow chemical neurotransmission. In contrast, small molecule neurotransmitters are predominantly found in small synaptic vesicles.
FN2e 60–61

19. **(C)** Of the neurotransmitters listed, only glutamate (excitatory) and GABA (inhibitory) are amino acids.
FN2e 67

20. **(E)** Approximately three fourths of all chemical messengers are believed to use G protein–coupled receptors to send neuronal signals. Such receptors are associated with heterotrimeric (α-, β-, and γ-subunits) G proteins that are loosely bound to the intracellular elements of the receptor protein. On stimulation of the receptor with a ligand, the α-subunit dissociates from the other two subunits and binds with adenylyl cyclase on the intracellular surface of the membrane. Increased adenylyl cyclase activity increases intracellular levels of the second messenger, cyclic adenosine monophosphate. The nicotinic cholinergic receptor is a classic example of a ligand-gated ion channel, not a G protein–coupled receptor.
FN2e 65–66

CHAPTER 5

Development of the Nervous System

1. A male newborn is noted to have a developmental defect that is characteristically seen when the anterior neuropore fails to close. Which of the following deficits is most likely the result of this developmental error?

- ○ (A) Myelomeningocele
- ○ (B) Anencephaly
- ○ (C) Chiari malformation
- ○ (D) Meningocele
- ○ (E) Encephalocele

2. A sonogram at 6 months of gestation reveals a male fetus with a malformation in the lumbosacral area; a small part of the neural plate is exposed, suggesting failure of the posterior neuropore to close. Which of the following represents the time at which the posterior neuropore closes?

- ○ (A) 20 days
- ○ (B) 22 days
- ○ (C) 26 days
- ○ (D) 30 days
- ○ (E) 35 days

3. A female infant is born with myelodysplasia, malformations related to those parts of the neural tube formed by secondary neurulation. Which of the following portions of the neuraxis is formed by secondary neurulation?

- ○ (A) Forebrain
- ○ (B) Cervical spinal cord
- ○ (C) Lumbar, sacral, and coccygeal segments of the spinal cord
- ○ (D) Sacral and coccygeal segments of the spinal cord
- ○ (E) Coccygeal segments of the spinal cord

4. In addition to contributing to the formation of the nucleus pulposus, what other important function does the notochord have?

- ○ (A) Formation of a congenital dermal sinus
- ○ (B) Formation of the somite

- ○ (C) Induction of the ectoderm to form the neural plate
- ○ (D) Induction of the neural plate to form the neural crest cells
- ○ (E) Induction of the mesoderm to form muscle cells

5. An apparently healthy 23-year-old woman has a spontaneous miscarriage early in her pregnancy. Examination of the embryo revealed that neurulation did not occur. Exposure to which of the following would result in a failure of neurulation?

- ○ (A) Folic acid
- ○ (B) Colchicine
- ○ (C) Glutamate
- ○ (D) Acetylcholine
- ○ (E) γ-Aminobutyric acid

6. A male newborn has a developmental defect in his occipital region that contains cerebrospinal fluid and brain tissue. Which of the following most likely represents the defect?

- ○ (A) Meningocele
- ○ (B) Meningoencephalocele
- ○ (C) Meningomyelocele (myelomeningocele)
- ○ (D) Syringobulbia
- ○ (E) Spina bifida occulta

7. A female newborn is born with a failure of the anterior neuropore to close. In its more severe form, this is anencephaly. Which of the following structures in the adult represents the position of the closed anterior neuropore?

- ○ (A) Interventricular foramen
- ○ (B) Hypothalamic sulcus
- ○ (C) Anterior commissure
- ○ (D) Lamina terminalis
- ○ (E) Rostrum of the corpus callosum

8. Which of the following structures contains the nuclei of cranial nerves related to the oral cavity, long

ascending and descending tracts, and is a secondary brain vesicle?

- ○ (A) Prosencephalon
- ○ (B) Mesencephalon
- ○ (C) Rhombencephalon
- ○ (D) Myelencephalon

9. A child is born with unusually close-set eyes (hypotelorism). MRI reveals that the forebrain is only partially separated into hemispheres and the falx cerebri is only partially formed. The hemispheres have some gyri and sulci, and the lateral ventricles are rudimentary. Which of the following most likely represents this developmental failure?

- ○ (A) Alobar holoprosencephaly
- ○ (B) Frontal encephalocele
- ○ (C) Semilobar holoprosencephaly
- ○ (D) Lissencephaly
- ○ (E) Schizencephaly

10. A male infant is born with abnormal development of the occipital bone and of the upper cervical vertebrae. This resulted in a failure of the bend in the developing neural tube, which signifies the junction of spinal cord with the medulla, to properly form. In the normal neonate, the junction of the spinal cord with the medulla is represented by which of the following?

- ○ (A) Cephalic flexure
- ○ (B) Cervical flexure
- ○ (C) Pontine flexure
- ○ (D) Primary fissure
- ○ (E) Secondary fissure

11. During development the somite gives rise to important structures that interface with neural elements. Which of the following structures, while not specifically a derivative of the somite, may be adversely affected by a failure of the somite to differentiate properly?

- ○ (A) Skeletal muscle
- ○ (B) Vertebrae
- ○ (C) Certain parts of the skin
- ○ (D) Posterior root ganglion
- ○ (E) Nucleus pulposus

12. During development of a male fetus, the neural crest cells fail to detach from the neural plate and to form their adult derivatives, some of which are neural elements. In spite of such an error in development, which of the following neural structures would most likely still be present in this infant?

- ○ (A) Ciliary ganglia
- ○ (B) Posterior root ganglia
- ○ (C) Cells of the basal plate
- ○ (D) Sympathetic chain ganglia
- ○ (E) Trigeminal ganglion

13. During the development of a female fetus, cells of the neural crest fail to detach and to form their adult derivatives, some of which are non-neural elements.

Which of the following non-neural structures would most likely be the least affected by this developmental error?

- ○ (A) Melanocytes
- ○ (B) Pia and arachnoid mater
- ○ (C) Chromaffin cells in the adrenal medulla
- ○ (D) Cartilages of the pharyngeal arches
- ○ (E) Dura mater

14. The sonogram of a developing fetus reveals a significant malformation of the cerebral cortex. The pediatrician concludes that there has been an interruption of cell (neuron) migration. Developing neurons within the CNS migrate on which of the following?

- ○ (A) Schwann cells
- ○ (B) Protoplasmic astrocytes
- ○ (C) Radial glia
- ○ (D) Oligodendroglia
- ○ (E) Fibrous astrocytes

15. In the developing fetus, the sulcus limitans separates the alar plate from the basal plate. In most areas of the CNS it disappears, but it is retained at some specific points. Which of the following structures are separated from each by the sulcus limitans in the adult?

- ○ (A) Hypothalamus from dorsal thalamus
- ○ (B) Precentral gyrus from postcentral gyrus
- ○ (C) Facial colliculus from the vestibular area
- ○ (D) Fornix from the corpus callosum
- ○ (E) Facial colliculus from the hypoglossal and vagal trigones

16. The functional component associated with the cell bodies located in visceromotor (autonomic) ganglia is

- ○ (A) GVE
- ○ (B) SVE
- ○ (C) GSE
- ○ (D) GVA
- ○ (E) SSA

17. A newborn has difficulty swallowing and suckling and has other motor problems of cranial nerve origin. Extensive tests suggest that the basal plate, and the nuclei derived therefrom, did not form properly. Which of the following is derived from the basal plate?

- ○ (A) Vestibular nuclei
- ○ (B) Solitary nuclei
- ○ (C) Oculomotor nucleus
- ○ (D) Spinal trigeminal nucleus
- ○ (E) Cochlear nuclei

18. The MRI of a male newborn reveals cerebral hemispheres devoid of gyri and sulci. The pediatrician concluded that there has been a profound failure of cell migration in the developing cerebral cortex. Which of the following most closely represents this defect?

- ○ (A) Pachygyria
- ○ (B) Schizencephaly
- ○ (C) Syringobulbia

○ (D) Microgyria
○ (E) Lissencephaly

19. Within a few days of birth it becomes clear that a female infant is having difficulty swallowing and crying. The physician concludes that this may relate to a failure of the neurons innervating muscles of the pharynx and larynx (including the vocalis) to properly form. Which of the following represents the most likely location of these neurons in the normal infant?

○ (A) Dorsal motor vagal nucleus
○ (B) Nucleus ambiguus
○ (C) Edinger-Westphal nucleus
○ (D) Inferior salivatory nucleus
○ (E) Superior salivatory nucleus

20. A female infant is born with malformations of the face related to abnormal development of the pharyngeal arches. These include abnormal patterns of muscles of facial expression and mastication. Which of the following functional components is associated with those cells that innervate skeletal muscles that originate from pharyngeal arches?

○ (A) GSE
○ (B) GVE
○ (C) SVE
○ (D) SVA
○ (E) GSA

21. The MRI of a male newborn reveals cerebral hemispheres that have areas of small irregular gyri (microgyri) intermixed with areas containing very large gyri (pachygyri). Which of the following would most likely explain these developmental defects?

○ (A) Failure of the anterior neuropore to close
○ (B) Stenosis of the cerebral aqueduct
○ (C) Agenesis of the corpus callosum
○ (D) Improper migration of neuroblasts on the radial glia
○ (E) Failure of microglia to invade the developing nervous system

22. The MRI of a female newborn reveals clefts in the hemisphere that create a channel between the ventricle and the subarachnoid space on the surface. This image also reveals abnormal gyri and sulci patterns. Which of the following most closely represents this developmental defect?

○ (A) Semilobar holoprosencephaly
○ (B) Schizencephaly
○ (C) Lissencephaly
○ (D) Agenesis of the corpus callosum
○ (E) Encephalocele

23. A child is born with a single midline eye and a misshapen, barely discernible nose. CT reveals a rim of cortical tissue lying closely apposed to the skull, with no evidence of separate hemispheres, a corpus callosum, or falx cerebri. This condition is best characterized as what?

○ (A) Anencephaly
○ (B) Alobar holoprosencephaly
○ (C) Meningomyelocele
○ (D) Semilobar holoprosencephaly
○ (E) Schizencephaly

24. The orientation of Purkinje cell dendritic trees in the cerebellum is dependent on the correct orientation and development of which of the following?

○ (A) Mossy fibers
○ (B) Climbing fibers
○ (C) Granule cells
○ (D) Subplate cells
○ (E) Oligodendrocytes

25. A 9-year-old girl presents to the ophthalmology clinic with difficulty in depth perception, which is causing difficulty in her ability to play goalie on the soccer team. Testing reveals normal vision in the right eye, but, when the right eye is covered, visual acuity is extremely low in the left eye and depth perception is nonexistent in the absence of size or other cues. The child is unable to perceive shapes in a random-dot stereogram. What is the most likely cause of these signs?

○ (A) Presbyopia
○ (B) Anencephaly
○ (C) Schizencephaly
○ (D) Amblyopia
○ (E) Congenital cataract

26. Exposure to which of the following during the first trimester of pregnancy can cause severe neurologic deficits?

○ (A) Cat feces
○ (B) Folic acid
○ (C) RGD sequences
○ (D) Myelodysplasia
○ (E) Notochord

27. A child is born with spina bifida and craniorachischisis. The mother's nutritional status and health are unremarkable. The only apparently significant feature of the mother's medical history is that she is epileptic and has been under long-term therapy to control a generalized seizure disorder. The mother has also been taking a single multivitamin supplement daily since her teens. There is no evidence of illegal drug use and no family history of dysraphic defects. Given these facts, which of the following is the most likely cause of this birth defect?

○ (A) High blood pressure
○ (B) Lack of folic acid
○ (C) Hypervitaminosis A
○ (D) Valproic acid toxicity
○ (E) Hirschsprung disease

Questions 28 and 29 are based on the following patient:

A 22-year-old woman is brought to the emergency department after a minor automobile collision. Although she does not have obvious injuries, she complains of a bilateral loss of pain and thermal sensations from her upper extremities. The MRI revealed several congenital craniospinal defects.

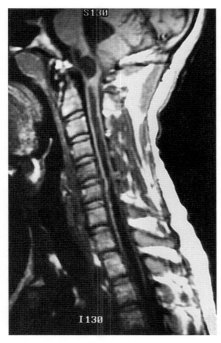

Figure 5–1

28.   Which of the following most specifically describes the developmental defect seen in this patient?

○ (A) Semilobar holoprosencephaly
○ (B) Myelomeningocele
○ (C) Anencephaly
○ (D) Spina bifida occulta
○ (E) Chiari I malformation

29.   This patient also has an acquired abnormality of the central nervous system that, when aggravated by trauma, is the probable cause of her somatosensory deficits. What is this defect?

○ (A) Tethered cord syndrome
○ (B) Hydrocephalus
○ (C) Syringomyelia
○ (D) Schizencephaly
○ (E) Agenesis of the corpus callosum

30.   A 29-year-old woman who has previously given birth to an infant with spina bifida aperta seeks counseling regarding measures to be taken before embarking on her second pregnancy. One simple, safe, and effective recommendation for such a patient would be what treatment?

○ (A) Megadoses of vitamin A
○ (B) Folic acid supplementation
○ (C) Anticonvulsant medicines such as carbamazepine
○ (D) Tubal ligation
○ (E) Amniocentesis to test for trisomy 21 (Down syndrome)

31.   A female child is born with a darkly pigmented patch on the lower back; closer examination reveals a tuft of sparse, dark hair in this region. A careful examination of the lumbosacral region reveals what appears to be a small opening exuding a colorless fluid. Which of the following represents the most likely cause of this finding?

○ (A) Spina bifida aperta
○ (B) Spina bifida occulta
○ (C) Anencephaly
○ (D) Craniorachischisis
○ (E) Dandy-Walker malformation

32.   Young patients who present with imperfect closure of the structures surrounding the neural tube, such as the meninges, and vertebral structures, as in spina bifida aperta, may have an increased frequency of which of the following?

○ (A) Appendicitis
○ (B) Megacolon
○ (C) Intraventricular hemorrhage
○ (D) Ectopia of the cerebellar tonsil
○ (E) Meningitis

ANSWERS

1.   **(B)** The lamina terminalis of the adult brain is generally regarded as the structure representing the location of the closed anterior neuropore. Failure of the anterior neuropore to close results in a profound defect in the brain (especially the forebrain), a largely absent skull, and facial abnormalities. Anencephaly is the most common brain defect (0.03% to 0.7% of births); most (95%) occur in families with histories of neural tube malformation. Affected infants are stillborn or usually die by 2 months of age.
FN2e 73

2.   **(C)** The posterior neuropore closes about 2 days after the anterior neuropore, which closes at about 24 days. Improper closure of the posterior neuropore, and malformation of the associated structures such as the vertebrae, meninges, and overlying skin, results in a variety of defects in the lumbosacral area.
FN2e 73

3.   **(D)** Secondary neurulation is the process that gives rise to the sacral and coccygeal levels of the spinal cord. The caudal eminence is a cell mass that appears at about

20 days, joins the caudal end of the neural tube, and enlarges. Its cavity joins the central canal of the neural tube. This eminence forms the sacral and coccygeal spinal cord.
FN2e 73

4.   **(C)** Substances in the notocord (inducing tissue) stimulate the overlying ectoderm (responding tissue) to form the neural plate. Formation of the vertebrae surrounding the spinal cord requires inductive signals from the notochord (to form vertebral bodies) and from the neural plate and tube (to form the vertebral arches). Remnants of notochord form parts of the nucleus pulposus.
FN2e 72–73

5.   **(B)** Colchicine disrupts microtubule formation and function. Because microtubules (and microfilaments) are essential to the folding process of the neural plate, exposure of an embryo to colchicine will result in a failure of neurulation. Deficiency of folic acid in the diet of pregnant women is associated with an increased risk of neural tube defects.
FN2e 73

6.   **(B)** A meninoencephalocele (this may also be called an encephalomeningocele) is a defect of the skull through which parts of the brain may protrude. Because cerebrospinal fluid within the subarachnoid space is found on the surface of the brain, this fluid and corresponding parts of the meninges are also found in this defect. These lesions are seen in about 1 in 5000 live births and in the United States are largely in the occipital area.
FN2e 73–75

7.   **(D)** The anterior neuropore closes at about 24 days. Its position in the adult is represented by the lamina terminalis. Failure of the anterior neuropore to close results in anencephaly.
FN2e 73

8.   **(D)** The myelencephalon (medulla oblongata) is one of two tertiary parts of the rhombencephalon, the other being the metencephalon. The mesencephalon is both a primary and secondary (tertiary) brain vesicle, and the prosencephalon is a primary brain vesicle.
FN2e 76–77

9.   **(C)** In semilobar holoprosencephaly there is the partial development of separate hemispheres especially in the occipital area. The falx cerebri is also partially formed. While individual lobes of the brain may be present, gyral and sulcal patterns are not normal. In general, the ventricles are large and not well formed.
FN2e 77

10.   **(B)** The cervical flexure, the gentle bend between the rhombencephalon and cervical spinal cord, begins at 22 to 30 days' gestation and progresses until 54 to 58 days' gestation. It is one of the two primary brain flexures, the other being the cephalic flexure.
FN2e 76–77

11.   **(D)** The posterior root ganglia are derived from neural crest cells that arise from the lateral margins of the neural plate. Although not a derivative of the somite, the development of the cells of the posterior root ganglia may be adversely affected by a failure of the dermatome to properly form. The other choices, either totally or in part, originate from portions of the somite (dermatome, sclerotome, and myotome).
FN2e 79–81

12.   **(C)** Basal plate cells (some of which are precursors of lower motor neurons) arise from the neural plate and would not be directly affected by a developmental failure of the neural crest. All peripheral ganglia, be they sensory (i.e., posterior root or trigeminal) or visceromotor/autonomic (i.e., ciliary, sympathetic chain) arise from neural crest cells.
FN2e 81–82

13.   **(E)** The primitive meninges (meninx primitiva) arise from mesenchyme (mesoderm) with some contributions from neural crest cells. However, the ectomeninx (future dura) is believed to originate from mesoderm with little or no neural crest contributions.
FN2e 79

14.   **(C)** Radial glia extend from the surface of the ventricle (or space of that particular portion of the brain) to the surface of the developing brain or spinal cord. Developing neurons migrate from the ventricular zone along the radial glia to take up their predetermined position in the adult.
FN2e 81, 85

15.   **(C)** The sulcus limitans is present in the spinal cord and in the floor of the rhomboid fossa in the embryo. However, in the adult it is present only in the floor of the fourth ventricle as a groove located lateral to the facial colliculus and the vagal and hypoglossal trigones. Motor structures are medial to the sulcus limitans and sensory structures (vestibular) are lateral.
FN2e 82–83

16.   **(A)** Cell bodies of visceromotor ganglia have the GVE functional component and their axons are postganglionic because they leave the ganglion to end in a visceral structure. GSE cells innervate skeletal muscle, and SVE cells (found only in certain cranial nerve nuclei) innervate striated muscles that originate from mesoderm located within the pharyngeal arches.
FN2e 81–82

17.   **(C)** The oculomotor nucleus is motor in function and originates from the basal plate. This nucleus provides innervation of four of the six main extraocular muscles. Sensory cranial nerve nuclei originate from the alar plate.
FN2e 82–84

18.   **(E)** Lissencephaly (smooth brain) describes a brain largely, or exclusively, devoid of gyri and sulci. The cells that should have formed the patterns characteristic of the cerebral cortex did not migrate properly on the radial glia, and the gyri and sulci were never formed. While the cortical patterns are altered, from the normal, in pachygyri, microgyri, and schizencephaly, the mere presence of gyri/sulci indicates that some cell migration did take place.
FN2e 86, 88

19. **(B)** The nucleus ambiguus is part of the special visceral efferent cell column of the brainstem. Cells of this nucleus primarily innervate the stylopharyngeus muscle, and muscles of the larynx and pharynx are innervated by the vagus nerve. One important muscle innervated by the vagus nerve is the vocalis, the small medial part of the thyroarytenoid muscle.
FN2e 81–82

20. **(C)** The motor nuclei (SVE functional component) of the brainstem that innervate muscles arising from mesoderm of the pharyngeal arches are the trigeminal (arch I), facial (arch II), and nucleus ambiguus (arches III and IV).
FN2e 83–84

21. **(D)** Abnormal migration of neuroblasts on the processes of radial glia may result in a variety of abnormal patterns of gyri/sulci. Exuberant migration may result in many small gyri (microgyri), a partial failure of migration in fewer but larger gyri (pachygryi), and a complete failure in a complete absence of sulci/gyri (lissencephaly). In many cases, the gyri/sulci formed do not resemble normal patterns.
FN2e 86

22. **(B)** Patients with schizencephaly have abnormal gyral/sulcal patterns and frequently have enlarged ventricles and other developmental defects. The clefts in these brains may result from localized cell migration failures or from microinfarcts during development with subsequent alterations in cell migration and tissue reabsorption.
FN2e 86–88

23. **(B)** The signs described in this question are consistent with alobar holoprosencephaly. As the name implies, this defect results in a single, globular brain mass with grossly enlarged ventricles; separate hemispheres fail to develop. There are frequently severe craniofacial abnormalities associated with this disorder.
FN2e 77

24. **(C)** Purkinje cell dendrites have a characteristic candelabra-like shape. They are extensively branched but only ramify in two dimensions. This characteristic shape is dependent on orientation perpendicular to the T processes of granule cells early in cerebellar development.
FN2e 84–85

25. **(D)** Amblyopia is a disease that results when information from one eye is "ignored" because it is miswired into the visual cortex. It can be corrected if it is detected before school age, but by 9 years of age the miswired connections can no longer be modified.
FN2e 88–89

26. **(A)** It is estimated that 80% of cats harbor asymptomatic *Toxoplasma spp.* infections. Exposure to contaminated cat feces by a pregnant woman can cause neurologic defects, especially if it occurs during the first trimester.
FN2e 77–78

27. **(D)** The antiseizure medications valproic acid and carbamazepine, among others, can cause dysraphic defects.
FN2e 73

28. **(E)** The Chiari malformation is characterized by ectopia (a congenital malposition) of the cerebellar tonsils through the foramen magnum and may be accompanied by cavitation of the spinal cord (syringomyelia) and/or of the medulla (syringobulbia).
FN2e 73–75

29. **(C)** Syringomyelia may be associated with the Chiari malformation and can be caused, or exacerbated, by trauma or increased intracranial pressure from any cause.
FN2e 73–74

30. **(B)** The MRC Vitamin Study of 1991 showed that in women who had previously given birth to an infant with dysraphic defects the incidence of further neural tube defects was reduced 70%, following folic acid supplementation, relative to untreated controls.
FN2e 73

31. **(A)** Spina bifida aperta is a dysraphic defect that often shows few external manifestations. However, pigmented patches and tufts of hair are often associated with otherwise minor dysraphic defects. In this case, the presence of a small, patent channel, which communicates with the lumbar cistern and leaks cerebrospinal fluid, is consistent with the diagnosis.
FN2e 74

32. **(E)** The patent aperture characteristic of spina bifida aperta or of a congenital dermal sinus may allow access of bacteria to the subarachnoid space, resulting in purulent meningitis.
FN2e 73–74, 109

CHAPTER 6

The Ventricles, Choroid Plexus, and Cerebrospinal Fluid

1. An 83-year-old man presents with mild dementia but no obvious motor or sensory deficits. An MRI reveals clearly enlarged ventricles (especially the lateral ventricles), widening of the cortical sulci, and enlargement of the deep parts of the sylvian (lateral) fissures over the insular cortex. There is no blood in the ventricles. Which of the following accurately describes the enlarged ventricles in this patient?

- (A) Obstructive hydrocephalus
- (B) Hydrocephalus ex vacuo
- (C) Congenital hydrocephalus
- (D) Posthemorrhagic hydrocephalus
- (E) Communicating hydrocephalus

2. A 19-year-old woman becomes ill rather suddenly with severe headaches, nausea and vomiting, and a progressively decreasing level of consciousness (all signs of increased intracranial pressure). MRI reveals a large pinealoma (pineoblastoma, an aggressive pineal tumor) that has blocked the cerebral aqueduct. The neurosurgeon explains to the family that the CSF must be drained immediately or she will die. Approximately how much CSF is produced in a 24-hour period in the average healthy adult?

- (A) 250 to 300 mL
- (B) 300 to 350 mL
- (C) 350 to 375 mL
- (D) 450 to 500 mL
- (E) 600 mL+

3. The epithelium of the choroid plexus sits on a basal lamina that is separated from the basal lamina of the capillary by a space. What is in this space?

- (A) CSF
- (B) Fibroblasts and collagen
- (C) Pia mater
- (D) Elastic fibers
- (E) Blood cells

4. The MRI of a 51-year-old man suffering from Huntington disease reveals the loss of a prominent structure associated with the lateral ventricle. Which of the following structures is found in the lateral wall of the anterior horn of the lateral ventricle?

- (A) Column of the fornix
- (B) Body of caudate nucleus
- (C) Head of caudate nucleus
- (D) Amygdaloid nucleus
- (E) Septum pellucidum

5. The MRI of a 13-year-old boy reveals a highly vascular tumor originating from the choroid plexus of the temporal horn of the lateral ventricle. Which of the following vessels is most likely the primary source of blood supply to this tumor?

- (A) Anterior choroidal artery
- (B) Medial posterior choroidal artery
- (C) Anterior inferior cerebellar artery

○ (D) Posterior inferior cerebellar artery
○ (E) Branches of M_1

6. A 4-year-old child complains to his mother of headaches (especially in the morning). He frequently vomits and is progressively more lethargic. An MRI reveals a tumor that originates from the choroid plexus of the fourth ventricle. Which of the following represents the primary blood supply to this part of the choroid plexus?

○ (A) Anterior inferior cerebellar artery
○ (B) Medial posterior choroidal artery
○ (C) Lateral posterior choroidal artery
○ (D) Anterior choroidal artery
○ (E) Posterior inferior cerebellar artery

7. The neuropathologist examines a tumor removed from the ventricular system of a 36-year-old woman. He observes cells that appear completely normal but they do not sit on a continuous basal lamina. These cells are most likely which of the following?

○ (A) Endothelial cells of the choroid plexus
○ (B) Endothelial cells lining arteries
○ (C) Ependymal cells
○ (D) Endothelial cells lining veins

8. A 23-year-old man presents with a fever of 102°F, headache, chills, and nausea and appears to be a bit confused. His symptoms began several days ago. He has been followed by an otolaryngologist for several weeks for a persistent and painful ear infection. A lumbar puncture yields a cloudy sample of CSF with a neutrophil count of 8500/mm³. This patient most likely has which of the following?

○ (A) A brain tumor
○ (B) Multiple sclerosis
○ (C) Arteriovenous malformation
○ (D) Acute bacterial meningitis
○ (E) Subarachnoid hemorrhage

9. An infant is delivered with anencephaly. A failure of which of the following structures to properly develop is associated with this catastrophic defect?

○ (A) Lamina terminalis
○ (B) Optic chiasm
○ (C) The mammillary bodies
○ (D) Anterior commissure
○ (E) Column of the fornix

10. The neuropathologist examining a tumor removed from the choroid plexus of a 49-year-old man discovers cells that appear to have developed from choroidal epithelium but lack apial surface specializations. Which of the following specializations is usually found on the apical surfaces of choroid epithelial cells?

○ (A) Cilia
○ (B) Stereocilia
○ (C) A smooth undulating membrane
○ (D) Microvilli
○ (E) Invaginations or crypts

11. The neuroradiologist examines the coronal and axial MRI of a 29-year-old woman with vague neurologic complaints. The radiologist notes that a structure seen in about 80% of patients that bridges the space of the third ventricle is absent in this patient. However, the vague neurologic problems are certainly not related to this observation. Which of the following structures is lacking in about 20% of human brains without an associated functional deficit?

○ (A) Anterior commissure
○ (B) Posterior commissure
○ (C) Massa intermedia
○ (D) Corpus callosum
○ (E) Optic chiasm

12. A 34-year-old woman who is morbidly obese presents with headache, papilledema, and visual deficits that interfere with daily living. Tests reveal an increase in intracranial pressure, but enlarged ventricles and effacement of the sulci are not seen on MRI. This patient is most likely suffering from which of the following?

○ (A) Aqueductal stenosis
○ (B) Communicating hydrocephalus
○ (C) Hydrocephalus ex vacuo
○ (D) Idiopathic intracranial hypertension
○ (E) Normal pressure hydrocephalus

13. A sample of CSF is taken, by lumbar puncture, from a 27-year-old woman who presents with vague neurologic complaints. Which of the following would most likely represent an abnormal condition in the CSF of this patient?

○ (A) 120 mg/dL protein
○ (B) Less than 5 lymphocytes per milliliter
○ (C) Lower K^+ and Ca^{2+} than blood plasma
○ (D) Higher Mg^{2+} and Cl^- than blood plasma

14. A sonogram of a 31-year-old woman who is 8 months pregnant reveals an enlarged fourth ventricle in the fetus. The attending physician concludes that the foramina of the fourth ventricle that open into the subarachnoid space and allow a circulation of CSF have not yet formed. Which of the following represent the approximate time when these foramina are usually patent?

○ (A) 2 weeks of gestation
○ (B) 1 month of gestation
○ (C) 1.5 months of gestation
○ (D) End of the first trimester
○ (E) End of the second trimester

15. The MRI of a 47-year-old woman reveals a small tumor blocking the interventricular foramen on the right side. Which of the two following structures most closely form the borders of the interventricular foramen?

○ (A) Periaqueductal gray matter and posterior commissure
○ (B) Column of fornix and anterior tubercle of thalamus
○ (C) Head of caudate and stria terminalis
○ (D) Septum pellucidum and head of caudate
○ (E) Septum pellucidum and column of fornix

16. Lumbar puncture of a 59-year-old man yields a sample of CSF containing large amounts of red blood

cells. Which of the following is the most likely explanation of these cells in the CSF of this patient?

- (A) Astrocytoma
- (B) Multiple sclerosis
- (C) Bacterial meningitis
- (D) Rupture of an intracranial aneurysm
- (E) Meningeal syphilis

17. The CT of a 51-year-old man reveals a calcified glomus choroideum. This large tuft of choroid plexus is found in which of the following locations?

- (A) Third ventricle
- (B) Atrium of lateral ventricle
- (C) Temporal horn of lateral ventricle
- (D) Anterior horn of lateral ventricle
- (E) Lateral recess of fourth ventricle

18. A 22-year-old woman undergoes a lumbar puncture to determine if she is suffering from a bacterial infection of the CNS. The attending physician assures the family that the 2-mL sample removed will not adversely affect the patient's clinical condition. Which of the following represents the amount of CSF found in the ventricles and subarachnoid spaces of the average adult human at any given moment?

- (A) 50 mL
- (B) 80 mL
- (C) 120 mL
- (D) 180 mL
- (E) 225 mL

19. A sample of CSF from a 36-year-old woman contains 75 lymphocytes per milliliter and elevated immunoglobulin G levels. This patient is most likely suffering from which of the following?

- (A) Acute subarachnoid hemorrhage
- (B) Meningioma
- (C) Syphilitic meningitis
- (D) Multiple sclerosis
- (E) Epidural hemorrhage

20. Production of CSF in any healthy adult is an active process that may proceed against a pressure gradient and with the expenditure of energy. Consequently, cells producing CSF contain many of which of the following structures?

- (A) Lysosomes
- (B) Mitochondria
- (C) Synaptic vesicles
- (D) Nuclei
- (E) Rough endoplasmic reticulum

21. The MRI of a 55-year-old man reveals a tumor of the pineal gland that has enlarged to about 2.5 cm in diameter and is compressing adjacent structures. Which of the following is a likely consequence of this tumor?

- (A) Enlargement of both lateral ventricles only
- (B) Communicating hydrocephalus
- (C) Enlargement of the entire ventricular system
- (D) Triventricular hydrocephalus
- (E) Hydrocephalus ex vacuo

22. A 44-year-old woman presents with symptoms of increased intracranial pressure, such as headache, nausea, and lethargy. MRI reveals a vascular tumor in the choroid plexus of the third ventricle that partially blocks the opening to the cerebral aqueduct. The blood supply to this tumor most likely originates from which of the following?

- (A) Anterior choroidal artery
- (B) Posterior inferior cerebellar artery
- (C) Lateral posterior choroidal artery
- (D) Medial posterior choroidal artery
- (E) Branches of P_4

23. An 18-year-old woman is brought to the emergency department by her parents. She has a severe headache and, according to her parents, she has become progressively more lethargic over the past several days and has had several bouts of vomiting. MRI reveals a tumor in the rostral portion of the third ventricle blocking the right and left interventricular foramina. The enlarged lateral ventricles in this patient are best described as

- (A) Aqueductal stenosis
- (B) Obstructive hydrocephalus
- (C) Communicating hydrocephalus
- (D) Idiopathic hydrocephalus
- (E) Normal pressure hydrocephalus

24. A 24-year-old man becomes acutely ill and presents to the emergency department in a depressed level of consciousness. MRI of his brain reveals enlarged ventricles as shown here; the fourth ventricle appears normal. Based on this information which of the following is the most likely site of the obstruction?

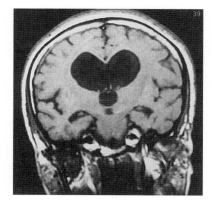

Figure 6–1

- (A) Right interventricular foramen
- (B) Left interventricular foramen
- (C) Both interventricular foramina
- (D) Cerebral aqueduct
- (E) Foramen of Magendie

25. A 66-year-old man presents with persistent headache and the physician orders a CT. This image is normal for a man the age of this patient, but the neuroradiologist notes that this patient has a "calcified glomus

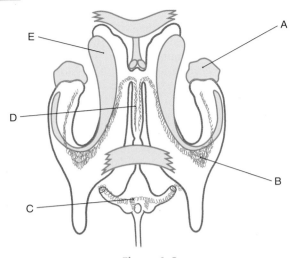

Figure 6–2

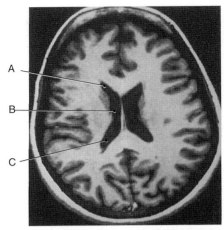

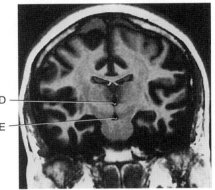

Figure 6–4

choroideum." Which of the above labeled structures is most likely calcified in this patient? (   )

26.   The CT of an 81-year-old woman shows slightly enlarged ventricles and subarachnoid cisterns. In addition, she has a calcified pineal gland that the physician indicates is not causing any neurological problems. Which of the following labeled structures is most likely calcified in this patient? (   )

28.   A 22-year-old man is brought to the emergency department after an automobile collision. Suspecting a head injury, the physician orders a CT, which reveals blood in the CSF in the subarachnoid spaces but not in the ventricles. Which of the following labeled areas would most likely contain bloody CSF in this patient? (   )

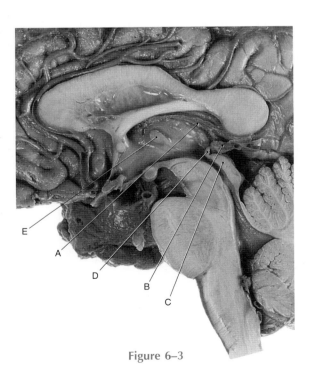

Figure 6–3

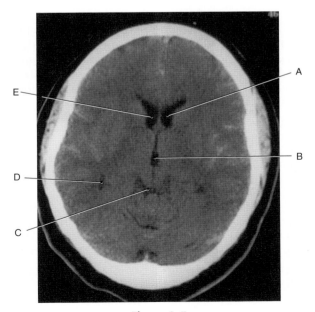

Figure 6–5

27.   A 43-year-old woman presents with headache and signs of increased intracranial pressure. MRI reveals a tumor in the body of the lateral ventricle. Which of the following labeled areas most closely represent this particular part of the ventricle? (   )

ANSWERS

1. **(B)** The enlarged ventricles in this patient are the result of an age-related decrease in the amount of the surrounding brain tissue with a corresponding increase in ventricle size. The enlarged ventricles are not due to increased pressure within the ventricles.
FN2e 106

2. **(D)** The volume of the ventricular system and the contiguous subarachnoid space is 120 to 140 mL in the average adult. The volume of CSF is replaced about 4 times every 24 hours. In this example the woman is suffering from acute hydrocephalus, which can be fatal within several hours of onset as CSF accumulates within the head. Reabsorption of CSF is an essential feature of maintaining intracranial pressure within a normal range.
FN2e 102

3. **(B)** The choroid plexus is basically a specialized epithelium sitting on a dense vascular network. A limited amount of connective tissue (fibroblasts and collagen) intervenes between the capillaries and choroid epithelium.
FN2e 101–102

4. **(C)** The caudate nucleus is characteristically found in the lateral wall of the lateral ventricle throughout, with the head in the anterior horn, the body in the body (or trunk), and the tail in the inferior (or temporal) horn. The septum pellucidum and column of the fornix are located medially in the anterior horn, and the amygdala is in the rostral wall of the inferior horn.
FN2e 96–98

5. **(A)** The anterior choroidal artery is a branch of the cerebral part of the internal carotid artery. This artery courses along the mesial temporal lobe and the trajectory of the optic tract and sends branches into the temporal horn (inferior horn) of the lateral ventricle. In addition to the choroid plexus of the temporal (inferior) horn, the anterior choroidal artery also serves the optic tract, inferior parts of the lenticular nucleus, the hippocampus, and other structures in this area.
FN2e 101, 123–124

6. **(E)** The blood supply to the choroid plexus within the fourth ventricle is through the posterior inferior cerebellar artery whereas that to the small tuft of choroid plexus sticking out of the foramen of Luschka is through the anterior inferior cerebellar artery.
FN2e 101–102, 127

7. **(C)** Ependymal cells sit on a glial limiting membrane formed by the processes of astrocytes. Occasionally, pieces of basal lamina, presumably arising from capillaries in the vicinity, may be found at the base of ependymal cells; these do not form a continuous basal lamina. Endothelial cells of arteries and veins and the endothelial cells of the choroid plexus sit on a continuous basal lamina.
FN2e 99–100

8. **(D)** All signs and symptoms of this patient plus the large amount of neutrophils in the CSF point to acute bacterial meningitis. Hemorrhage from an arteriovenous malformation typically involves the brain substance, less commonly the ventricles and the subarachnoid space. A brain tumor would shed proteins into the CSF, and multiple sclerosis would result in increased immunoglobulin in the CSF.
FN2e 102–103

9. **(A)** The lamina terminalis extends from the upper rostral edge of the optic chiasm to the lower aspect of the anterior commissure. It forms the rostral wall of the third ventricle on the midline and is regarded as the point at which the anterior neuropore closes. The other choices all form the floor of the third ventricle.
FN2e 97

10. **(D)** The apical surface of choroid epithelial cells have many microvilli. This structural feature, as well as the fact that these cells contain many mitochondria, relate to their high level of secretory activity.
FN2e 101

11. **(C)** The massa intermedia is a result of the two anlage of the dorsal thalami opposing each other close enough that they touch on the midline, resulting in a bridge of tissue extending across the space of the third ventricle. This results in a fusion of the two anlage of the dorsal thalamus, the point of fusion represented by the massa intermedia of the adult. In about 20% of individuals this does not happen.
FN2e 96, 98, 221

12. **(D)** Idiopathic intracranial hypertension (also called pseudotumor cerebri) is seen in obese women of child-bearing age. Although there is an increase in intracranial pressure, no such evidence may be seen on MRI. Treatment may include a weight loss program, shunting, or fenestration of the optic nerve sheath to prevent further loss of vision.
FN2e 106

13. **(A)** Excessively high levels (20 to 50 mg/dL is normal) of protein would not be seen in normal CSF. Increased levels of protein in CSF may be indicative of tumor, tissue damage, bacterial meningitis, or tuberculosis. The other choices are characteristic of CSF from a normal healthy individual.
FN2e 102–103

14. **(D)** The choroid plexus is being formed and being invaded by blood vessels before the end of the first trimester. However, the only naturally occurring openings between the ventricular system and the subarachnoid space are those of the fourth ventricle. These openings are established at 10 to 12 weeks.
FN2e 95

15. **(B)** The column of the fornix is located rostromedial to the interventricular foramen and the anterior tubercle of the thalamus (overlying the anterior nuclei of the thalamus) and is located caudolateral to the foramen. These relationships are frequently obvious in axial MRI.
FN2e 97

16. **(D)** Red blood cells in a sample of CSF, in the absence of other elements such as increased levels of

protein, white blood cells, or bacteria, are indicative of a rupture of an aneurysm into the subarachnoid space. Other causes of red blood cells in the CSF may be a traumatic tap or intermittent bleeding from an aneurysm or arteriovenous malformation.
FN2e 102–103

17. **(B)** The atrium of the lateral ventricle is that point where the body, posterior horn, and temporal horn of the lateral ventricle converge. The glomus choroideum, which frequently contains calcifications (a convenient landmark on CT), is the enlarged portion of the choroid plexus in the atrium.
FN2e 97

18. **(C)** The amount of CSF within the ventricles and subarachnoid space is somewhat variable and partially dependent on body size. It may range from 70 to 150 mL but averages 120 to 140 mL.
FN2e 102

19. **(D)** Elevated lymphocytes (normally there are usually fewer than 5 cells/mL) and especially elevated levels of immunoglobulin G are characteristic of patients with multiple sclerosis.
FN2e 102–103

20. **(B)** Epithelial cells of the choroid plexus produce CSF under normal conditions and will also produce CSF against a pressure gradient. That is, CSF is produced even when the pressure in the ventricular system is increased. Choroidal cells contain many mitochondria, which are the energy source for this activity.
FN2e 101–102

21. **(D)** Tumors of the pineal gland may compress the cerebral aqueduct with a resultant enlargement of the third ventricle and both lateral ventricles. Triventricular hydrocephalus refers to the fact that three ventricles are simultaneously involved.
FN2e 99, 104

22. **(D)** The medial posterior choroidal artery originates from P_2, arches around the brainstem, and enters the caudal aspect of the third ventricle to serve the choroid plexus. En route, this vessel gives rise to branches to the brainstem and to a small caudomedial portion of the thalamus.
FN2e 101, 233–234

23. **(B)** Blockage of the flow of CSF within the ventricular system may result in obstructive hydrocephalus. Ventricular spaces upstream to the blockage will enlarge and the patient will experience signs and symptoms of increased intracranial pressure. Colloid cysts at the interventricular foramen are one cause of obstructive hydrocephalus.
FN2e 104–105

24. **(D)** This image reveals enlarged lateral ventricles (they are symmetrically enlarged) and a clearly enlarged third ventricle. Obstruction of the cerebral aqueduct results in enlargements of all ventricular spaces upstream to the blockage. Obstruction of the interventricular foramen (or foramina) will result in enlargement of the lateral ventricle (or ventricles) but not of the third ventricle.
FN2e 104–106

25. **(B)** The large tuft of choroid plexus in the atrium of the lateral ventricle is the glomus choroideum, commonly called the glomus. In older individuals this part of the choroid plexus may become calcified, in which case it is obvious in CT. The atrium of the lateral ventricle is that point at which the body of the lateral ventricle, posterior horn of the lateral ventricle, and inferior (temporal) horn of the lateral ventricle converge.
FN2e 97

26. **(B)** The pineal gland is located superior to the midbrain portion of the brainstem (and immediately caudad to the third ventricle). It is located inferior to the splenium of the corpus callosum on the midline. Large tumors of the pineal may compress the midbrain, obstruct the cerebral aqueduct, and interrupt the flow of CSF.
FN2e 97–99

27. **(B)** The body of the lateral ventricle is rostrally continuous with the anterior horn of the lateral ventricle and caudally continuous with the atrium. This part of the ventricular system is especially obvious on axial MRI or CT.
FN2e 96–97, 104–105

28. **(C)** The quadrigeminal cistern (superior cistern) is an enlarged part of the subarachnoid space. It is located posterior (dorsal) to the superior and inferior colliculi and, in addition to the colliculi, contains the root of the trochlear nerve, pineal gland, great cerebral vein, and portions of the posterior cerebral, quadrigeminal, and choroidal arteries.
FN2e 99, 104–105, 117–119

CHAPTER 7

The Meninges

1.   The mother of a 6-month-old girl expresses concern to the pediatrician about a red dimpled, hyperpigmented area and a small tuft of hair on her daughter's lumbosacral area. The physician expresses a small amount of purulent material from a small opening at the dimple and concludes that this patient has a dermal sinus (congenital dermal sinus or dermal sinus tract). Which of the following is also indicative of this lesion?

○ (A) Increased blood pressure
○ (B) Chronic increase in intracranial pressure
○ (C) Tethered cord syndrome
○ (D) Recurrent meningitis
○ (E) Enlarged ventricles on MRI

2.   The MRI of a 56-year-old woman reveals an aneurysm on the posterior cerebral artery as it passes through the ambient cistern. The aneurysm is large and completely fills this cistern. Which of the following structures would most likely be damaged by this aneurysm?

○ (A) Trochlear nerve
○ (B) Trigeminal nerve
○ (C) Pontine veins
○ (D) Great cerebral vein (of Galen)
○ (E) Basilar artery

3.   In the developing human, the meninges originate from the endomeninx and the ectomeninx. A failure of the ectomeninx to properly develop will most adversely affect which of the following?

○ (A) Pia mater
○ (B) Arachnoid mater
○ (C) Dura mater
○ (D) Denticulate ligament
○ (E) Filum terminale internum

4.   A 23-year-old man presents with recurring headaches that have become more severe over the past 2 weeks. These headaches are most prominent in frontal and parietal areas but do not involve the back of the head or the neck. This would suggest that they originate from

supratentorial portions of the cerebral dura. Which of the following is the most consistent nerve supply to this particular portion of the dura matter?

○ (A) Vagus nerve
○ (B) V_1 only of trigeminal nerve
○ (C) Facial nerve
○ (D) Vagus and facial nerves
○ (E) V_1, V_2, and V_3 of trigeminal nerve

5.   Which of the following is not a naturally occurring biologic space associated with the cerebral meninges but actually represents an artifactual space resultant to trauma or some type of pathologic process?

○ (A) Spinal epidural space
○ (B) Subarachnoid space
○ (C) Subdural space
○ (D) Lumbar cistern
○ (E) Dorsal cerebellomedullary cistern

6.   A 39-year-old woman presents with ataxia accompanied by a visual problem. Recognizing this as an unusual combination of deficits, the physician orders an MRI, which reveals a large tumor, probably a meningioma, impinging on both the cerebellum and the occipital lobe. Which of the following represents the most likely location of this tumor?

○ (A) Falx cerebri
○ (B) Falx cerebelli
○ (C) Tentorium cerebelli
○ (D) Diaphragma sellae
○ (E) Filum terminale internum

7.   A 22-year-old man is brought to the emergency department after an automobile collision. A CT reveals a skull fracture that has resulted in a tear of the middle meningeal artery. This important dural vessel most consistently arises from which of the following?

○ (A) Occipital artery
○ (B) Ethmoidal arteries

35

○ (C) Maxillary branch of the external carotid artery
○ (D) Ascending pharyngeal artery
○ (E) Vertebral arteries

8. During development of the human fetus, spaces normally appear within the endomeninx. A failure of these spaces to develop normally would most likely result in the absence of which of the following?

○ (A) Subpial space
○ (B) Subarachnoid space and cisterns
○ (C) Subdural space
○ (D) Epidural space
○ (E) Venous sinuses

9. A 47-year-old man presents with headache and bilateral weakness and numbness of both lower extremities. Realizing this is an unusual combination of deficits the physician orders an MRI. This image reveals a 2.5 × 3.0-cm tumor impinging on the somatomotor and somatosensory cortices of both cerebral hemispheres. Which of the following represents the most likely location of this tumor?

○ (A) Falx cerebri
○ (B) Falx cerebelli
○ (C) Tentorium cerebelli
○ (D) Diaphragma sellae
○ (E) Filum terminale externum

10. A 61-year-old woman presents with headaches that have slowly worsened over the last year. She has no other symptoms. MRI reveals a grape-size tumor on the tentorium cerebelli. Her physician suggests that the headaches may relate to this tumor. Which of the following most likely gives rise to the tentorial nerve that innervates the tentorium cerebelli?

○ (A) Facial nerve
○ (B) C2 spinal nerve
○ (C) Maxillary branch of the trigeminal nerve
○ (D) Ophthalmic branch of the trigeminal nerve
○ (E) Vagus nerve

11. In the normal healthy patient, the occurrence of many tight (occluding) junctions prohibits the movement of cerebrospinal fluid (CSF) out of the subarachnoid space. Which of the following portions of the meninges characteristically has many tight junctions?

○ (A) Meningeal dura
○ (B) Periosteal dura
○ (C) Dural border cell layer
○ (D) Pia mater
○ (E) Arachnoid barrier cell layer (arachnoid mater)

12. The MRI of a 14-year-old girl reveals a small tumor in the posterior fossa located on the surface of the cerebellum and invading the overlying dura and inner table of the skull. This patient complains of pain and headache. Which of the following represents the most consistent nerve supply to the infratentorial portion of the dura mater?

○ (A) C1 to C3 spinal nerves plus vagal branches
○ (B) Facial nerve only
○ (C) C1 to C3 spinal nerves only
○ (D) C1 to C3 spinal nerves plus facial branches
○ (E) Vagus nerve only

13. The neuropathologist examines a tumor from a 31-year-old man and concludes that it is a meningioma. Which of the following layers of the meninges is the primary source of the cells that give rise to this type of tumor?

○ (A) Periosteal dura mater
○ (B) Meningeal dura mater
○ (C) Arachnoid mater
○ (D) Pia mater
○ (E) Dura, arachnoid, and pia equally

14. A 37-year-old man becomes acutely ill with fever, chills, nausea, and a painful stiff neck. Suspecting meningitis, the physician orders a lumbar puncture, which contains many white blood cells and organisms. Which of the following is the most common causative agent of bacterial meningitis in adults?

○ (A) *Haemophilus influenzae*
○ (B) *Listeria monocytogenes*
○ (C) group B *Streptococcus*
○ (D) *Escherichia coli*
○ (E) *Streptococcus pneumoniae*

15. The neuropathologist examines a tumor from a 62-year-old woman that was removed from the falx cerebri near the crista galli. This tumor contains elongated fibroblasts and copious amounts of extracellular collagen. Which of the following layers of the meninges is most obviously represented in this tumor?

○ (A) Arachnoid barrier cell layer
○ (B) Pia mater
○ (C) Dural border cell layer
○ (D) Meningeal and periosteal layers of the dura mater
○ (E) Arachnoid trabecular layer

16. The endomeninx will give rise to which of the following portions of the adult meninges?

○ (A) Pia mater only
○ (B) Arachnoid mater only
○ (C) Dura mater
○ (D) Leptomeninges
○ (E) Dura + arachnoid

17. In the normal adult, the brain does not "float" but is suspended by the arachnoid trabeculae within the CSF of the subarachnoid space. Which of the following represents the approximate weight of a 1400-gram brain (if weighed in air) when it is suspended in CSF?

○ (A) 130 to 140 grams
○ (B) 80 to 125 grams
○ (C) 40 to 50 grams
○ (D) 10 to 20 grams
○ (E) 0 gram; the brain has no weight in CSF

18. The MRI of a 47-year-old emaciated woman with widely metastatic cancer reveals a blood clot in the venous sinus located along the point where the falx cerebri attaches to the tentorium cerebelli. Which of the following represents the most likely location of this obstruction to venous flow?

○ (A) Straight sinus
○ (B) Transverse sinus
○ (C) Inferior sagittal sinus
○ (D) Sigmoid sinus
○ (E) Superior petrosal sinus

19. A 16-year-old girl becomes acutely ill with nausea and vomiting, fever, and headache. A lumbar puncture confirms the physician's initial interpretation of bacterial meningitis. Which of the following portions of the meninges is most commonly involved in meningitis?

○ (A) Arachnoid mater only
○ (B) Pia mater only
○ (C) Arachnoid plus pia (leptomeninges)
○ (D) Periosteal dura mater
○ (E) Meningeal dura mater
○ (F) Dura, arachnoid, and pia

20. A 3-week-old girl presents with hydrocephalus, bulging fontanelles, and dilated scalp. An angiogram reveals a large vein of Galen malformation. Which of the following represents the most likely location of this vascular malformation?

○ (A) Interpeduncular cistern
○ (B) Superior (quadrigeminal) cistern
○ (C) Dorsal cerebellomedullary cistern
○ (D) Ambient cistern
○ (E) Prepontine cistern

21. A 31-year-old woman is brought to the emergency department after an automobile collision; she is unresponsive. MRI reveals a large collection of blood in the area of the dural border cell layer. Which of the following is most characteristic of this particular layer of the meninges?

○ (A) A layer of friable cells is located at the external surface of the periosteal dura.
○ (B) A layer of mesothelial cells lines a patent (permanently open) space at the dura-arachnoid interface.
○ (C) A cell layer is found between the pia mater and the surface of the brain in the subpial space.
○ (D) A layer of cells may be dissected open, under certain conditions, by blood or CSF, with the result being a space-occupying lesion.
○ (E) A layer of cells is found at the interface of the periosteal layer of the dura with the meningeal layer of the dura.

22. The angiogram of a 49-year-old man reveals an aneurysm of the basilar bifurcation; this patient has decreased movement in his left eye and a dilated pupil. Which of the following represents the most likely space into which this aneurysm is protruding?

○ (A) Ambient cistern
○ (B) Interpeduncular cistern
○ (C) Superior (quadrigeminal) cistern
○ (D) Prepontine cistern
○ (E) Chiasmatic cistern

23. Lesions commonly called "subdural hematomas" or "subdural hygromas" are actually accumulations of blood or fluid (such as CSF) within which of the following?

○ (A) Meningeal dura mater cell layer
○ (B) Periosteal dura mater cell layer
○ (C) Dural border cell layer
○ (D) Arachnoid barrier cell layer
○ (E) Pia mater

24. The MRI of a 67-year-old man who fell off his barn roof reveals an epidural (or extradural) hematoma. Which of the following labeled regions of the meninges represents the most likely location of this hematoma? (   )

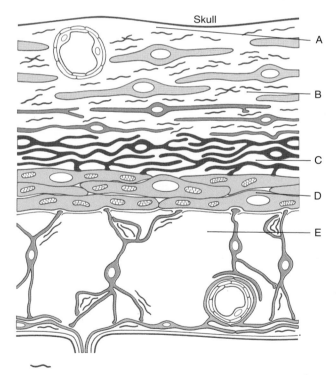

Figure 7–1

25. A 43-year-old man suddenly developed a severe headache that felt like a "bolt of lightning" while he was exercising. This was followed immediately by vomiting and a depressed level of consciousness. CT reveals blood in the cisterns at the base of the brain. Which of the following labeled areas of the meninges represents the most

likely location of the blood in this patient? See Figure 7–2 at right. (   )

26.   A man of unknown age is found by a passerby at the intersection of two rural roads. He is transported to the emergency department where the examination reveals a broken right humerus, some skin abrasions, and scratches on the right side of his head. CT shows a subarachnoid hemorrhage. Which of the following is the most common cause of blood in the subarachnoid space?

○ (A)   Rupture of an aneurysm
○ (B)   Leaking from an aneurysm
○ (C)   Leaking from an arteriovenous malformation
○ (D)   Trauma
○ (E)   Hypertension

27.   A 19-year-old woman presents with headache and a slurring of speech. MRI reveals an arteriovenous malformation, the venous side of which is the superior anastomotic vein (of Trolard). Which of the following labeled sinuses in Figure 7–3 below, associated with meningeal reflections, receives venous blood predominately from this vein? (   )

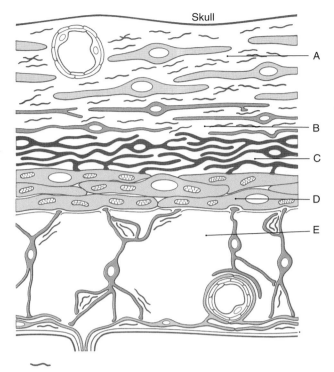

Figure 7–2

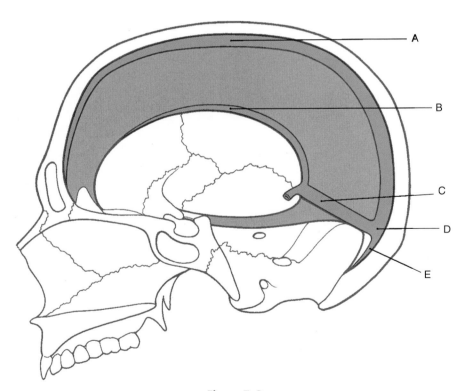

Figure 7–3

28.   A 59-year-old woman presents with medial deviation of her left eye; that is, this eye is deviated toward the midline and cannot be abducted on attempted gaze to the left. MRI reveals a tumor filling a cistern and compressing the root of a cranial nerve. Which of the following labeled cisterns is the most likely location of this tumor? (   )

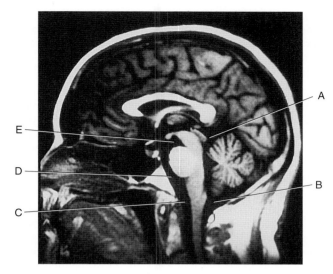

Figure 7–4

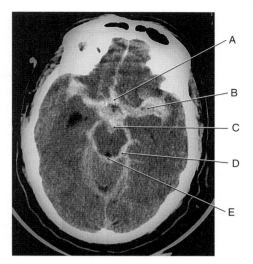

Figure 7–6

29. A 62-year-old woman presents with visual deficits involving both eyes. The physician orders MRI enhanced with gadolinium, which reveals a tumor filling a cistern and compressing structures within this cistern. Which of the following labeled cisterns is the most likely location of this tumor? (   )

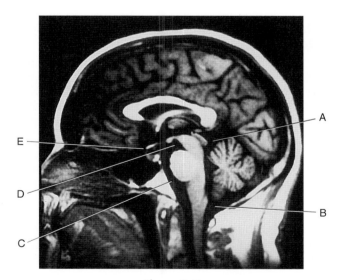

Figure 7–5

30. A 64-year-old man is brought to the emergency department by his son after experiencing a severe headache and being nauseated. In the emergency department, he is sensitive to light and has a stiff neck. The left eye is largely immobile and has a dilated pupil. CT reveals blood in the subarachnoid space. The mass effect of an aneurysm at which of the following locations would most likely account for the largely immobile eye and dilated pupil? (   )

31. A collection of CSF between the arachnoid barrier cell layer and the dura (within the dural border cell layer) resultant to a tear of the arachnoid results in a

- ○ (A) "Subdural" hemorrhage
- ○ (B) Syringomyelia
- ○ (C) Subarachnoid hemorrhage
- ○ (D) Hygroma
- ○ (E) Empyema

ANSWERS

1. **(E)** The spinal dermal sinus tract extends from the skin surface to the meninges, in some cases penetrating the dura, and may end as a small tumor (dermoid or epidermoid) adjacent to the spinal cord. This provides a direct route for bacteria to access the central nervous system and may result in recurrent bouts of meningitis in young patients.
FN2e 108–109

2. **(A)** The ambient cistern is that portion of the subarachnoid space located along the lateral aspect of the midbrain. It contains the trochlear nerve (innervation of the ipsilateral superior oblique muscle), parts of the posterior cerebral, superior cerebellar, and quadrigeminal arteries, and the basal vein (of Rosenthal).
FN2e 118

3. **(C)** The ectomeninx gives rise, in general, to the dura of the adult whereas the endomeninx gives rise to the pia and arachnoid (leptomeninges). The denticulate ligament and filum terminale internum are specializations of the pia.
FN2e 108–109

4. **(E)** Branches of the maxillary (V_2) and mandibular (V_3) nerves innervate the dura of the anterior and middle fossae. The tentorium cerebelli is innervated by the tentorial nerve, a branch of the ophthalmic (V_1) nerve. The

vagus nerve may provide a few sensory branches to the dura of the posterior fossa; the facial nerve does not provide sensory branches to the dura.
FN2e 110–111

5.   **(C)** In the living and healthy individual the arachnoid is attached to the dural border cell layer; there is no naturally occurring "subdural space." Trauma, such as a tear in a bridging vein, may result in the extravasated blood dissecting open the dural border cell layer, producing what is commonly called a "subdural" hematoma or hemorrhage.
FN2e 115–116

6.   **(C)** The tentorium cerebelli is insinuated between the cerebellum and occipital lobes. It is attached to the posterior clinoid process, the petrous portion of the temporal bone, the inner aspect of the occipital bone, and the falx cerebelli on the midline at the position of the straight sinus.
FN2e 111–113

7.   **(C)** The middle meningeal artery arises from the maxillary artery, enters the skull via the foramen spinosum, and usually divides into frontal and parietal branches. This vessel is liable to damage in fractures of the squamous part of the temporal bone or the parietal bone. Such injuries may result in an epidural (extradural) hematoma on the convexity of the hemisphere.
FN2e 111

8.   **(B)** The endomeninx, in general, gives rise to the arachnoid and pia (the leptomeninges). The spaces that appear in this layer early in development will coalesce to form the subarachnoid space and the contiguous cisterns.
FN2e 108–109

9.   **(A)** The falx cerebri is the largest of the meningeal reflections. It has a large sinus (superior sagittal) in its edge attached to the inner surface of the skull and is the only dural reflection to have a sinus in its free edge. Tumors originating from the falx cerebri may bilaterally affect the medial surfaces of both cerebral hemispheres.
FN2e 112–113

10.   **(D)** The tentorial nerve is a recurrent branch of the ophthalmic nerve that leaves the nerve just distal to the ganglion and courses caudad to the tentorium cerebelli sometimes in close association with the trochlear nerve.
FN2e 11

11.   **(E)** Tight junctions are found in the arachnoid barrier cell layer. Relatively few cell junctions are found in the periosteal and meningeal dura (these layers contain a great deal of collagen) or in the pia mater. The dural border cell layer has few cell junctions, has small extracellular spaces, and is a structurally weak cell layer at the dura-arachnoid interface.
FN2e 113–114

12.   **(A)** The innervation of the infratentorial dura is through small meningeal branches of the C1 (when this root is present) to C3 posterior roots and possibly through small filaments from the vagus nerve.
FN2e 111–112

13.   **(C)** Meningiomas arise primarily from meningothelial cap cells or arachnoid cap cells. These cells are most commonly found in the arachnoid trabeculae, along the cribriform plate, at the points where cranial nerves enter the foramina and in association with arachnoid villi.
FN2e 115

14.   **(E)** Bacterial meningitis is most commonly caused by *Streptococcus pneumoniae* in adults. Group B *Streptococcus* and *Escherichia coli* are common causative agents in neonates. Other causative agents in adults are *Neisseria meningitidis*, *Listeria monocytogenes*, and *Haemophilus influenzae*.
FN2e 120

15.   **(D)** Extracellular collagen is found in large amounts in the periosteal and meningeal dura and in sparse amounts in association with trabecular cells in the subarachnoid space and occasionally between the pia mater and surface of the brain (the subpial space). Extracellular collagen is not characteristic of other meningeal layers.
FN2e 110

16.   **(D)** In general the endomeninx gives rise to the leptomeninges (pia and arachnoid). Cavitations within the endomeninx give rise to the subarachnoid space and cisterns.
FN2e 108–109

17.   **(C)** The brain loses most (95% to 97%) of its weight in CSF, but not all. Witness the fact that when an unfixed brain is removed from a fresh cadaver and placed in fluid (e.g., saline, formalin solution) it will slowly sink and then flatten on one side. The brain is suspended in its fluid envelope by the arachnoid trabeculae.
FN2e 114

18.   **(A)** The straight sinus is located in the junction formed by the falx cerebri as it attaches to the upper surface of the tentorium cerebelli on the midline. Rostrally, the straight sinus is continuous with the great cerebral vein (of Galen) and caudad with the sinus confluens.
FN2e 112–113

19.   **(C)** Bacterial infections of the meninges are, for the large part, located in the subarachnoid space. Consequently, the leptomeninges are the layers of the meninges involved, hence the clinical term *leptomeningitis*.
FN2e 120

20.   **(B)** In addition to the great cerebral vein and the root of the trochlear nerve, the superior (or quadrigeminal) cistern also contains portions of the posterior cerebral, quadrigeminal, and medial posterior choroidal arteries. As the trochlear nerve passes around the lateral aspect of the midbrain it courses through the ambient cistern.
FN2e 118, 133–134

21.   **(D)** The dural border cell layer is a friable layer of cells located at the dura-arachnoid interface. This layer has small extracellular spaces, few cell junctions, and no extracellular collagen. It is easily disrupted and can be dissected open by blood from ruptured or torn vessels, resulting in what has classically been called a "subdural" hematoma.
FN2e 113–114

22.   **(B)** The juxtaposition of the basilar bifurcation and the root of the oculomotor nerve within the interpeduncular fossa explain why an aneurysm of basilar bifurcation may result in changes of pupil diameter or a paralysis of most eye movement, both on the ipsilateral side.
FN2e 117–118

23.   **(C)** Because the dural border cell layer (DBCL) is a structurally weak plane at the dura-arachnoid interface, a tear in the arachnoid membrane may result in a hygroma (CSF dissecting open and collecting within the DBCL). A tear of a vein bridging from the surface of the brain to the superior sagittal sinus may result in blood dissecting open the DBCL ("subdural" hematoma).
FN2e 115–116

24.   **(A)** An epidural or extradural hematoma results from a fracture of the skull that usually causes an injury to the middle meningeal or accessory meningeal arteries. The combination of the injury to the skull and the tearing of the vessel(s) results in a stripping of the periosteal dura from the inner table of the skull and an accumulation of blood.
FN2e 115–116

25.   **(E)** The cisterns are enlarged portions of the subarachnoid space; most are located on the base of the forebrain and brainstem and around the brainstem. Blood in the cisterns will also enter the subarachnoid space, and blood in the subarachnoid space will also enter cisterns as these spaces are contiguous.
FN2e 119–120

26.   **(D)** The most common cause of blood in the subarachnoid space (subarachnoid hemorrhage) is trauma. Blood may also originate from leaking aneurysms or arteriovenous malformations. After trauma, the most common cause of subarachnoid hemorrhage is the rupture of intracranial aneurysms. Hypertension is a risk factor for subarachnoid hemorrhage.
FN2e 119–120

27.   **(A)** As its name ("superior") implies, the superior anastomotic vein drains into the superior sagittal sinus. On the lateral aspect of the hemisphere, the superior and inferior anastomotic veins and the superficial middle cerebral vein all interconnect with each other.
FN2e 111–113, 130

28.   **(D)** The prepontine cistern is located on the anterior aspect of the basilar pons and contains the abducens nerve, the basilar artery, and small pontine veins. A tumor invading this cistern could compromise the abducens nerve, which innervates the lateral rectus muscle on that side.
FN2e 117–118

29.   **(E)** The chiasmatic cistern is an enlarged part of the subarachnoid space located around the optic chiasm and immediately adjacent to parts of the optic nerve. This cistern also contains a segment of the ophthalmic artery. Expanding lesions of the pituitary may invade the chiasmatic cistern and damage the optic chiasm.
FN2e 117–118

30.   **(C)** The lack of most eye movement and a dilated pupil, both in the left eye, indicate damage to the root of the oculomotor nerve. This cranial nerve exits the inferior surface of the midbrain and passes through the interpeduncular fossa, which, in this patient, contains extravascular blood.
FN2e 117–119

31.   **(D)** A hygroma is a collection of CSF within a disrupted dural border cell layer, hemorrhage is a collection of blood, and empyema is a collection of purulent material. An empyema may occur in bacterial meningitis.
FN2e 115–116, 120

CHAPTER 8

A Survey of the Cerebrovascular System

1. A 69-year-old man presents with a left homonymous hemianopsia and with some behavioral modifications that interfere with daily functions. MRI reveals a lesion on the right side involving about the lower third of the lenticular nucleus especially at caudal levels, the optic tract, and portions of the amygdaloid nucleus and the hippocampal formation. Which of the following vessels is most likely occluded in this patient?

○ (A) Medial striate artery
○ (B) Lateral striate artery(ies)
○ (C) Anterior choroidal artery
○ (D) Thalamoperforating artery(ies)
○ (E) Thalamogeniculate artery(ies)

2. The angiogram of a 37-year-old hypertensive man reveals a small (berry) aneurysm at the point where the second intracranial branch of the cerebral part of the internal carotid artery originates. Which of the following is usually the second branch of the cerebral part of the internal carotid artery?

○ (A) Posterior communicating artery
○ (B) Ophthalmic artery
○ (C) Anterior choroidal artery
○ (D) Anterior communicating artery
○ (E) Central artery of the retina

3. During the neurologic examination of a 37-year-old woman, the physician notices that she is almost completely blind in her left eye. The funduscopic examination suggests that the central artery of the retina has been occluded. Which of the following is the most likely origin of this vessel?

○ (A) Internal carotid artery
○ (B) A_1 segment
○ (C) M_1 segment
○ (D) Anterior choroidal artery
○ (E) Ophthalmic artery

4. A 69-year-old man with hypertension is brought to the emergency department by his wife and son. He complained of a severe headache, became nauseated, and felt light headed. MRI reveals a hemorrhagic lesion involving the head of the caudate nucleus and adjacent portions of the anterior limb of the internal capsule. A little blood is seen in the lateral ventricle on the same side. Hemorrhage from which of the following vessels would most likely account for this lesion?

○ (A) Medial posterior choroidal artery
○ (B) Lateral striate arteries
○ (C) Anterior choroidal artery
○ (D) Medial striate artery
○ (E) Ophthalmic artery

5. The brain weighs about 2% of the total body weight but consumes about what percent of the total oxygen used by the body?

○ (A) About 5%
○ (B) About 10%
○ (C) About 20%
○ (D) About 30%
○ (E) About 40%

6. The MRI of a 25-year-old college student reveals an aneurysm on the large branch of A_2 that is located immediately above the corpus callosum. Which of the following most likely represents this vessel?

○ (A) Frontopolar branches
○ (B) Callosomarginal artery
○ (C) Pericallosal artery
○ (D) Orbital branch
○ (E) Parieto-occipital artery

Questions 7 and 8 are based on the following patient:

A 19-year-old man presents with headaches that wax and wane. He is unable to concentrate on his college classes. His roommate has also noticed changes in his personality. MRI reveals the lesion shown below. The neurologist concludes that this lesion has large arteries feeding the malformation and large venous structures draining it.

42

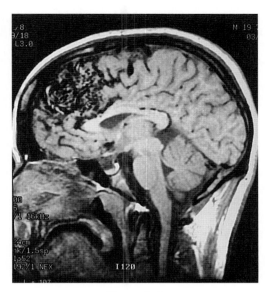

Figure 8–1

7. Which of the following most likely represents the major artery(ies) feeding this lesion?

○ (A) Branches of A_1
○ (B) Branches of A_2
○ (C) Medial striate arteries
○ (D) Branches of M_4
○ (E) Anterior choroidal artery

8. Which of the following most likely represents the major venous structure(s) drawing this lesion?

○ (A) Inferior sagittal sinus
○ (B) Straight sinus
○ (C) Internal cerebral veins
○ (D) Superior sagittal sinus
○ (E) Basal vein of Rosenthal

9. A 67-year-old man presents with a pronounced weakness of the right side of the body, a loss of discriminative touch and vibratory sense on the right side of the body, and a deviation of the tongue to the left on attempted protrusion. The neurologist concludes that there is a vascular lesion involving the corticospinal tract, medial lemniscus, and hypoglossal nerve. Which of the following vessels is most likely occluded to result in these deficits?

○ (A) Anterior spinal branches to the right
○ (B) Anterior spinal branches to the left
○ (C) Vertebral branches on the left
○ (D) Vertebral branches on the right
○ (E) PICA branches on the left

10. The MRI of a 39-year-old woman reveals a cyst in the orbital area of the frontal lobe. This cyst is drained by the anterior cerebral vein that joins the basal vein (of Rosenthal). Which of the following represents the venous structure that receives blood from the basal vein?

○ (A) Inferior sagittal sinus
○ (B) Straight sinus

○ (C) Great cerebral vein (of Galen)
○ (D) Internal cerebral vein
○ (E) Confluence of sinuses

11. The vascular structure found along the attachment of the falx cerebri to the tentorium cerebelli is the

○ (A) Sigmoid sinus
○ (B) Superior sagittal sinus
○ (C) Inferior petrosal sinus
○ (D) Transversus sinus
○ (E) Straight sinus

12. The neurologist treating a 34-year-old woman for intractable headaches orders an MRI. An incidental finding in this patient is an unusually small vertebral artery. This artery is located in which of the following cisterns?

○ (A) Lateral cerebellomedullary
○ (B) Dorsal cerebellomedullary
○ (C) Prepontine
○ (D) Ambient
○ (E) Interpeduncular

13. A 73-year-old man presents with a visual field deficit. A careful examination reveals a homonymous hemianopsia resulting from a lesion in the primary visual cortex. If this is assumed to be a vascular event, which of the following vessels is most likely involved?

○ (A) Posterior parietal artery
○ (B) Calcarine artery
○ (C) Lateral striate (lenticulostriate) artery(ies)
○ (D) Thalamoperforating artery
○ (E) Parieto-occipital artery

14. The MRI of a 44-year-old man reveals a small aneurysm on the M_3 segment. This aneurysm is most likely located on which of the following?

○ (A) Base of the hemisphere medial to the limen insulae
○ (B) Insular cortex
○ (C) Inner aspect of the parietal operculum
○ (D) Frontal cortex
○ (E) Parietal cortex

15. After aneurysm surgery on a 61-year-old woman, the neurosurgeon discovers that the clip had inadvertently occluded an especially important branch of P_1; in fact, the patient will not wake up. Which of the following is a branch of P_1?

○ (A) Anterior choroidal artery
○ (B) Thalamogeniculate artery
○ (C) Lateral posterior choroidal artery
○ (D) Thalamoperforating artery
○ (E) Medial posterior choroidal artery

16. A 27-year-old man is brought to the emergency department after a motorcycle accident. Suspecting a basilar skull fracture, the attending physician orders a CT, which reveals a fracture through the jugular foramen. In addition to the sigmoid sinus, which of the following

venous structures might also be involved in this injury, owing to its location relative to the jugular foramen?

○ (A) Superior petrosal sinus
○ (B) Transverse sinus
○ (C) Inferior petrosal sinus
○ (D) Confluence of sinuses
○ (E) Straight sinus

17. A 4-month-old infant presents with hydrocephalus, bulging fontanelles, and dilated veins in the scalp and face. An angiogram reveals a type of arteriovenous malformation called a vein of Galen malformation. Which of the following most likely represents the principal feeding artery to this lesion?

○ (A) Calcarine
○ (B) Vertebral
○ (C) Posterior cerebral
○ (D) Posterior inferior cerebellar
○ (E) Parietal branches of M_4

18. Angiography in a 64-year-old woman reveals a laterally expanding lesion within the cavernous sinus. Further tests confirm that this lesion is an aneurysm of the internal carotid artery. Which of the following is affected first by this expanding lesion owing to its approximation to the internal carotid artery?

○ (A) The maxillary nerve
○ (B) The trochlear nerve
○ (C) The mandibular nerve
○ (D) The oculomotor nerve
○ (E) The abducens nerve

19. The CT of a 73-year-old man reveals a hemorrhage into the putamen, globus pallidus, and adjacent parts of the posterior limb of the internal capsule. The physician concludes that this lesion is a result of rupture of lenticulostriate arteries. Which of the following represents the primary site of origin of these vessels?

○ (A) A_1
○ (B) M_1
○ (C) M_2
○ (D) M_3
○ (E) M_4

20. A 19-year-old man presents with visual deficits that have become more severe with time. MRI reveals a small arteriovenous malformation in the primary visual cortex on the right side. Which of the following is the most likely source of the arterial branches serving this malformation?

○ (A) A_2
○ (B) M_3
○ (C) P_2
○ (D) P_4
○ (E) M_4

21. A neurologist explains to the family of a 52-year-old woman that she has an aneurysm of the vertebrobasilar system. Which of the following represents the most common location of aneurysms found within the vertebrobasilar system?

○ (A) Branch point of PICA from the vertebral artery
○ (B) Branch point of the anterior spinal artery from the vertebral artery
○ (C) Branch point of the posterior spinal artery from the vertebral artery
○ (D) Junction of the vertebral arteries
○ (E) Basilar bifurcation

22. A 9-year-old girl has a serious bacterial infection on her face. By the time she is brought to the physician's office she has signs of bacterial meningitis (elevated temperature, stupor, ill appearance, rigid neck). Which of the following represents the most likely route through which this infection could access the central nervous system?

○ (A) Internal cerebral vein(s)
○ (B) Anterior cerebral vein(s)
○ (C) Sphenoparietal sinus
○ (D) Superficial middle cerebral vein(s)
○ (E) Ophthalmic vein(s)

23. A 49-year-old woman presents with headache and nausea. MRI reveals a tumor originating from the choroid plexus in the atrium of the lateral ventricle. Which of the following represents the primary source of arterial blood to this portion of the choroid plexus?

○ (A) Internal carotid artery
○ (B) P_1
○ (C) P_2
○ (D) P_3
○ (E) M_1

24. The MRI of a 62-year-old woman reveals a large lesion in the head of the caudate nucleus. The physician notes that this structure is served primarily by the medial striate artery. Which of the following represents the most common origin of this vessel?

○ (A) A_1
○ (B) A_1/A_2 intersection and proximal A_2
○ (C) A_2
○ (D) M_1
○ (E) The anterior communicating artery

25. A 58-year-old woman presents to the emergency department nauseated, confused, and complaining of a severe headache. CT reveals a lesion in the lenticular nucleus that spares its most inferior part but extends slightly into portions of the adjacent posterior limb of the internal capsule. Which of the following vessels is most likely involved in this lesion?

○ (A) Medial striate artery(ies)
○ (B) Anterior choroidal artery
○ (C) Lateral striate arteries
○ (D) Thalamoperforating artery
○ (E) Lateral posterior choroidal artery

26. A 47-year-old man with untreated high blood pressure presents to the emergency department with nausea and a severe headache. The neurologic examination reveals a lack of all movement in the right eye (extraocular muscles are served by cranial nerves III, IV, and VI) and abnormal sensory sensations over the right forehead (the area served by the ophthalmic nerve). Taking

all these deficits together, which of the following is the most likely location of the lesion causing these deficits?

○ (A) Orbital fissure
○ (B) At the bifurcation of A_1 and M_1 from the internal carotid artery
○ (C) Midbrain
○ (D) Cavernous sinus
○ (E) Genu of the internal capsule

27. An 89-year-old man with morbid obesity and untreated hypertension presents with motor and sensory deficits involving the right side of the face, right upper extremity, and portions of the trunk. MRI reveals hemorrhage from those vessels serving the primary motor and sensory cortices. Which of the following labeled vessels in Figure 8–2 below, is the most likely source of this hemorrhage? (   )

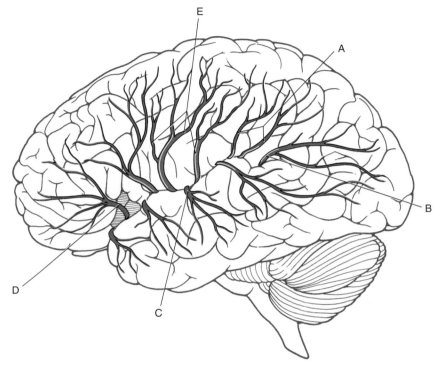

Figure 8–2

28. A 55-year-old woman presents with a homonymous hemianopia suggesting a lesion of visual structures at, or caudad to, the optic tract. MRI reveals an aneurysm on the vessel(s) serving the primary visual cortex. Which of the following labeled blood vessels in Figure 8–3 below, is the most likely the site of this aneurysm? (   )

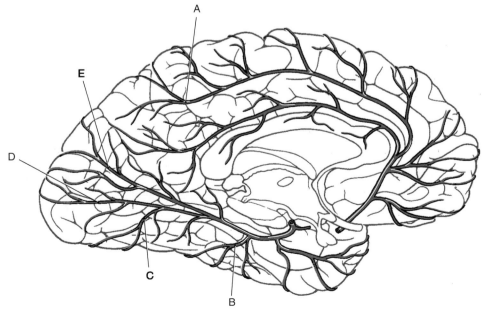

Figure 8–3

29.   A 60-year-old man passes out at his job and is transported to the emergency department. The initial examination reveals very low blood pressure (hypotension). When the patient recovers, the neurologist determines that he has profound weakness of his right lower extremity; the neurologist concludes that this patient has had a watershed infarct. A lesion in which of the following labeled areas in Figure 8–4 below, each representing a lesion, would most likely explain this patient's deficit? (   )

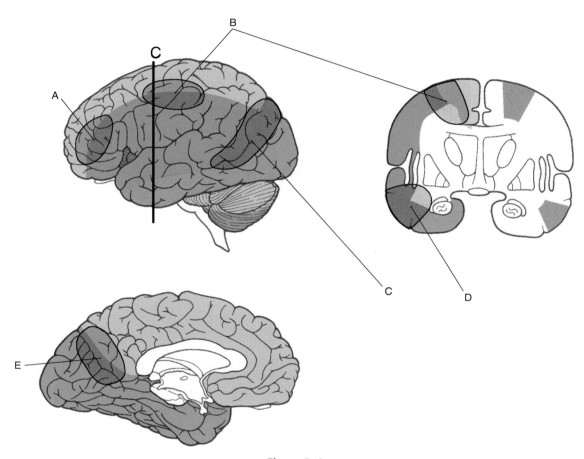

Figure 8–4

30.   A 73-year-old man complains to his physician that his left "leg" is weak and seems to be numb. The physical examination reveals loss of most pain and thermal sensation and proprioception from the weak lower extremity. MRI reveals hemorrhage from those vessels serving the somatosensory and somatomotor cortices for the lower extremity. Which of the following labeled vessels (see Figure 8–5) is the most likely source for the patient's hemorrhage? (   )

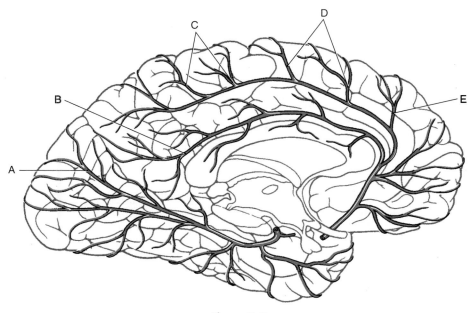

Figure 8–5

31. A 32-year-old woman becomes acutely ill with fever, pain in the orbits, and diplopia. The neurologist discovers that she has a severe maxillary sinus infection that has spread into her nose and onto the face. The examining physician concludes that this patient has a venous thrombosis. Based on their location and venous connection, which of the following is the most likely venous structure involved in this patient?

○ (A) Straight sinus
○ (B) Transverse sinus
○ (C) Vein of Labbé
○ (D) Cavernous sinus
○ (E) Superior sagittal sinus

32. A 2-year-old boy presents after the sudden onset of fever, vomiting, and a headache. The examination reveals a middle ear infection that has spread into the mastoid air cells. MRI shows a venous thrombosis with possible CNS infection. Which of the following is the most likely venous structure involved in this patient?

○ (A) Straight sinus
○ (B) Transverse sinus
○ (C) Cavernous sinus
○ (D) Deep middle cerebral vein
○ (E) Internal cerebral vein

ANSWERS

1. **(C)** The left homonymous hemianopsia (a loss of the temporal visual field in the left eye and the nasal visual field in the right eye) is indicative of a lesion of the optic tract. In addition to the optic tract, the anterior choroidal artery also serves internal structures of the temporal lobe (amygdaloid nucleus and hippocampus), including the choroid plexus of the temporal horn.
FN2e 123–124

2. **(A)** The three major branches of the cerebral part of the internal carotid artery are the ophthalmic artery (usually first), the posterior communicating artery (usually second), and the anterior choroidal artery (usually third). The superior hypophyseal arteries arise from the internal carotid in the general area of ophthalmic and posterior communicating arteries. These vessels supply the stalk and anterior lobe of the pituitary and portions of the optic nerve and chiasm.
FN2e 123–124

3. **(E)** The central artery of the retina arises from the ophthalmic artery just distal to the optic foramen. It enters the optic nerve 10 to 15 mm caudad to the bulb. Because of this pattern, an occlusion of the ophthalmic artery close to its origin may result in significant visual deficits in the ipsilateral eye.
FN2e 123

4. **(D)** The junction of the anterior cerebral artery (ACA) with the anterior communicating artery is called the anterior communicating artery complex. A_1 is proximal to this point, and A_2 is distal. Actually, the "complex" consists of the anterior communicating artery and the immediately contiguous portions of both A_1 and A_2. The medial striate artery originates from the ACA at its junction or just distal to its junction with the anterior communicating artery in 60% to 65% of individuals. The medial striate serves, primarily, the head of the caudate nucleus, anterior limb of the internal capsule, and adjacent parts of the putamen.
FN2e 123–125

5. **(C)** The brain requires a constant flow of oxygenated blood. Even though the brain represents only a

small portion of total body weight, it consumes a disproportionately large amount of oxygen. Interruption of the blood supply to the brain will result in syncope and, within a few minutes, permanent brain damage or death.
FN2e 122

6. **(C)** The pericallosal artery, part of the A$_2$ segment of the anterior cerebral artery, is located in the area of the callosal sulcus and within the callosal cistern on the medial surface of the hemisphere. Choices A, B, and D are the other main branches of A$_2$.
FN2e 123–124

7. **(B)** This lesion is an arteriovenous malformation located within the territory of A$_2$, most likely in territories of frontopolar and callosomarginal branches. These branches of A$_2$ are the primary arterial inputs to this lesion.
FN2e 123–124

8. **(D)** This arteriovenous malformation is located in the medial aspect of the frontal lobe adjacent to the midline. The superior sagittal sinus is immediately adjacent to this lesion and also receives the superficial cortical veins from this area of the cerebral cortex.
FN2e 123, 130–131

9. **(B)** The anterior spinal artery is located in the anterior median fissure (between the pyramids). It gives rise to penetrating branches that alternate to the right and left. These penetrating branches (to the left in this question) serve corticospinal fibers in the pyramid (weakness of body), the medial lemniscus (discriminative touch/vibratory sense loss) and nucleus, and exiting fibers of the hypoglossal nerve (deviation of the tongue).
FN2e 124–125, 129

10. **(C)** The great cerebral vein (of Galen) receives venous blood from the internal cerebral veins (which are important venous structures and sometimes quite obvious in MRI), the posterior vein of the corpus callosum, and the basal vein (of Rosenthal) and continues into the rostral end of the straight sinus.
FN2e 131–133

11. **(E)** The straight sinus is triangular when viewed in cross section. It extends from the great cerebral vein to the confluence of sinuses. En route, it receives superior cerebellar veins from the superior surface of the cerebellum. Its channels at the confluence are variable; the straight sinus is usually continuous with the left transverse sinus.
FN2e 130

12. **(A)** The lateral cerebellomedullary cistern also contains the origin of the posterior inferior cerebellar artery; the roots of cranial nerves IX, X, XI, and XII; and small medullary veins
FN2e 125

13. **(B)** The calcarine artery is located within, or adjacent to, the calcarine sulcus. Primary visual cortex (area 17) is located on the upper (cuneus) and lower (lingual gyrus) banks of the calcarine sulcus.
FN2e 124, 127–128

14. **(C)** The M$_3$ segment is that portion of the middle cerebral artery that is located in the inner aspect of the

opercula (frontal, parietal, or temporal). The M$_2$ segments are those branches on the insular cortex, and the M$_4$ segments are the cortical branches on the convexity of the hemisphere.
FN2e 125

15. **(D)** In addition to the thalamoperforating artery, small branches arise from P$_1$ that enter the interpeduncular fossa (at the posterior perforated substance), the quadrigeminal artery, and a few small circumflex branches that course around the crus cerebri to lateral aspects of the midbrain.
FN2e 127

16. **(C)** The inferior petrosal sinus, along with the larger sigmoid sinus, joins the internal jugular vein at the jugular foramen. In addition, some small arteries and cranial nerves IX, X, and XI also pass through the jugular foramen.
FN2e 131–132

17. **(C)** A vein of Galen malformation is usually seen in newborns or infants. The predominant feeder artery is the posterior cerebral.
FN2e 133–134

18. **(E)** The abducens nerve is laterally adjacent to the cavernous portion of the internal carotid within the sinus. An expanding lesion would first involve the abducens nerve and then the oculomotor, trochlear, ophthalmic division of V, (V$_1$), and maxillary division of V (V$_2$). The latter four nerves are located in the lateral portions of the sinus from upper to lower in the order listed here.
FN2e 132

19. **(B)** The first segment of the middle cerebral artery (M$_1$) gives rise to lenticulostriate arteries, an uncal artery (to the uncus), and small anterior temporal and polar temporal branches.
FN2e 124

20. **(D)** The P$_4$ segment of the posterior cerebral artery consists of the parieto-occipital and calcarine arteries. The calcarine branch of P$_4$ serves the primary visual cortex; this area of cortex borders on the calcarine sulcus (the lower edge of the cuneus and the upper edge of the lingual gyrus).
FN2e 127–128

21. **(E)** About 15% of all intracranial aneurysms are located in the vertebrobasilar system. The majority of these are at the bifurcation of the basilar artery (also called the basilar apex) where they may impinge on the oculomotor nerve.
FN2e 127

22. **(E)** The veins of the upper portion of the face and the orbit communicate with the ophthalmic veins, which, in turn, drain into the cavernous sinus. Bacteria from facial or orbital infections may access the central nervous system via these veins.
FN2e 131–132

23. **(C)** The medial (83% of patients) and lateral (51% of patients) posterior choroidal arteries usually arise from the P$_2$ segment of the posterior cerebral artery. The next

most common origin for the lateral posterior choroidal artery is the P_3 segment (30%).
FN2e 127–128

24. **(B)** The medial striate artery (also called the artery of Heubner) arises from the junction of A_1 with A_2 (this is the point where the anterior communicating artery joins the anterior cerebral) or from A_2 just distal to the anterior communicator in about 65% of cases. The junction of the anterior communicating artery with the A_1–A_2 intersection is called the anterior communicating artery complex.
FN2e 123–124, 129

25. **(C)** The lateral striate arteries (also called the lenticulostriate) are branches of the first major part of the middle vertebral artery (M_1 segment). These vessels serve the superior portions of the lenticular nucleus (its inferior parts are served by branches of the anterior choroidal artery) and portions of the medially adjacent posterior limb of the internal capsule. The head of the caudate nucleus is served by the medial striate artery.
FN2e 125, 127, 129

26. **(D)** The abducens, oculomotor, and trochlear nerves and the ophthalmic and maxillary nerves (branches of the trigeminal nerve) pass through the cavernous sinus. The abducens nerve is close to the internal carotid artery, while the remaining nerves are located in the lateral aspect of the sinus from superior to inferior.
FN2e 132

27. **(E)** The central (Rolandic) and postcentral arteries are those M_4 branches that serve the area of the precentral (somatomotor) and postcentral (somatosensory) gyri. The areas of cortex for the lower extremity are in the territory served by A_2 branches of the anterior cerebral artery.
FN2e 125–126

28. **(D)** The calcarine artery, a branch of P_4, serves the primary visual cortex, which is located in either bank of the calcarine sulcus. The other branch of P_4, the parieto-occipital artery, is located in the parieto-occipital sulcus and does not serve the primary visual cortex.
FN2e 124, 127–128

29. **(B)** Watershed infarcts occur under conditions of systemic hypotension or hypoperfusion where the territories of major vessels interface and perhaps overlap slightly. The resulting infarct damages not only cells in the area but fibers passing through the damaged area. In this case, the lesion is located at the interface of the territories served by anterior and middle cerebral arteries in the mid rostrocaudal region of the hemisphere and involves the fibers exiting the somatomotor cortex for the lower extremity.
FN2e 128, 390

30. **(C)** The paracentral and internal parietal branches of the callosomarginal artery serve the areas of the anterior and posterior paracentral gyri. These gyri represent, respectively, the somatomotor and somatosensory cortices for the contralateral lower extremity.
FN2e 123–124, 262, 390

31. **(D)** The cavernous sinus is connected rostrally to the orbit and face by the ophthalmic veins and their branches. Infection on the face or in the orbit may spread into the central nervous system via these connections and may result in a septic lesion within the cavernous sinus. Caudad, the cavernous sinus connects with the transverse and sigmoid sinuses via the superior and inferior petrosal sinuses.
FN2e 130–132

32. **(B)** The transverse sinus (also called the lateral sinus by some clinicians and in some clinical texts) is immediately posterior to the petrous portion of the temporal bone. In addition to receiving venous blood from the confluence of sinuses, the transverse sinus has small venous connections from adjacent structures of the posterior fossa.
FN2e 130–132

CHAPTER 9

The Spinal Cord

Questions 1 through 3 are based on the following patient:

A 47-year-old man complains of slowly progressing weakness of both "legs." On examination he has a flaccid paralysis of both lower extremities, muscle fasciculations, hypotonia, and areflexia. In addition, there is loss of pain and temperature sensations over the anterior aspect of both lower extremities and most of the feet but sparing the little toes.

1. The flaccid paralysis, fasciculations, hypotonia, and areflexia in this patient are most likely the result of damage to what structures?

- ○ (A) Lateral corticospinal tracts
- ○ (B) Posterior (dorsal) roots
- ○ (C) Anterior (ventral) horn cells and alpha motor neurons
- ○ (D) Reticulospinal/vestibulospinal tracts
- ○ (E) Afferent fibers involved in monosynaptic reflexes

2. The loss of pain and thermal sensations in this patient is most likely the result of damage where?

- ○ (A) To the posterior (dorsal) horn cells
- ○ (B) To the anterolateral system on the right
- ○ (C) To the anterolateral system on the left
- ○ (D) To the anterolateral systems bilaterally
- ○ (E) To the anterior (ventral) white commissure

3. Based on information collected in the examination of this patient, which of the following is the most likely cause of his deficits?

- ○ (A) Tabes dorsalis
- ○ (B) Hemisection of the spinal cord (Brown-Séquard syndrome)
- ○ (C) Small syringomyelia at T12-L5
- ○ (D) Large syringomyelia at T12-L5
- ○ (E) Large syringomyelia at T1-T12

4. A 54-year-old construction worker presents with pain and weakness in the left upper extremity. The examining neurologist suspects a herniated cervical disc impinging on the posterior and anterior roots of the spinal cord. Which of the following is characteristic of the posterior and anterior roots?

- ○ (A) *Each* is accompanied by a radicular artery *and* a spinal medullary artery.
- ○ (B) All exit above (rostral to) their respectively numbered vertebra.
- ○ (C) Posterior roots are motor and anterior roots are sensory in their function.
- ○ (D) There is no dermatome associated with the coccygeal root(s).
- ○ (E) Roots C1 to C7 exit above (rostral to) their respectively numbered vertebrae and beginning with T1 these roots exit below (caudad to) their respectively numbered vertebrae.

5. A newborn presents with a defect that represents a failure of the entire vertebral arches and the adjacent spinal portion of the neural plate to close properly. Which of the following is most representative of this development defect?

- ○ (A) Meningomyelocele
- ○ (B) Frontal encephalocele
- ○ (C) Spina bifida occulta
- ○ (D) Rachischisis
- ○ (E) Meningocele

6. A 44-year-old morbidly obese, hypertensive, and diabetic man presents with signs and symptoms indicative of an occlusion of the anterior spinal artery at levels C4 to C8. Which of the following structures would most likely be spared in this lesion?

- ○ (A) Hypothalamospinal fibers
- ○ (B) Posterior columns of the spinal cord
- ○ (C) Anterior (ventral) horns
- ○ (D) Medial portions of the lateral corticospinal tracts
- ○ (E) Portions of the posterior horns

7. Which of the following is a structure from which preganglionic sympathetic axons most likely originate?

○ (A) Lamina II, the substantia gelatinosa
○ (B) Lamina VI, lateral portions
○ (C) Lamina IX cell clusters
○ (D) Lamina VII, intermediolateral cell column
○ (E) Lamina VIII

8. A 26-year-old man presents with a tethered cord syndrome. This defect is related to an error in secondary neurulation involving the caudal eminence. Which of the following levels of the spinal cord originates from the caudal eminence?

○ (A) Coccygeal only
○ (B) Coccygeal + sacral
○ (C) Sacral only
○ (D) Sacral + lumbar
○ (E) Coccygeal + sacral + lumbar

9. A 26-year-old woman presents with a unilateral lesion of the lateral funiculus at C4 as a result of a fall. The lesion is located posterior to the level of the denticulate ligament. The most obvious deficit seen in this patient is a weakness of the upper and lower extremities on the side of the lesion. Damage to which of the following tracts would most likely explain this deficit in this patient?

○ (A) Posterior spinocerebellar tract
○ (B) Spinocervical fibers
○ (C) Hypothalamospinal fibers
○ (D) Anterolateral system
○ (E) Lateral corticospinal tract

10. The caudal end of the spinal cord (conus medullaris) is anchored to the inner aspect of the spinal dural sac by which of the following?

○ (A) Filum terminale externum
○ (B) Filum terminale internum
○ (C) Coccygeal ligament
○ (D) Denticulate ligament
○ (E) Arachnoid trabeculae

11. A 49-year-old man presents with intractable pain. The neurosurgeon proposes to transect pain fibers as they enter the spinal cord at the posterior root entry zone (dorsal root entry zone). Which of the following represents the most likely location of this zone?

○ (A) Anterolateral sulcus
○ (B) Anterior median fissure
○ (C) Posterior median sulcus
○ (D) Posterior intermediate sulcus
○ (E) Posterolateral sulcus

12. The neuropathologist examines the spinal cord from a 62-year-old man who died of the consequences of amyotrophic lateral sclerosis. The pathologist tells the resident "this is the posterior horn." Which of the following is the most distinct and characteristic structure of the posterior horn?

○ (A) Posteromarginal nucleus (lamina I)
○ (B) Substantia gelatinosa (lamina II)
○ (C) Nucleus proprius (laminae III, IV)
○ (D) Intermediolateral cell column (lamina VII)
○ (E) Clarke nucleus (lamina VII)

13. The neurosurgeon is preparing to conduct a surgical procedure on a 51-year-old cancer patient to relieve intractable pain. Which of the following is a characteristic of the posterior root entry zone (dorsal root entry zone) that is particularly relevant to this procedure?

○ (A) It is located along the posterior intermediate sulcus.
○ (B) Large-diameter proprioceptive fibers and the small-diameter exteroceptive fibers are intermixed at this zone.
○ (C) Large-diameter proprioceptive fibers are located laterally and the small-diameter exteroceptive fibers are located medially at this zone.
○ (D) The large-diameter proprioceptive fibers are located medially and the small-diameter exteroceptive fibers are located laterally at this zone.
○ (E) Only small diameter exteroceptive fibers are found in this zone; there are no large-diameter fibers.

14. An 82-year-old woman presents with a degenerative disease affecting the large neuronal cell bodies located in lamina IX of the spinal cord, as well as neurons in the nuclei of cranial nerves III, IV, VI, and XII. Which of the following represents the functional component associated with these lamina IX cells?

○ (A) SVE
○ (B) GSE
○ (C) GVE
○ (D) GSA
○ (E) GVA

15. During a surgical procedure to remove a small tumor from the posterior surface of the spinal cord in a 27-year-old man, the neurosurgeon is careful to spare the large-diameter, heavily myelinated fibers of the posterior root entry zone. Which of the following sensations will most likely be spared?

○ (A) Sensations of pain
○ (B) Sensations of temperature
○ (C) Sensations of nondiscriminative touch
○ (D) Sensations of pressure, discriminative touch, and vibratory sense
○ (E) Sensations of interoceptive pain

16. A 21-year-old woman presents with a left spinal cord hemisection at C3. In addition to characteristic motor and sensory deficits, she has ptosis, miosis, anhidrosis, and enophthalmos on the left side. These latter deficits indicate an interruption of descending input from higher levels of the neuraxis to the intermediolateral cell column. Damage to which of the following fibers would most likely account for this observation?

○ (A) Raphespinal fibers
○ (B) Corticospinal fibers

○ (C) Spinospinal fibers
○ (D) Vestibulospinal fibers
○ (E) Hypothalamospinal fibers

17.   A 47-year-old male smoker presents with lung cancer that has penetrated the pleura and invaded the sympathetic chain. Surgical removal of this tumor results in the transection of the gray communicating rami at three levels. Which of the following fiber populations would most likely be affected by the damage of these rami?

○ (A) GVA + GVE preganglionic
○ (B) GVA only
○ (C) GVA + GVE postganglionic
○ (D) GVE postganglionic only
○ (E) SVA only

18.   The laminae of Rexed (spinal laminae of the gray matter) that collectively form the posterior horn of the spinal cord are

○ (A) I, II
○ (B) I–V
○ (C) I–VI
○ (D) II–V
○ (E) II–VII

19.   During the neurologic evaluation of a 47-year-old man with peripheral neuropathy, the physician discovers (via electrophysiologic tests) that those fibers conducting proprioceptive information are especially affected by the disease. Which of the following represent the conduction velocity of fibers conveying proprioceptive information?

○ (A) 0.5 to 25 m/sec
○ (B) 40 to 60 m/sec
○ (C) 60 to 80 m/sec
○ (D) 70 to 120 m/sec
○ (E) Greater than 125 m/sec

20.   A 46-year-old man presents with waxing and waning muscle weakness that affects his extremities as well as extraocular muscles. Tests reveal that this is a neurotransmitter disease associated with lower motor neurons in the anterior horn and in cranial nerve nuclei and with their terminals in skeletal muscle. Which of the following represents the neurotransmitter associated with these motor neurons and their terminals?

○ (A) Glutamate
○ (B) Dopamine
○ (C) Aspartate
○ (D) Glycine
○ (E) Acetylcholine

21.   A 47-year-old woman presents with pain radiating down the lateral aspect of the right upper extremity and into the thumb. MRI reveals a protruding intervertebral disc that is extending into the intervertebral foramen at which of the following levels?

○ (A) C3–4 interspace
○ (B) C4–5 interspace
○ (C) C5–6 interspace
○ (D) C6–7 interspace
○ (E) C7-T1 interspace

22.   Interoceptive information is conveyed by receptors concerned with nociceptive input and stretch-pressure information. These receptors are located in what tissues?

○ (A) Tendons and ligaments
○ (B) Cardiac muscle only
○ (C) Skeletal muscle
○ (D) Smooth muscles and glands of the skin
○ (E) Visceral structures of the gut and thorax

23.   An elderly man from a rural setting complains that his "leg" and "arm" are weak and he really "couldn't move them much for a long time." Damage to which of the following fiber populations in the spinal cord would most likely explain these symptoms?

○ (A) Raphespinal fibers
○ (B) Lateral corticospinal tract/fibers
○ (C) Spinospinal fibers
○ (D) Rubrospinal fibers
○ (E) Fastigiospinal fibers

24.   During a surgical procedure to remove a tumor from the spinal cord of a 29-year-old woman, the posterior roots and their ganglia at two adjacent levels are removed with the tumor. This was because the tumor completely encased these structures. Which of the following functional components is associated with cell bodies of the posterior root ganglia?

○ (A) GSA only
○ (B) GSA + GVA
○ (C) GVA only
○ (D) GSA + GSE
○ (E) GVA + GVE

25.   A 23-year-old man is brought to the emergency department from an accident site. He has burns on his hands and forearms resulting from his opening the door of a burning truck to rescue the driver. He was able to get the door open owing to the modulation (inhibition) of pain transmission at spinal levels. Which of the following fibers is most likely involved in the modulation of nociceptive (pain) information at spinal levels?

○ (A) Raphespinal fibers
○ (B) Hypothalamospinal fibers
○ (C) Vestibulospinal fibers
○ (D) Spinospinal fibers
○ (E) Fastigiospinal fibers

26.   During the neurologic examination on a 7-year-old boy, the physician taps the patellar tendon and elicits a simple knee-jerk reflex that is also called the quadriceps stretch reflex. This is one example of a tendon reflex. Which of the following is characteristic of this type of reflex?

○ (A) Is a three-neuron reflex; the afferent receptor is the Golgi tendon organ and the afferent endings are neuromuscular junctions
○ (B) Requires glutaminergic (excitatory) input to extensor and flexor motor neurons
○ (C) Relies on nociceptive input to the primary sensory ending
○ (D) Causes withdrawal on the ipsilateral limb and extension of the contralateral limb

○ (E) Is a two-neuron reflex; the afferent receptor is the muscle spindle and the efferent endings are neuromuscular junctions

27. A 19-year-old man presents with a gradually increasing weakness of his left lower extremity and sensory loss on his left upper extremity. The sensory deficit is most obvious as a loss of discriminative touch and pain sense in the left hand and forearm. MRI reveals an extramedullary tumor (a tumor outside the spinal cord). Which of the following labeled areas (see Figure 9–1), each representing a region potentially involved by the tumor, contains the tracts/fibers that when damaged would give rise to the deficits seen in this patient? ( )

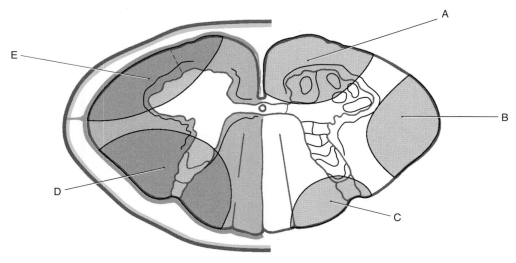

Figure 9–1

28. A 17-year-old girl is walking through the woods and steps on a sharp metal object that penetrates her shoe and lacerates the plantar surface of her foot. She withdraws the injured foot but continues to stand using the other lower extremity. Which of the following reflexes contain the circuits that provide for this reaction in this patient?

○ (A) Tendon reflex
○ (B) Crossed extension reflex
○ (C) Withdrawal reflex
○ (D) Inverse myotatic reflex
○ (E) Nociceptive reflex

29. A 39-year-old construction worker falls about 20 feet, injuring his cervical spinal cord. He presents to the emergency department with a loss of voluntary motor control in the right upper and lower extremities and a loss of pain and thermal sense in the same extremities on the left. Which of the labeled areas shown below (see Figure 9–2), each representing a lesion, contains the tracts/fibers that when injured would give rise to the deficits seen in this patient? ( )

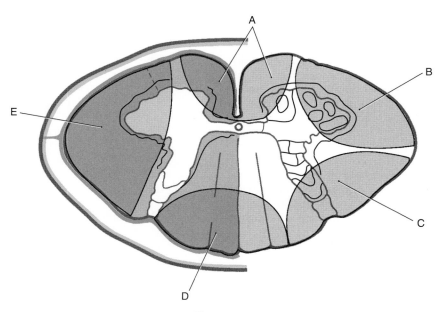

Figure 9–2

30. A 43-year-old man presents to his physician's office with difficulty walking. During the examination the physician notices a gait disturbance, especially how the patient places his left foot forcibly to the floor when taking a step. The physician concludes that there is an interruption in proprioceptive input from the left lower extremity. Which of the following labeled areas (see Figure 9–3) of the spinal cord contain the fibers that, if injured, would most likely give rise to the deficits experienced by this patient? (   )

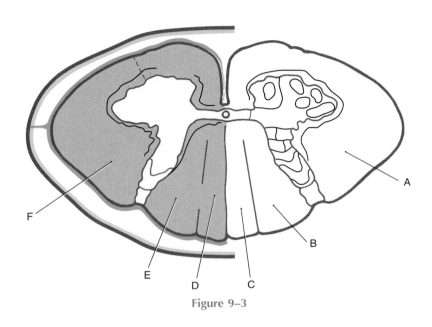

Figure 9–3

31. During the neurologic examination of a 47-year-old man, the physician uses a pin to activate the pathway of the flexor reflex, also called the withdrawal reflex or nociceptive reflex. Which of the following is characteristic of the pathway constituting this reflex?

○ (A) The heavily myelinated primary sensory fibers terminate directly (monosynaptic) on motor neurons innervating extensor muscles.

○ (B) The lightly myelinated primary sensory fibers terminate on interneurons that inhibit motor neurons innervating both extensor and flexor muscles.

○ (C) The lightly myelinated primary sensory fibers terminate on interneurons that inhibit motor neurons innervating extensor muscles and on interneurons that excite motor neurons innervating flexor muscles.

○ (D) The lightly myelinated primary sensory fibers terminate on interneurons that inhibit motor neurons innervating flexor muscles and on interneurons that excite motor neurons innervating extensor muscles.

○ (E) The heavily myelinated primary sensory fibers terminate on interneurons that inhibit motor neurons innervating extensor muscles and on interneurons that excite motor neurons innervating flexor muscles.

32. A 43-year-old man presents with weakness of the abdominal muscles. He has noticed that when he exercises he does not seem to sweat much on the same side as the weakness. Which of the following labeled areas, each representing a lesion, contain the fibers, tracts, or cell bodies that would explain the deficits experienced by this patient? (   )

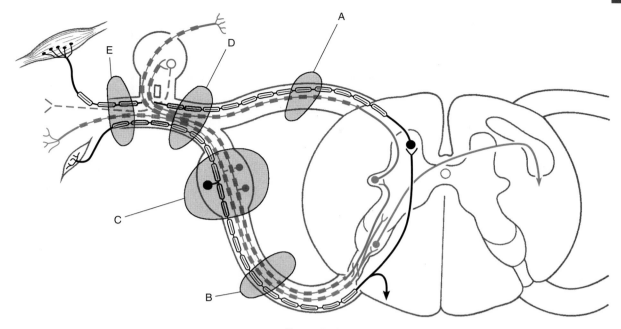

Figure 9-4

33.   A 21-year-old man is brought to the emergency department after an automobile collision. The examination reveals that he has damage to his spinal cord at levels C3 to C7, resulting in characteristic motor and sensory losses. In addition, he has a Horner syndrome (ptosis, miosis, anhidrosis), indicating damage to fibers descending from the hypothalamus to the visceromotor cells of the intermediolateral cell column. Which of the following labeled areas includes the location of the hypothalamospinal fibers? (   )

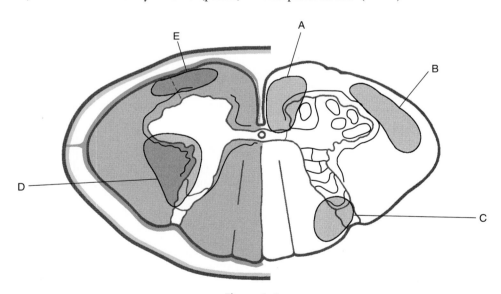

Figure 9-5

ANSWERS

1.   (C) These deficits are characteristic of damage to alpha motor neurons (the large lower motor neurons) of the ventral horn when viewed in concert with the sensory losses. Both lower extremities are involved; therefore, both anterior horns are involved in the lesion.
FN2e 145, 388

2.   (E) Bilateral loss of pain and thermal sensations with sparing of some levels caudad to the loss is indicative of a lesion of the fibers crossing in the anterior white commissure. If the lesion involved the entire anterolateral system there would be a loss of pain and thermal sensations on the contralateral side (side opposite the lesion) or complete loss of these sensations caudad to the lesion with no sacral sparing (bilateral lesion).
FN2e 144, 148–149

3. **(D)** The bilateral weakness of the lower extremities indicates involvement of much of the anterior horn in lumbar levels. The loss of pain and temperature sensations over much of the lower extremities (with sacral sparing) points to anterior white commissure damage. A large syrinx (a cavity within the spinal cord) in lower thoracic and lumbar levels explains this patient's deficits.
FN2e 143–144, 280

4. **(E)** Spinal roots C1 through C7 exit above their respective vertebrae; roots T1 and below exit caudal to their respective vertebrae; and the C8 root exits between the C7 and T1 vertebrae. The relationship between the exiting roots and the corresponding vertebrae is an important element in the diagnosis of root disease or trauma involving the roots.
FN2e 139–140

5. **(D)** A failure of the portion of the neural plate that forms the spinal cord to close is rachischisis, a type of spinal dysraphism. A failure of the rostral portion (brain) of the neural tube to close results in anencephaly. A complete failure of the neural tube to close (spinal cord + brain) is sometimes called craniorachischisis or craniorachischisis totalis. All of these developmental defects are catastrophic and not compatible with life.
FN2e 138–139

6. **(B)** The blood supply to the posterior columns is through penetrating branches of the posterior spinal artery. The main trunk of the posterior spinal artery lies medial to the posterior root entry zone; these penetrating branches serve the ipsilateral side of the cord.
FN2e 142

7. **(D)** The intermediolateral cell column is the nucleus of origin for GVE preganglionic sympathetic fibers that exit through the anterior root. These fibers may pass to paravertebral ganglia (sympathetic chain ganglia) or to prevertebral ganglia (such as the celiac or superior mesenteric); at both of these locations the prevertebral axons will terminate on postganglionic GVE neurons.
FN2e 144–145

8. **(B)** Coccygeal and sacral levels S2 through S5 of the spinal cord originate from the caudal eminence. This mass of tissue forms caudad to the neural tube and then forms a cavity that joins with the cavity (central canal) of the neural tube.
FN2e 75, 138–139

9. **(E)** The most obvious deficit in this patient would be an ipsilateral paralysis of upper and lower extremities reflecting damage to the lateral corticospinal tract. Although other tracts/fibers such as the posterior spinocerebellar and rubrospinal tracts would be included in the lesion, the motor deficits would be the overwhelmingly obvious problem.
FN2e 148–149

10. **(B)** The filum terminale internum (also called the pial part of the filum terminale) extends from the conus medullaris caudad to attach to the inner aspect of the dural sac. This structure is composed primarily of pia, traverses the lumbar cistern, and is surrounded by the anterior and posterior roots forming the cauda equina.
FN2e 116–117, 140

11. **(E)** The posterior root entry zone is located at the posterolateral sulcus. The clinical significance of this zone is reflected by the fact that heavily myelinated fibers enter the medial portion of the entry zone while the lightly myelinated fibers enter the lateral portions of the entry zone.
FN2e 139–140, 143–144

12. **(B)** The substantia gelatinosa is prominent at all levels of the spinal cord. It is light in myelin-stained sections, indicating an almost complete lack of myelinated fibers. It appears much like a broad inverted U at cervical and lumbosacral levels, and a narrow inverted V at thoracic levels.
FN2e 141–143

13. **(D)** Large-diameter, rapidly conducting fibers are medially located and small-diameter, slowly conducting fibers are located lateral within this zone. This is the anatomic basis for the DREZ (dorsal root entry zone) operation in which the laterally located small diameter fibers (which conduct pain and thermal sense) are transected to relieve pain, but the medially located proprioceptive fibers are preserved.
FN2e 143–144

14. **(B)** The large alpha motor neurons forming lamina IX of the anterior horn innervate skeletal (striated) muscle arising from mesoderm. Consequently, their functional component is GSE. These cells use acetylcholine as their neurotransmitter.
FN2e 143–145

15. **(D)** Heavily myelinated, rapidly conducting fibers of the posterior root have their cell bodies of origin in the posterior root ganglia. The central processes of these fibers enter the posterior columns and branch into the spinal gray matter (as reflex collaterals). Information conveyed by these fibers is interpreted by the nervous system as sensations of pressure, discriminative touch, stretch, and vibratory sense, collectively called proprioception/position sense.
FN2e 143–144

16. **(E)** Hypothalamospinal projections arise from the paraventricular nucleus and the lateral and posterior hypothalamic areas and descend through the posterior regions of the lateral funiculus of the spinal cord to synapse in the intermediolateral cell column. Interruption of these fibers will result in a Horner syndrome on the ipsilateral side.
FN2e 148–149, 487

17. **(D)** Postganglionic GVE fibers arise from cell bodies in the sympathetic chain ganglia, join the spinal nerve via gray ramus (gray because these fibers are unmyelinated) and distribute to the periphery on branches of the spinal nerve. These postganglionic fibers will innervate smooth muscle, glandular epithelium, or a combination of these two visceral tissues.
FN2e 144–145

18. **(C)** The posterior horn is composed of laminae I through VI, the intermediate zone of lamina VII, and the anterior horn of laminae VIII and IX. At some levels, portions of lamina VII extend into the geographic confines of the anterior horn. Area X (frequently, and mis-

takenly, called lamina X) is a small region immediately around the central canal.
FN2e 141–142

19. **(D)** Proprioceptive information enters the spinal cord on heavily myelinated, large-diameter fibers that form the medial division of the posterior root. These rapidly conducting fibers either ascend as the posterior columns or send collaterals into the gray matter as reflex collaterals.
FN2e 148–149

20. **(E)** Acetylcholine is found in many areas of the CNS and loss of acetylcholine cells has been linked to some diseases such as myasthenia gravis.
FN2e 145–146

21. **(C)** Pain radiating distally on the lateral aspect of the upper extremity and into the thumb indicates involvement of the C6 sensory root. This root exits through the C5–6 intervertebral space; cervical roots C1 through C7 exit above their respective vertebrae with the C8 root exiting between the C7 and T1 vertebrae.
FN2e 140

22. **(E)** Interception/interoceptive refers to sensory input from visceral structures (structures composed of smooth muscle, cardiac muscle, or glandular epithelium or a combination of these tissues). These GVA fibers relay information that is more poorly localized, when compared with somatic inputs, and may be involved in the phenomenon of referred pain.
FN2e 144, 297–298

23. **(B)** Damage to upper motor neurons, such as the corticospinal tract, will initially result in weakness and/or paralysis. In many cases, as time progresses over days, weeks, or months, the weak or paralyzed limb may become rigid and hyperreflexive and there may be increased muscle tone.
FN2e 148–149

24. **(B)** The posterior root ganglion contains large unipolar cell bodies generally associated with large-diameter, heavily myelinated (GSA proprioceptive) fibers and smaller unipolar cell bodies generally associated with smaller-diameter lightly myelinated (GSA—exteroceptive, pain and thermal sense; GVA—interoceptive) fibers.
FN2e 143–144

25. **(A)** Raphespinal fibers originate from the nucleus raphe magnus of the medulla and medulla-pons junction, descend in the posterior part of the lateral funiculus, and terminate on interneurons that presynaptically inhibit primary sensory fibers in the posterior horn.
FN2e 149, 291–292

26. **(E)** The knee-jerk (one example of several tendon reflexes) is also called a monosynaptic myotatic reflex. It requires an afferent fiber and its receptor (in this case a muscle spindle) and an efferent neuron that directly innervates the muscle from which the stimulus arose.
FN2e 146–147

27. **(D)** The loss of discriminative touch in the upper extremity indicates damage to the fasciculus cuneatus on the left side, and the weakness of the left leg indicates involvement of lateral portions of the corticospinal tract. The intervening position of the posterior horn and the pain fibers in the posterior root account for the loss of pain sensation. In addition, patients with lesions impinging on the posterior roots may perceive pain sensations as coming from the area of the extremity innervated by those roots; this is the result of mechanical pressure on the roots.
FN2e 143–144, 148–149

28. **(B)** The fact that this patient withdrew the injured foot but continued to stand on the uninjured lower extremity indicated that (a) on the injured side, the flexor muscles are excited and the extensor muscles are inhibited and (b) on the uninjured side the extensor muscles are excited and the flexor muscles are inhibited.
FN2e 147–148

29. **(E)** The loss of voluntary motor activity on the right specifies a lesion on the right involving the corticospinal tract. The pain and thermal losses on the left indicate damage to the anterolateral system on the right because these fibers cross at about the level of their origin in the spinal cord.
FN2e 148–150

30. **(C)** Loss of proprioception from the lower extremity on the left is indicative of a lesion to fibers of the gracile fasciculus on the left. The patient will slap his foot to the floor with each step in an attempt to create proprioceptive input. Primary sensory fibers from the left lower extremity are located in the ipsilateral fasciculus gracilis. Although somewhat unsteady, the patient does not have muscle weakness or paralysis.
FN2e 148–149

31. **(C)** This reflex functions to protect the body from further damage by withdrawing the extremity from the source of the nociceptive input (inhibit extensors, excite flexors). While the reflex is taking place at spinal levels, second-order neurons cross in the anterior white commissure and ascend via the anterolateral system to eventually reach a level of conscious perception.
FN2e 146–147

32. **(A)** Damage to the anterior (ventral) root involves the axons of lower (alpha) motor neurons innervating the skeletal muscles of the trunk wall. The same lesion will injure sympathetic preganglionic general visceral efferent fibers (GVE) that are en route to the sympathetic chain and from there as postganglionic fibers to sweat glands in the body wall. All other lesions shown here also involve sensory fibers, but the patient has no sensory losses.
FN2e 143–145

33. **(D)** Hypothalamospinal fibers are located in the lateral funiculus of the spinal cord adjacent to the spinal cord gray matter. These fibers are frequently involved in lesions of the spinal cord, such as the Brown-Séquard syndrome (functional hemisection of the spinal cord).
FN2e 141, 148–149

An Overview of the Brainstem and the Medulla Oblongata

1. A 56-year-old woman is brought to the neurologist with headache, nausea, and lethargy. MRI reveals that all ventricles are enlarged, owing to an intraventricular tumor blocking the egress of cerebrospinal fluid from the ventricular system into the subarachnoid space. Which of the following most likely represents the point(s) of blockage of cerebrospinal fluid flow in this patient?

○ (A) Interventricular foramina
○ (B) Cerebral aqueduct and interventricular foramina
○ (C) Foramen of Magendie
○ (D) Foramen of Luschka
○ (E) Foramina of Magendie and Luschka

2. A 7-year-old boy complains of a headache, especially in the morning. He is frequently nauseated and has developed difficulty speaking and swallowing. On examination, his tongue consistently deviates to the left when protruded. The MRI ordered by the pediatric neurologist reveals an ependymoma that has invaded the floor of the fourth ventricle. Involvement of which of the following labeled areas, each representing a lesion, by this tumor would most likely lead to this motor deficit? (   )

3. A 4-year-old girl is brought to the emergency department having become acutely ill over the last 4 hours. When examined, she is limp, is stuporous, and only responds to deep painful stimulation. CT is suggestive of a large arteriovenous malformation that the pediatric neurologist explains to the parents has bled into the "brainstem." Which of the following would most likely represent those regions of the brain where hemorrhage is found in this patient?

○ (A) Midbrain
○ (B) Midbrain + pons
○ (C) Midbrain + pons + cerebellum
○ (D) Midbrain + pons + medulla
○ (E) Midbrain + pons + medulla + cerebellum

4. A 61-year-old woman complains of a headache accompanied by nausea. She has an ataxic gait and is deaf in the right ear. An occlusion of which of the following vessels would damage structures that would most likely explain the deficits experienced by this patient? (   )

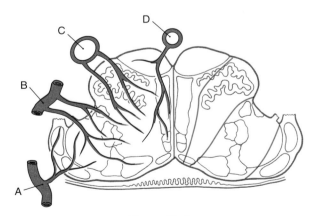

Figure 10–2

5. Soon after birth, an apparently healthy infant experiences difficulty swallowing and, when attempting to cry, makes only weak, airy sounds. The pediatric neurologist

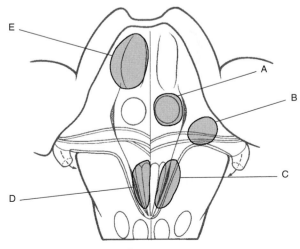

Figure 10–1

concludes that the neurons that form the special visceral efferent nucleus of the medulla failed to form properly and failed to innervate their target tissues. Based on the deficits experienced by this patient, which of the following nuclei of the medulla is most likely involved in this developmental failure?

○ (A) Nucleus ambiguus
○ (B) Dorsal motor nucleus of the vagus
○ (C) Solitary tract and nucleus
○ (D) Hypoglossal nucleus
○ (E) Medial and spinal vestibular nuclei

6.   During a surgical procedure to remove an ependymoma from the fourth ventricle of a 7-year-old boy, the surgeon notes that the tumor has invaded the floor of the medullary portion of the ventricle just lateral to the sulcus limitans. Which of the following nuclei is most likely to be involved in this lesion?

○ (A) Dorsal motor nucleus of the vagus
○ (B) Facial motor nucleus
○ (C) Inferior and spinal vestibular nuclei
○ (D) Hypoglossal nucleus
○ (E) Abducens nucleus

7.   A 64-year-old man presents with the sudden onset of difficulty speaking and swallowing. He is ataxic and has a loss of pain and temperature sensations on the left side of the face and the right side of the body. This patient's MRI reveals a lesion in the medulla (see Figure 10–3).

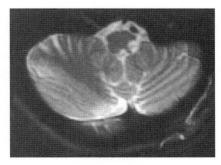

Figure 10–3

This lesion most likely resulted from occlusion of which of the following vessels?

○ (A) Labyrinthine artery
○ (B) Anterior spinal artery
○ (C) Basilar artery
○ (D) Anterior inferior cerebellar artery
○ (E) Posterior inferior cerebellar artery

8.   A 13-year-old girl is brought to a pediatric neurologist by her mother. She has developed trouble talking and swallowing. On examination, the palate elevates symmetrically but the tongue protrudes to the right. MRI reveals a small tumor in the subarachnoid space adjacent to the medulla. Based on the girl's signs and symptoms, which of the following labeled areas (see Figure 10–4), most likely represents the location of this tumor? (   )

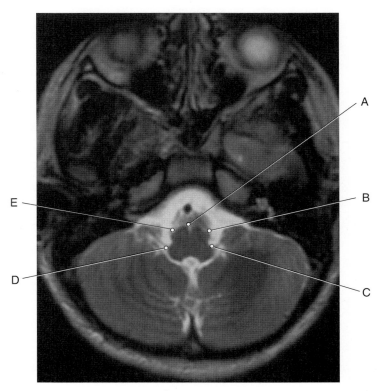

Figure 10–4

9. An 89-year-old woman presents with loss of sensation (vibratory sense and discriminative touch) affecting the left upper extremity. MRI reveals a small infarct in the medulla. Damage to which of the following labeled structures would most likely result in this woman's sensory loss? (   )

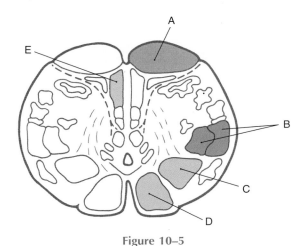

Figure 10–5

10. Which of the following labeled structures contains motor fibers that innervate muscles originating from head mesoderm and, therefore, have a general somatic efferent functional component? (   )

11. A 62-year-old woman presents with difficulty tasting food. The neurologic examination suggests that the peripheral nerves conveying taste are intact and that the lesion is centrally located in the medulla. Which of the following medullary structures is most likely involved in a lesion that results in a decrease, or loss, of taste sensation?

- ◯ (A) Gracile nucleus
- ◯ (B) Dorsal motor nucleus of the vagus
- ◯ (C) Spinal trigeminal nucleus and tract
- ◯ (D) Solitary tract and nucleus
- ◯ (E) Nucleus ambiguus

Questions 12 through 14 are based on the following patient:

A 72-year-old man presents with loss of pain and thermal sensation on the right side of the face and on the left side of the body. Before arriving at the emergency department, he complained of a severe headache, became nauseated, and briefly lost consciousness. The MRI reveals a lesion in the medulla.

12. Involvement of which of the following structures of the medulla would most likely explain the sensory deficits (loss of pain and thermal sensations) affecting this patient's face?

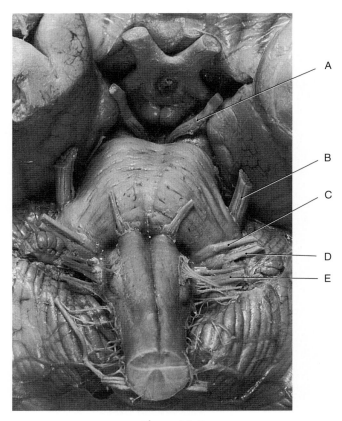

Figure 10–6

- (A) Solitary tract and nucleus
- (B) Spinal trigeminal tract and nucleus
- (C) Nucleus ambiguus
- (D) Hypoglossal nucleus
- (E) Gracile nucleus

13.   Damage to which of the following medullary structures would most likely be responsible for the sensory deficits (loss of pain and thermal sensation) affecting this patient's body?

- (A) Medial lemniscus
- (B) Posterior columns
- (C) Medial longitudinal fasciculus
- (D) Hypothalamospinal fibers
- (E) Anterolateral system

14.   Assuming this patient's deficits are the result of a vascular lesion, occlusion of penetrating branches of which of the following vessels would most likely result in this lesion?

- (A) Posterior spinal artery
- (B) Posterior inferior cerebellar artery
- (C) Vertebral artery
- (D) Anterior spinal artery
- (E) Anterior inferior cerebellar artery

15.   A 9-year-old girl presents with headache, lethargy, emesis, and ataxia. MRI reveals a large tumor within the fourth ventricle that the pediatric neurosurgeon concludes can be removed. Which of the following landmarks in the rhomboid fossa would the surgeon use to determine the border of the pons with the medulla?

- (A) Rostral aspect of the facial colliculus
- (B) Caudal aspect of the facial colliculus
- (C) Rostral aspect of the striae medullares
- (D) Caudal aspect of the striae medullares
- (E) Rostral aspect of the vagal and hypoglossal trigones

16.   A 6-year-old, previously healthy boy suddenly develops episodic emesis. In between bouts of vomiting he feels fine. MRI reveals a small tumor in the medullary portion of the fourth ventricle at caudal levels. Compression of which of the following structures is most likely the cause of this patient's symptoms?

- (A) Vestibular area
- (B) Area postrema
- (C) Striae medullares
- (D) Vagal trigone
- (E) Hypoglossal trigone

17.   Which of the following areas labeled in this MRI of the medulla indicates the position of corticospinal fibers? (   )

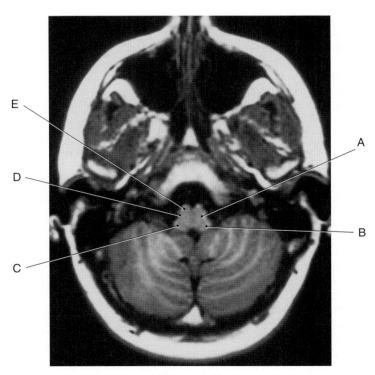

Figure 10–7

18.   A 71-year-old woman presents with a loss of vibratory sense, discriminative touch, and proprioception on the right side of the body. MRI reveals a small vascular lesion. Which of the following structures is most likely involved in a lesion that would result in this woman's deficits? (   )

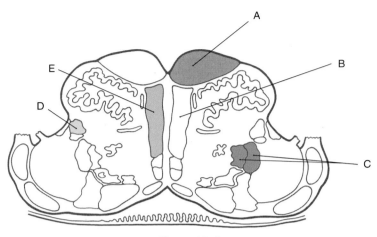

Figure 10–8

19.   A 47-year-old hypertensive man presents with weakness of the left upper and lower extremities. MRI reveals a lesion of the right side of the brainstem involving those descending fibers that influence motor neurons in the anterior horn of the spinal cord on the left side. Which of the following represents the point at which the fibers injured in this patient cross the midline?

○ (A) Anterior white commissure
○ (B) Sensory decussation
○ (C) Anterior (ventral) tegmental decussation
○ (D) Motor (pyramidal) decussation
○ (E) Posterior (dorsal) tegmental decussation

20.   A 52-year-old man presents with a meningioma (a tumor of the meninges) originating from the clivus and involving the cranial nerves of the pons-medulla junction. His signs and symptoms are unique to involvement of these nerves. Which of the following cranial nerves (CNs) is most likely involved in this tumor?

○ (A) CNs V and VI
○ (B) CNs IX, X, and XI
○ (C) CNs V and VII
○ (D) CNs VI and XII
○ (E) CNs VI, VII, and VIII

21.   A 6-year-old boy presents to the neurosurgeon's office with headache and vomiting. MRI reveals a large tumor blocking the flow of cerebrospinal fluid from the fourth ventricle into the subarachnoid cisterns. After carefully studying the MRI, the neurosurgeon determines that he can remove the tumor by dissecting from the cisterna magna (dorsal cerebellomedullary cistern) into the fourth ventricle. Which of the following represents the opening between the fourth ventricle and the cisterna magna?

○ (A) Interventricular foramen
○ (B) Foramen of Magendie
○ (C) Foramen of Luschka
○ (D) Foramen caecum of medulla oblongata

22.   Which of the following represents that part of the spinal trigeminal nucleus located between upper cervical levels of the spinal cord and the obex?

○ (A) Pars oralis
○ (B) Pars interpolaris
○ (C) Pars caudalis
○ (D) Pars opercularis
○ (E) Pars triangularis

23.   A 41-year-old woman presents with a 6-month history of headache, tinnitus, and diminished hearing. Enhanced MRI reveals a tumor of the cerebellopontine angle that involves two cranial nerves. Which of the following cranial nerves is most likely affected by this tumor?

○ (A) Abducens and hypoglossal
○ (B) Facial and vestibulocochlear
○ (C) Glossopharyngeal and vagus
○ (D) Abducens and facial
○ (E) Trochlear and oculomotor

24.   A 71-year-old man presents to the neurologist's office complaining that his "left leg feels funny." The examination reveals a loss of proprioception and vibratory sense from the patient's left lower extremity. Which of the following structures is most likely involved in the lesion that results in these deficits?

○ (A) Reticular nuclei
○ (B) Spinal trigeminal nucleus

○ (C) Accessory cuneate nucleus
○ (D) Cuneate nucleus
○ (E) Gracile nucleus

25. A 59-year-old man with poorly controlled hypertension presents with loss of proprioception, vibratory sense, and discriminative touch on the right upper and lower extremities. MRI reveals a small lesion of the posterior column nuclei on the right side, most probably a vascular lesion. Which of the following arteries represents the most specific branch of the vertebrobasilar system that serves the posterior column nuclei?

○ (A) Vertebral artery
○ (B) Posterior spinal artery
○ (C) Posterior inferior cerebellar artery
○ (D) Anterior spinal artery
○ (E) Anterior inferior cerebellar artery

26. The MRI of a 69-year-old woman reveals a tumor in the posterior fossa resulting in significant compression of the medulla. Which of the following deficits could appear suddenly in this patient and would signal potential medullary failure?

○ (A) Agnosia
○ (B) Paralysis of the lower extremities
○ (C) Complete loss of pain and thermal sense from the body
○ (D) Central apnea
○ (E) Blindness

27. Which of the following nuclei of the brainstem is the source of raphespinal fibers that provide for inhibition of pain transmission in the posterior horn of the spinal cord?

○ (A) Nucleus raphae pallidus
○ (B) Nucleus raphae magnus
○ (C) Nucleus raphae obscurus
○ (D) Nucleus raphae pontis
○ (E) Superior central nucleus

28. An 81-year-old man admitted to the intensive care unit for uncontrolled hypertension has a relatively sudden onset of central apnea. CT reveals hemorrhage in medial portions of the cerebellum that is resulting in compression of the medulla. Damage to which of the following structures in the medulla would most likely result in the breathing difficulties experienced by this patient?

○ (A) Solitary tract and nucleus
○ (B) Spinal trigeminal tract and nucleus
○ (C) Nucleus raphae magnus
○ (D) Dorsal motor nucleus of the vagus
○ (E) Ventrolateral reticular area

29. A 49-year-old man with a family history of high blood pressure presents with bilateral loss of proprioception, discriminative touch, and vibratory sense of his lower extremities. MRI reveals a small medullary lesion presumably of vascular origin. Which of the following labeled areas, each representing a lesion, includes the

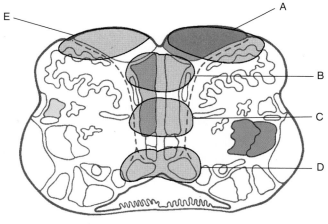

Figure 10–9

structures that when damaged would most likely give rise to the deficits experienced by this patient?

Questions 30 through 33 are based on the following patient:

A 73-year-old woman is brought to the emergency department by her son after developing hoarseness and nausea. The neurologic examination reveals a weak gravelly voice, a Horner syndrome on the left, and a loss of pain and thermal sensation on the right side of the body and on the left side of the face. MRI shows a small hemorrhage on the left side of the medulla.

30. The loss of pain and thermal sensation on the right side of the body is most likely the result of damage to which of the following?

○ (A) Medial lemniscus
○ (B) Spinal trigeminal tract
○ (C) Anterolateral system
○ (D) Anterior (ventral) trigeminothalamic tract
○ (E) Internal arcuate fibers

31. The loss of pain and thermal sensation of the left side of the face suggests that this lesion involves the spinal trigeminal tract and nucleus. In addition to the trigeminal nerve, which of the following cranial nerves (CNs) also contain primary sensory fibers that enter the spinal trigeminal tract and nucleus?

○ (A) CNs VII and VIII
○ (B) CNs IX, X, and XII
○ (C) CNs VI, VII, and VIII
○ (D) CNs VII, IX, and X
○ (E) CNs VIII and IX

32. The hoarseness in this patient suggests that this lesion has involved motor neurons that innervate laryngeal muscles, especially the vocalis muscle. Which of the following cranial nerves most likely conveys these fibers?

○ (A) Hypoglossal
○ (B) Vagus
○ (C) Glossopharyngeal
○ (D) Spinal accessory
○ (E) Facial

33. This patient has a Horner syndrome on the same side (left) as the facial sensory loss. Damage to which of the following fibers would most likely result in this sign?

○ (A) Hypothalamospinal fibers
○ (B) Reticulospinal fibers
○ (C) Vestibulospinal fibers
○ (D) Spinohypothalamic fibers
○ (E) Reticulothalamic fibers

34. A 67-year-old woman presents with loss of vibratory sensation and discriminative touch on the left side of the body. MRI indicates a small lesion of the gracile and cuneate nuclei. Which of the following represents the axons that arise from these nuclei and course toward the midline where they eventually cross as the sensory decussation?

○ (A) Posterior (dorsal) tegmental decussation
○ (B) Pyramidal decussation
○ (C) Anterior (ventral) tegmental decussation
○ (D) Internal arcuate fibers
○ (E) Anterior white commissure

ANSWERS

1. **(E)** Both exit routes out of the fourth ventricle, the foramina of Magendie and Luschka, must be occluded to effectively block the flow of cerebrospinal fluid from the ventricular system into the subarachnoid space. Blockage of these foramina will cause enlargement of all ventricular spaces upstream to the occlusion.
FN2e 95, 153–154

2. **(D)** Ependymomas are one of the most common fourth ventricular tumors in children. They typically originate from the floor of the fourth ventricle and may produce cranial nerve deficits associated with their point of invasion in the rhomboid fossa. The vagal and hypoglossal trigones are located in the caudal portion of the rhomboid fossa. The hypoglossal nucleus, innervating the ipsilateral musculature of the tongue, is located internal to the hypoglossal trigone. Injury to these motor neurons will result in deviation of the tongue toward the side of the lesion on protrusion.
FN2e 153–154, 396–399

3. **(D)** The brainstem consists of the rhombencephalon (pons and medulla) plus the midbrain but excludes the cerebellum; this latter structure is commonly referred to as suprasegmental. Regardless of the source, injury to the brainstem is frequently catastrophic, resulting in permanent disability or death.
FN2e 152

4. **(A)** The anterior inferior cerebellar artery serves the cochlear nuclei, some of the adjacent restiform body, and a large portion of the inferior aspect of the cerebellar hemisphere (excluding most of the nuclei). Occlusion of vessels serving the cochlear nuclei will result in ipsilateral deafness. The ataxia is a reflection of combined injury to the restiform body and cerebellum.
FN2e 169–170

5. **(A)** The motor neurons of the nucleus ambiguus innervate muscles that arise from the third (stylopharyngeus) and fourth (muscles of larynx and pharynx, including the vocalis) pharyngeal arches. This nucleus contributes motor fibers primarily to the glossopharyngeal and vagus nerves.
FN2e 164–166

6. **(C)** The inferior and spinal vestibular nuclei are located in the floor of the medullary part of the rhomboid fossa. These are sensory nuclei and are, therefore, located lateral to the sulcus limitans. The rostral edge of the striae medullares of the fourth ventricle is regarded as the border between medullary and pontine portions of the rhomboid fossa.
FN2e 154–157, 164

7. **(E)** The posterolateral area of the medulla is served by penetrating branches of the posterior inferior cerebellar artery. Included in the territory of this vessel are the nucleus ambiguus, spinal trigeminal tract and nucleus, the ascending fibers of the anterolateral system, and descending hypothalamospinal fibers.
FN2e 170–171

8. **(E)** The hypoglossal nerve exits the preolivary fissure, the groove between the pyramid and the olivary eminence. The lesion involves the right exiting hypoglossal root because the tongue deviates to the right.
FN2e 161–162

9. **(C)** Vibratory sense and discriminative touch are conveyed by the cuneate fasciculus (for the upper extremity) in the spinal cord and by the cuneate nucleus in the medulla. Both of these structures convey sensory information that has originated from the ipsilateral side of the body.
FN2e 164–165

10. **(A)** The oculomotor nerve innervates most of the extraocular muscles; these muscles arise from head mesoderm, not from the pharyngeal arches. Cranial nerves V, VII, and X innervate muscles that arise in pharyngeal arches I, II, and IV and have a special visceral efferent functional component. Cranial nerve VIII is sensory.
FN2e 156, 161

11. **(D)** Taste fibers are transported centrally on cranial nerves VII, IX, and X. The central processes of these fibers contribute to the formation of the solitary tract, once they enter the medulla, and synapse on the surrounding solitary nuclei.
FN2e 156–157, 165–166

12. **(B)** The central processes of fibers from the face conveying pain and thermal sensations form the spinal trigeminal tract and terminate in the medially adjacent spinal trigeminal nucleus. Although cranial nerve V is the main source of these fibers, cranial nerves VII, IX, and X also make small contributions to this tract and nucleus.
FN2e 156–157

13. **(E)** Pain and thermal sense from the body is conveyed through fibers of the anterolateral system. Some of the fibers in this system terminate in the medullary reticular formation (as spinoreticular fibers) whereas others continue to more rostral levels of the neuraxis as spinothalamic fibers.
FN2e 163, 164–166

14. **(B)** The posterolateral area of the medulla that contains the spinal trigeminal tract and nucleus and the fibers of the anterolateral system is served by branches of the posterior inferior cerebellar artery. A number of other important structures are also located in the territory served by this vessel.
FN2e 169–171

15. **(C)** The junction of the medulla with the pons in the floor of the fourth ventricle is regarded as a line along the rostral edge of the striae medullares. This line extends into the lateral recess and along the caudal aspect of the inferior and middle cerebellar peduncles.
FN2e 154

16. **(B)** The area postrema is an emetic center in the wall of the fourth ventricle at the level of the obex; this is the point at which the central canal in the caudal medulla flares open into the fourth ventricle.
FN2e 166

17. **(E)** The elevation on the anterior surface of the medulla adjacent to the midline is the pyramid. This structure contains corticospinal fibers that originate from the ipsilateral motor cortex and terminate in the contralateral spinal cord.
FN2e 162–163, 165–166

18. **(B)** The medial lemniscus of the medulla contains the fibers conveying proprioception, discriminative touch, and vibratory sense from the gracile and cuneate nuclei to higher levels of the neuraxis. The cells of the gracile and cuneate nuclei give rise to axons that cross the midline to form the medial lemniscus on the opposite side. Consequently, the left medial lemniscus is conveying information from the right side of the body.
FN2e 162–164

19. **(D)** The lesion in this patient involves corticospinal fibers at some point in the brainstem. These fibers descend through the midbrain and pons and enter the pyramid of the medulla. They cross to the opposite side in the pyramidal decussation, also called the motor decussation. This explains why a lesion of these fibers on one side of the brainstem will result in weakness on the contralateral side of the body.
FN2e 162–164

20. **(E)** The cranial nerves of the pons-medulla junction are, from medial to lateral, the abducens (VI), facial (VII, including the intermediate nerve), and the vestibulocochlear (VIII). The VI is motor, the VII is mixed, and the VIII is, for our purposes, sensory.
FN2e 152

21. **(B)** The foramen of Magendie is located in the caudal roof of the fourth ventricle and opens from the fourth ventricle into the dorsal cerebellomedullary cistern (also called the cisterna magna). This foramen is frequently used by neurosurgeons to gain midline access to the fourth ventricle.
FN2e 153

22. **(C)** The most caudal portion of the spinal trigeminal nucleus, the pars caudalis, extends from the upper cervical levels of the spinal cord (for our purposes we will regard this as C1–C2) to a cross-sectional level of the medulla at the obex. This portion of the spinal trigeminal nucleus is the main cell group for the relay of pain and thermal sensations from the face to the contralateral thalamus.
FN2e 157, 284–286

23. **(B)** The cranial nerves of the cerebellopontine angle are the facial (VII) and the vestibulocochlear (VIII). These nerves are located adjacent to each other, enter the internal acoustic meatus along with the labyrinthine artery, and may be affected by tumors of the cerebellopontine angle, such as a vestibular schwannoma or a meningioma.
FN2e 160–161

24. **(E)** The gracile nucleus (frequently called the nucleus gracilis) is located on the posterior (dorsal) aspect of the medulla immediately caudad to the obex. It receives information from the ipsilateral lower extremity and projects to the contralateral thalamus through the internal arcuate fibers and the medial lemniscus.
FN2e 163–165

25. **(B)** The posterior column nuclei and immediately adjacent structures such as the rostral portion of the posterior columns are served by the posterior spinal artery. In about 75% of brains, this artery is a branch of the posterior inferior cerebellar artery, and, in about 25%, it originates from the vertebral artery.
FN2e 125, 169–170

26. **(D)** The sudden onset of apnea (the absence of breathing) reflects compression of the medulla; central apnea specifically signifies apnea caused by medullary compromise. Pressure increases in the posterior fossa may cause herniation of the cerebellar tonsils downward through the foramen magnum, resulting in pressure on the medulla and producing central apnea.
FN2e 168–169

27. **(B)** Raphespinal fibers originate from cells of the nucleus raphae magnus, which is located in the rostral medulla and extends slightly into the caudal pons. These fibers terminate on interneurons that, in turn, presynaptically inhibit primary sensory fibers in the posterior horn that convey pain and thermal information. Raphespinal fibers also project into the spinal trigeminal nucleus.
FN2e 168–169, 291–292

28. **(E)** Cells located in the lateral portion of the reticular formation of the medulla, specifically in the ventrolateral reticular area, influence respiration. Damage to this area of the medulla through compression, or other lesions, may slow respiration or, in acute situations, may produce sudden apnea.
FN2e 168–169

29. **(B)** The modalities of proprioception, discriminative touch, and vibratory sense from the lower extremi-

ties are conveyed by fibers located in the anterior (ventral) portions of the medial lemniscus. Bilateral loss of these sensations indicates bilateral damage to this part of the medial lemniscus. These areas of the medial lemniscus are in the territory of the anterior spinal artery.
FN2e 162–164

30.   **(C)** Pain and thermal sensation from the body are conveyed on fibers of the anterolateral system (ALS); these fibers originate in the contralateral posterior horn of the spinal cord. The ALS is located in the lateral area of the medulla immediately adjacent to the spinal trigeminal tract and nucleus and within the territory of the posterior inferior cerebellar artery.
FN2e 162–163, 166, 171

31.   **(D)** Pain and thermal sensation from the surface of the ear, from the skin lining the external auditory meatus, and from the external surface of the eardrum are conveyed centrally on fibers of the facial (VII), glossopharyngeal (IX), and vagus (X) nerves.
FN2e 157, 284, 286

32.   **(B)** The nucleus ambiguus contains SVE motor neurons that travel on the vagus nerve to innervate laryngeal muscles including the vocalis muscle. These muscles originate from the third pharyngeal arch, hence their functional component of SVE.
FN2e 156, 164

33.   **(A)** Hypothalamospinal fibers arise in the ipsilateral hypothalamus and descend through the lateral medullary area to eventually terminate in the intermediolateral cell column in upper thoracic levels (about T1 to T3). Interruption of these fibers at any location along this route may result in the deficits collectively known as the Horner syndrome.
FN2e 170

34.   **(D)** The axons of neurons in the gracile and cuneate nuclei course anteromedially as the internal arcuate fibers to cross the midline as the sensory decussation. Once crossed, these axons collect to form the medial lemniscus and pass rostrally toward the ventral posterolateral nucleus of the thalamus.
FN2e 164

CHAPTER 12

The Pons and Cerebellum

Questions 1 through 5 are based on the following patient:

A 74-year-old woman with poorly controlled hypertension presents with an inability to abduct the right eye, a left-sided paralysis of the upper and lower extremities, and a loss of proprioception, discriminative touch, and vibratory sense on the left side of the body. The patient's family indicates that these symptoms appeared suddenly after she had eaten dinner and were accompanied by nausea and dizziness.

1. Which of the following represents the best localizing sign in this patient?

- ○ (A) Paralysis of the upper extremity
- ○ (B) Loss of proprioception
- ○ (C) Paralysis of the lower extremity
- ○ (D) Loss of discriminative touch and vibratory sense
- ○ (E) Inability to abduct right eye

2. The descending motor fibers influencing upper and lower extremities on the left and the cranial nerve fibers innervating the lateral rectus muscle on the right are adjacent to each other at which of the following locations?

- ○ (A) Basilar pons at rostral levels
- ○ (B) Pyramid at mid olivary levels
- ○ (C) Basilar pons at caudal levels
- ○ (D) Crus cerebri
- ○ (E) Posterior limb of the internal capsule

3. Damage to which of the following structures would most likely explain the loss of proprioception and vibratory sense?

- ○ (A) Central tegmental tract
- ○ (B) Medial longitudinal fasciculus
- ○ (C) Ventral trigeminothalamic fibers
- ○ (D) Medial vestibular nuclei
- ○ (E) Medial lemniscus

4. The historical findings of a sudden onset of this patient's symptoms most likely indicates what disorder?

- ○ (A) Meningitis
- ○ (B) Meningioma
- ○ (C) Intramedullary astrocytoma
- ○ (D) Hemorrhage into the brain
- ○ (E) Traumatic injury

5. The alternating pattern of the deficits seen in this patient is also called a crossed deficit. This is a pattern of a deficit on one side of the body and on the opposite side of the face and is generally indicative of a lesion where?

- ○ (A) Cerebral cortex
- ○ (B) Internal capsule
- ○ (C) Cerebellum
- ○ (D) Brainstem
- ○ (E) Spinal cord

6. A 69-year-old woman presents with motor deficits indicative of a lesion in the cerebellum. MR angiography reveals an interruption of blood supply to the cerebellar nuclei. Which of the following vessels is most likely to be occluded?

- ○ (A) Superior cerebellar artery
- ○ (B) Anterior inferior cerebellar artery
- ○ (C) Posterior inferior cerebellar artery
- ○ (D) Posterior cerebral artery
- ○ (E) Long circumferential pontine arteries

7. The MRI of a 29-year-old man reveals a meningioma impinging on the brainstem at the point where the basilar pons is continuous with the middle cerebellar peduncle. Which of the following structures is located at the junction of these structures and would most likely be damaged by this tumor?

- ○ (A) Exit of the facial nerve
- ○ (B) Exit of the trigeminal nerve
- ○ (C) Exit of the glossopharyngeal nerve
- ○ (D) Position of the restiform body
- ○ (E) Exit of the abducens nerve

8. A 42-year-old man has developed tinnitus and hearing loss in his left ear. Enhanced MRI reveals a tumor in the area of the cerebellopontine angle and extending into the internal acoustic meatus. Which of the following structures would most likely also be damaged by this tumor?

○ (A) Trochlear nerve
○ (B) Trigeminal nerve
○ (C) Glossopharyngeal nerve
○ (D) Facial nerve
○ (E) Abducens nerve

9. Which of the following areas labeled in this MRI of the pons indicates the position of corticospinal fibers? (   )

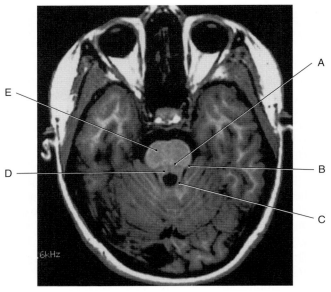

Figure 12–1

10. Which of the following functional components is associated with the abducens nucleus?

○ (A) GSA
○ (B) SVE
○ (C) GSE and GVE
○ (D) GSE
○ (E) SVE and GVE

11. During testing of the gag reflex of a 27-year-old woman, the physician discovers that the stylopharyngeus muscle does not respond. Which of the following nuclei contain the motor neurons innervating this muscle?

○ (A) Superior salivatory nucleus
○ (B) Inferior salivatory nucleus
○ (C) Gigantocellular reticular nucleus
○ (D) Nucleus raphae magnus
○ (E) Nucleus ambiguus

12. A 49-year-old woman presents to her physician's office with deafness and ringing in the right ear. The subsequent examination reveals an occlusion of the labyrinthine artery. Which of the following is the most likely source of this particular artery?

○ (A) Superior cerebellar artery
○ (B) Vertebral artery
○ (C) Anterior inferior cerebellar artery
○ (D) Posterior inferior cerebellar artery
○ (E) Paramedian branch of the basilar artery

13. A 19-year-old man presents with a severe headache and motor disturbances. MRI reveals an arteriovenous malformation that involves wide areas of the cerebellar cortex. It is likely that this lesion has partially compromised the efferent neurons of the cerebellar cortex. Which of the following represents this particular cell type?

○ (A) Granule cell
○ (B) Basket cell
○ (C) Golgi cell
○ (D) Purkinje cell
○ (E) Stellate cell

14. The MRI of a male newborn reveals several developmental defects related to the posterior fossa. Among these was a failure of the first fissure to appear in the cerebellar plate. Which of the following fissures is most likely lacking in this patient?

○ (A) Primary fissure
○ (B) Secondary fissure
○ (C) Posterolateral fissure
○ (D) Horizontal fissure
○ (E) Precentral fissure

15. A 58-year-old man with poorly controlled hypertension and atherosclerosis presents to his internist's office with headache, nausea, and double vision (diplopia). The neurologic examination reveals an inability to abduct the left eye. An occlusion of which of the following vessels, or an infarct in which of the following vascular territories, would explain the deficits seen in this patient? (   )

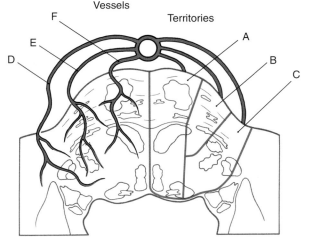

Figure 12–2

16. A male newborn is noted to have developmental defects that indicate a failure of the second pharyngeal arch to develop. Motor neurons in which of the following nuclei would be most affected by this developmental error?

❍ (A) Trigeminal motor nucleus
❍ (B) Facial motor nucleus
❍ (C) Superior salivatory nucleus
❍ (D) Nucleus ambiguus
❍ (E) Dorsal motor nucleus of the vagal nerve

Questions 17 through 22 are based on the following patient:

A 64-year-old man develops subtle slurring of speech, combined with loss of pain and thermal sensation on the right side of the face and left side of the body. A careful examination reveals that he has paralysis of facial muscles on the right side involving upper and lower portions of the face. Masticatory muscles appear to function normally, and there is no deviation of the tongue on protrusion.

17. In this patient, paralysis of the facial muscles most likely indicates involvement of which of the following structures?

❍ (A) Genu of the internal capsule (cortionuclear fibers)
❍ (B) The crus cerebri (corticonuclear fibers)
❍ (C) The root of the facial nerve in the subarachnoid space
❍ (D) The facial nerve in the internal auditory meatus
❍ (E) The facial motor nucleus or facial nerve fibers within the brainstem

18. The loss of pain and thermal sense on the left side of the body is most likely caused by involvement of which of the following structures?

❍ (A) Anterior white commissure
❍ (B) Anterolateral system
❍ (C) Ventral posterolateral nucleus of the thalamus
❍ (D) Posterior limb of the internal capsule
❍ (E) Medial lemniscus

19. The loss of pain and thermal sensation on the right side of the face is most likely caused by involvement of which of the following structures?

❍ (A) Root of the trigeminal nerve
❍ (B) Spinal trigeminal nucleus, pars oralis
❍ (C) Spinal trigeminal nucleus, pars caudalis
❍ (D) Spinal trigeminal tract
❍ (E) Ventral trigeminothalamic fibers

20. Based on the combination of deficits noted in this patient, this lesion is best localized to which of the following?

❍ (A) Medulla oblongata at mid olivary levels
❍ (B) Lateral areas of the pons at caudal levels
❍ (C) Lateral areas of the pons at mid to rostral levels
❍ (D) Subarachnoid space at the pons-medulla junction
❍ (E) Ventral and medial midbrain involving the crus cerebri

21. The lesion in this patient is best described as being located where?

❍ (A) On the patient's right
❍ (B) On the patient's left
❍ (C) Bilateral (lesion on both right and left)
❍ (D) Insufficient information to decide laterality

22. Assuming this to be a vascular lesion, which vessel(s) is(are) most likely involved?

❍ (A) Paramedian branches of the basilar artery
❍ (B) Posterior inferior cerebellar artery
❍ (C) Superior cerebellar artery
❍ (D) Short and long circumferential branches of the basilar artery
❍ (E) Anterior spinal artery

23. Which of the following areas labeled in this MRI of the pons indicates the position of the medial lemniscus? ( )

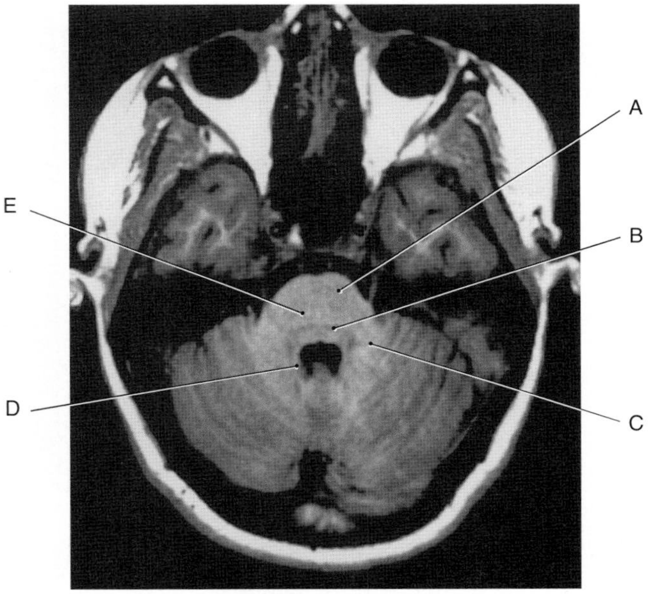

Figure 12–3

24. A newborn has difficulty sucking a pacifier. Examination reveals that those striated muscles innervated by the trigeminal motor nucleus did not form properly. Which of the following is the source of these muscles in the normal infant?

❍ (A) First pharyngeal arch
❍ (B) Second pharyngeal arch
❍ (C) Third pharyngeal arch
❍ (D) Fourth pharyngeal arch

25. A 5-year-old boy presents with headache and signs of increased intracranial pressure. MRI reveals a tumor

in the fourth ventricle. At surgery, the neurosurgeon finds that the tumor has infiltrated an important oval-shaped structure located medial to the sulcus limitans in the floor of the fourth ventricle immediately rostral to the stria medullares. Which of the following most likely represents this structure?

○ (A) Facial colliculus
○ (B) Vestibular area
○ (C) Vagal trigone
○ (D) Hypoglossal trigone
○ (E) Medial eminence of fourth ventricle

26.   MRI of a 57-year-old man reveals a small vascular lesion in the pons that involves corticospinal fibers and portions of the medial lemniscus. Which of the following arteries serve these structures within the pons? See Figure 12–4 at right. (   )

27.   A 49-year-old woman has weakness of the facial muscles on the left side of her face; pain and thermal sensation is normal. Assuming this to be a small lesion at the pons-medulla junction, which of the following structures is most likely involved? See Figure 12–5 below. (   )

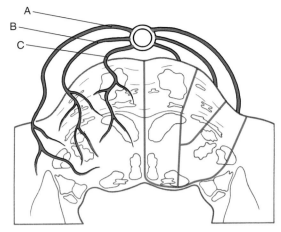

Figure 12–4

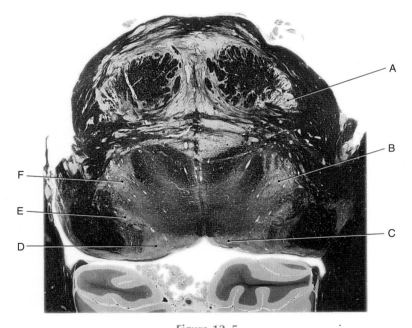

Figure 12–5

28.   A 37-year-old man complains of changes in his perception of sound. Although not deaf in either ear, his perception of sound localization has changed. MRI reveals a tumor in the mid to rostral pons. Which of the following structures is concerned with the transmission of auditory information?

○ (A) Lateral lemniscus
○ (B) Medial lemniscus
○ (C) Central tegmental tract
○ (D) Anterolateral system
○ (E) Posterior (dorsal) longitudinal fasciculus

29.   The visceromotor (autonomic) preganglionic fibers that distribute with the peripheral branches of the facial nerve originate where?

○ (A) Facial motor nucleus
○ (B) Inferior salivatory nucleus
○ (C) Superior salivatory nucleus
○ (D) Nucleus ambiguus
○ (E) Edinger-Westphal nucleus

30. A 72-year-old man presents with a loss of proprioception, vibratory sensation, and discriminative touch suggesting a lesion of the medial lemniscus. Which of the following structures is most likely involved in this lesion? ( )

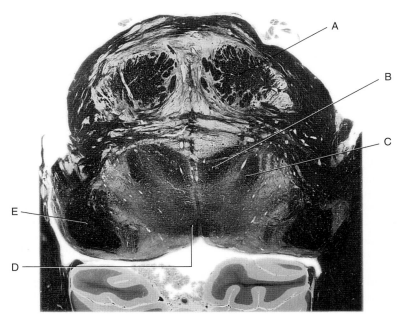

Figure 12–6

31. A 6-year-old girl is brought to the pediatric neurologist by her mother. The neurologic examination reveals an inability to abduct the right eye and weakness of muscles around the oral cavity and eye. MRI reveals a tumor in the fourth ventricle. Damage to which of the following structures would most likely explain the deficits seen in this patient?

○ (A) Vagal trigone
○ (B) Vestibular area
○ (C) Hypoglossal trigone
○ (D) Facial colliculus
○ (E) Medial eminence of fourth ventricle

32. A 69-year-old woman presents with weakness of the masticatory muscles on the right side and loss of pain and thermal sense from the same side of the face. The latter finding suggests that primary sensory fibers are most likely involved in the lesion along with motor structures. Which of the following labeled areas, each representing a lesion, contains the tracts and/or fibers that, when damaged, would give rise to the deficits seen in this patient? See Figure 12–7 below. ( )

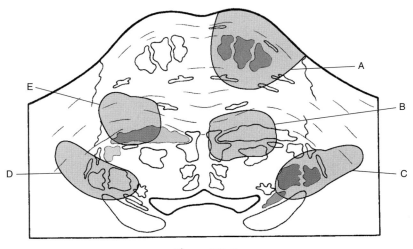

Figure 12–7

ANSWERS

1. **(E)** Long tract signs (A–D), even in combination, could indicate a lesion at several different levels of the neuraxis. However, the inability to abduct the right eye points to involvement of the abducens nerve or nucleus. Because only the right eye will not abduct (no movement deficits are mentioned for the left eye), it is likely that abducens fibers within the brainstem, or at its exit point, are damaged.
FN2e 8–9, 178–180

2. **(C)** Weakness/paralysis of the extremities suggests damage to corticospinal fibers. Injury to corticospinal fibers, in combination with the abducens palsy, would put this lesion in the caudal basilar pons. It is true that corticospinal fibers are found in the crus cerebri and pyramid, but damage at these levels would probably include roots of the oculomotor and hypoglossal nerves, respectively, not the abducens.
FN2e 178, 180

3. **(E)** The medial lemniscus is located immediately posterior (dorsal) to the corticospinal fibers in medial portions of the pons. These fibers convey information interpreted by the brain as proprioception and vibratory sense.
FN2e 178–179

4. **(D)** The clinical neurologic examination includes a detailed history and examination. Although the examination is most useful in determining the location of the pathologic process, the history is particularly useful in determining the type of pathologic process. The symptoms experienced by this patient appeared suddenly, suggesting either a vascular event or trauma. There was no history of trauma, and the other choices would result in symptoms that would appear slowly over time.
FN2e 122, 123, 287

5. **(D)** Alternating, or crossed deficits, refer to damage to a long tract serving contralateral structures (ascending or descending) and to a closely adjacent cranial nerve serving ipsilateral structures (root, nucleus). In this example the corticospinal fibers and the root of the abducens nerve are adjacent to each other in the basilar pons. Crossed deficits are generally characteristic of lesions in the brainstem.
FN2e 9, 179–180

6. **(A)** The superior cerebellar artery serves the superior surface of the cerebellum (including the anterior lobe) and, through penetrating branches, most of the cerebellar nuclei located in the white matter of the cerebellum. A few branches of the anterior inferior cerebellar artery serve a small caudal portion of the dentate nucleus.
FN2e 184–185

7. **(B)** On the lateral aspect of the pons, the exiting fibers of the trigeminal nerve signify the interface of basilar pons (anterior/ventral to the exit) with the middle cerebellar peduncle (posterior/dorsal to the exit). In addition, the part of the pons rostral to the exit of V may be called the pretrigeminal pons and that part caudal to the exit, the post-trigeminal pons.
FN2e 174–175

8. **(D)** The cerebellopontine angle is formed by the junction of the cerebellum, pons, and medulla. Cranial nerves VII and VIII are commonly regarded as the nerves at this location, although it should be noted that nerves IX and X are immediately caudal to the exit of VII in the postolivary sulcus. Vestibular schwannoma is the most common tumor found in this location. *Acoustic neuroma* is an inaccurate historical term. This tumor is actually a schwannoma that arises from the superior division of the vestibular nerve. An acoustic origin of this lesion is uncommon. Neuromas are post-traumatic lesions.
FN2e 174–175

9. **(E)** Corticospinal fibers at this level are located in the basilar pons adjacent to the midline. The exiting fibers of the abducens nerve are located immediately lateral to the corticospinal fibers in the basilar pons at the pons-medulla junction.
FN2e 175, 178–180

10. **(D)** Lower motor neurons of the abducens nucleus innervate the lateral rectus muscle on the ipsilateral side. This muscle originates from head mesoderm in the area of the orbit and, therefore, is assigned a general somatic efferent (GSE) functional component.
FN2e 154–156, 174–175

11. **(E)** The stylopharyngeus muscle originates from the mesoderm of the third pharyngeal arch and is innervated by SVE motor neurons located in the nucleus ambiguus. These fibers are carried by the glossopharyngeal nerve.
FN2e 154–156, 174–175

12. **(C)** In about 75% of individuals the labyrinthine artery originates from the anterior inferior cerebellar artery. This latter artery also serves the inferior and lateral aspect of the cerebellar hemisphere and caudal and middle portions of the middle cerebellar peduncle, and sends some penetrating branches into the pontine tegmentum at caudal pontine levels.
FN2e 126, 185

13. **(D)** Purkinje cells send their inhibitory GABAergic axons to terminate in the cerebellar nuclei and in the vestibular nuclei, both on the ipsilateral side. These projections are topographically organized. The other cortical cells are interneurons with synaptic relationships only in the cortex.
FN2e 184

14. **(C)** The posterolateral fissure appears between the flocculonodular lobe and the remaining portions of the cerebellum and extends from the midline (separating lobule IX from lobule X, the nodulus) to the lateral margins of the cerebellum (separating lobule HIX from lobule HX, the flocculus).
FN2e 85, 184–185

15. **(A)** The inability to abduct the left eye suggests a lesion of the abducens root or nucleus on the patient's left side. The exiting roots of the abducens nerve and most of the abducens nucleus are located within the territory served by the paramedian branches of the basilar artery.
FN2e 183–184

16. **(B)** The mesoderm of the second pharyngeal arch gives rise to the muscles of facial expression plus the stapedius, buccinator, stylohyoid, platysma, and the pos-

terior belly of the digastric. These muscles are innervated by the SVE motor neurons in the facial nucleus.
FN2e 154–156, 178–179

17. **(E)** Two points need to be considered. First, paralysis of the upper and lower portions of the face suggests a lesion of the root or nucleus of the facial nerve. Second, loss of pain and thermal sense on the left side of the body indicated involvement of the anterolateral system. The facial nucleus/root (serving the ipsilateral face) and the anterolateral system (serving the contralateral body) are located in close proximity in the lateral pons. The facial muscle paralysis is the best localizing sign in this patient.
FN2e 178–180

18. **(B)** Pain and thermal sensations from the body (specifically the contralateral side) are transported via the anterolateral system. These fibers are located in anterolateral (ventrolateral) portions of the brainstem throughout its extent; in the pons these fibers are in anterolateral areas of the tegmentum.
FN2e 178–180

19. **(D)** Loss of pain and thermal sensations from the face could suggest a lesion of the root of the trigeminal nerve or of the spinal trigeminal tract, the latter being the central processes of primary sensory axons entering the brainstem on the trigeminal nerve. However, when combined with the loss of pain and thermal sensations on the body and the paralysis of facial muscles, the lesion localizes to the internal pons; the trigeminal nerve is excluded.
FN2e 178–180

20. **(B)** The combination of an alternating sensory loss (face on one side, body on the other side) and a paralysis of facial muscles (nucleus or root of VII) localizes this lesion to lateral portions of the caudal pons. A lesion in the lateral pons at more rostral levels would result in a paralysis of masticatory muscles, a symptom not experienced by this patient.
FN2e 178–180

21. **(A)** The sensory loss on the right side of the patient's face coupled with the paralysis of muscles of facial expression on the right indicate a lesion on the patient's right side. The paralysis of facial muscles is the best localizing sign in this patient.
FN2e 8–9, 12–13, 178–180

22. **(D)** The lateral part of the pontine tegmentum at more caudal levels is served by short and long circumferential pontine arteries. This region of the brainstem also receives a supplemental blood supply from the anterior-inferior cerebellar artery.
FN2e 183–184

23. **(B)** The medial lemniscus in the pons, especially at mid to rostral levels, is located at the interface of the tegmentum of the pons with the basilar pons. At this position it is horizontally oriented from medial to lateral.
FN2e 181–182

24. **(A)** The muscles of mastication plus the tensor tympani, tensor veli palatini, mylohyoid, and anterior belly of the digastric arise from mesenchyme of the first pharyngeal arch. These muscles are innervated by the SVE lower motor neurons located in the trigeminal motor nucleus.
FN2e 154–156, 174–175

25. **(A)** The facial colliculus is located medial to the sulcus limitans (and the superior fovea) and just rostral to the stria medullares of the fourth ventricle. This colliculus is located in the caudal part of the pontine portion of the fourth ventricle and contains the abducens nucleus (GSE cells that innervate the ipsilateral lateral rectus muscle) and the internal genu of the facial nerve (SVE fibers that innervate the muscles of facial expression on the ipsilateral side).
FN2e 154, 178

26. **(C)** The corticospinal tract is located in medial portions of the basilar pons. The medial lemniscus is located at the interface of the basilar pons with the tegmental pons. These structures are within the region of the pons that is served by the paramedian branches of the basilar artery.
FN2e 183–184

27. **(B)** The motor facial nucleus is located in the anterolateral pontine tegmentum just rostral to the pons-medulla junction. The axons of these SVE cell bodies arch medially, pass around the abducens nucleus (internal to the facial colliculus), and course anterolaterally to exit the brainstem at the pons-medulla junction.
FN2e 178–180

28. **(A)** Fibers conveying auditory information in the brainstem originate from cells of the posterior (dorsal) and anterior (ventral) cochlear nuclei. Some of these fibers will decussate in the trapezoid body and then turn rostrally as a component of the lateral lemniscus. This bundle is conveying auditory signals from both ears.
FN2e 180

29. **(C)** The superior salivatory nucleus gives rise to GVE preganglionic parasympathetic fibers that join the facial nerve lateral to the internal genu; these fibers do not arch through the internal genu. These preganglionic fibers distribute to the pterygopalatine and submandibular ganglia in which the postganglionic cells are located.
FN2e 156

30. **(B)** The medial lemniscus in the pons is obliquely oriented at the pons-medulla junction and becomes more horizontally oriented at midpontine levels. This structure conveys information from the contralateral side of the body.
FN2e 178–181

31. **(D)** The abducens nucleus (innervating the ipsilateral lateral rectus muscle) and the internal genu of the facial nerve (innervating the ipsilateral muscles of facial expression) are located immediately internal to the elevation of the facial colliculus. Indeed, these structures participate in forming this elevation.
FN2e 178–179

32. **(D)** This lesion involves the trigeminal motor nucleus on the right side of the patient at about midpontine levels. Incoming sensory fibers of the trigeminal nerve enter the pons at this level and turn caudad to form the spinal trigeminal tract. Therefore, injury to this level of the pons would most likely also involve these primary sensory fibers.
FN2e 178, 181, 286

CHAPTER 13

The Midbrain

1. A 32-year-old woman presents with double vision (diplopia). The left eye is deviated laterally and slightly inferiorly. The left pupil is dilated and does not constrict to bright light. MR angiography reveals an aneurysm. An aneurysm found at which of the following locations would most likely explain the deficits experienced by this patient? (   )

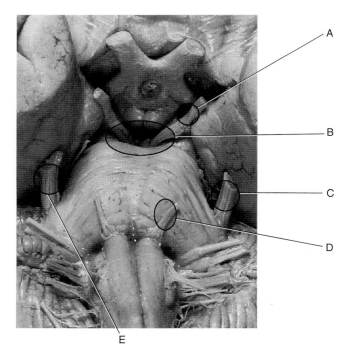

Figure 13–1

2. A 67-year-old man presents to the emergency department with a headache and nausea. MRI reveals a tumor in the quadrigeminal cistern. Which of the following structures would most likely be affected by this tumor?

- ○ (A) Abducens nerve
- ○ (B) Trochlear nerve
- ○ (C) V_1
- ○ (D) Oculomotor nerve
- ○ (E) Brachium of the superior colliculus

3. During the neurologic examination of a 16-year-old boy the physician discovers the absence of the pupillary light reflex. Injury to which of the following structures would most likely interrupt the pathway from the optic tract to the pretectal nuclei?

- ○ (A) Brachium of the inferior colliculus
- ○ (B) Posterior commissure
- ○ (C) Brachium of the superior colliculus
- ○ (D) Optic chiasm
- ○ (E) Supraoptic commissure

4. A 44-year-old man presents with a small vascular lesion that affects that area of the midbrain involved in the modulation of pain transmission in the medulla and spinal cord through descending projections. Which of the following structures of the midbrain is most likely involved in this lesion?

- ○ (A) Red nucleus
- ○ (B) Oculomotor nucleus
- ○ (C) Central nucleus of the inferior colliculus
- ○ (D) Periaqueductal gray matter
- ○ (E) Anterior (ventral) trigeminothalamic tract

Questions 5 and 6 are related to the following patient:

A 39-year-old woman with hypertension complains to her family physician that "I can't hear as good as I used to. . . ." She is referred to an audiologist who finds that she is not deaf in either ear, although her perception of sounds, and to a certain extent her ability to localize sound, is altered.

5.   Which of the following midbrain structures is most likely involved in a lesion that would result in the deficits experienced by this patient?

○ (A) Superior colliculus
○ (B) Brachium of the superior colliculus
○ (C) Inferior colliculus
○ (D) Crus cerebri
○ (E) Periaqueductal gray matter

6.   The MRI in this patient reveals a small infarct in the midbrain. Occlusion of branches of which of the following vessels would most likely result in this patient's lesion and deficits?

○ (A) Thalamoperforating artery
○ (B) Medial posterior choroidal artery
○ (C) Superior cerebellar artery
○ (D) Penetrating branches of P_1
○ (E) Quadrigeminal artery

7.   A 52-year-old man presents with a dilated pupil in the left eye. MRI/MRA reveals an aneurysm pressing on the root of the left oculomotor nerve within the subarachnoid space. Which of the following represents the specific fibers damaged by this tumor that would result in the deficits experienced by this patient?

○ (A) GSE
○ (B) GVE preganglionic parasympathetic
○ (C) SVE
○ (D) GVE preganglionic sympathetic
○ (E) GVE postganglionic parasympathetic

8.   A 71-year-old man presents to his neurologist with a tremor that predominately affects his upper extremities. The neurologist concludes that this patient is suffering a neurodegenerative disease that is related to a progressive loss of dopamine-containing cells. The greatest concentration of dopamine-containing cells is found in which of the following midbrain structures?

○ (A) Substantia nigra, pars reticulata
○ (B) Red nucleus
○ (C) Posterior raphe nucleus
○ (D) Substantia nigra, pars lateralis
○ (E) Substantia nigra, pars compacta

9.   Which of the following structures represents the point at which rubrospinal fibers cross the midline of the brainstem?

○ (A) Motor decussation
○ (B) Anterior (ventral) tegmental decussation
○ (C) Decussation of the internal arcuate fibers
○ (D) Posterior (dorsal) tegmental decussation
○ (E) Central tegmental tract

10.   An 82-year-old woman presents with weakness of the upper and lower extremities on the right. MRI reveals a small lesion in the midbrain suggestive of a focal hemorrhage into the substance of the brainstem. Damage to which of the following labeled structures below would most likely result in the deficit seen in this patient? (   )

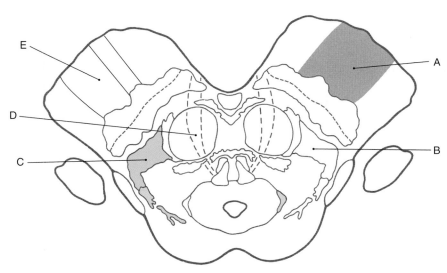

Figure 13–2

11.   A 61-year-old woman is brought to the neurologist's office by her son. She had been complaining of a "funny feeling" on the left side of her body. The neurologic examination reveals a loss of pain and thermal sensation and of discriminative touch and vibratory sense on the left side of her body. Which of the following areas, each representing a lesion, contains tracts or nuclei that, if damaged, would likely give rise to the deficits experienced by this patient? See Figure 13–3. (   )

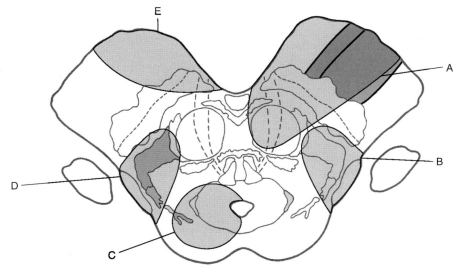

Figure 13–3

Questions 12 to 14 are based on the following patient:

A 74-year-old woman presents to the emergency room with a headache and lethargy. The neurologic examination reveals a paralysis of most movements of the left eye and a profound weakness of the upper and lower extremity on the right side of the body. The left eye will abduct and appears to be in a "down and out" position. The woman has no sensory losses. Her family noted that her symptoms appeared suddenly while watching the evening news.

12. Which of the following midbrain structures is most likely damaged in this patient, to result in the weakness of the extremities?

○ (A) Corticospinal fibers on the right
○ (B) Rubrospinal fibers
○ (C) Corticospinal fibers on the left
○ (D) Rubrospinal fibers on the left
○ (E) Corticonuclear fibers on the left

13. Which of the following midbrain structures is most likely damaged in this patient, to result in the paucity of eye movement?

○ (A) Abducens root fibers
○ (B) Trochlear root fibers
○ (C) Trigeminal nerve in the cavernous sinus
○ (D) Oculomotor root fibers
○ (E) Optic nerve fibers

14. In addition to the deficits described for this patient, a careful neurological examination would most likely reveal which of the following?

○ (A) Dilation of the left pupil
○ (B) Constriction of the left pupil
○ (C) Dilation of the right pupil
○ (D) Constriction of the right pupil
○ (E) Dilation of right and left pupils

15. Which of the following structures is functionally related to the visual and visuomotor systems? (   )

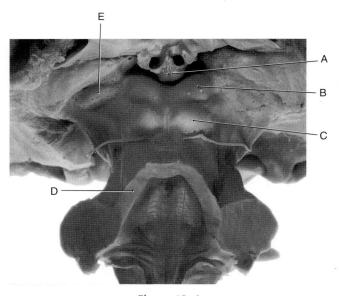

Figure 13–4

16. A 59-year-old woman develops a severe headache associated with complete paralysis of the right upper and lower extremities. MRI reveals a hemorrhagic lesion in the midbrain on the right side that includes the crus cerebri and substantia nigra. Which of the following terms most specifically includes only these two parts of the midbrain?

○ (A) Cerebral peduncle
○ (B) Tegmentum
○ (C) Tectum
○ (D) Basis pedunculi
○ (E) Basal pons

17. A 62-year-old, hypertensive, diabetic man is watching television with his family, suddenly moans, and falls

forward out of his chair and onto the floor. He is unconscious on arrival of the paramedics. After several days in the neuroscience intensive care unit he is comatose with slow respirations, dilated pupils and an electroencephalogram that is characteristic of a sleep state. A lesion in which of the following midbrain structures would most likely explain the depressed level of consciousness experienced by this patient?

○ (A) Substantia nigra
○ (B) Reticular formation
○ (C) Red nucleus
○ (D) Periaqueductal gray matter
○ (E) Tectum

18. A 31-year-old woman with a past diagnosis of multiple sclerosis presents to the emergency department with new onset of paralysis of most movements of the left eye and weakness of her extremities on the right. MRI reveals a vascular lesion in the midbrain. In addition to fibers of the oculomotor nerve and corticospinal fibers, which of the following fibers is most likely involved in this lesion?

○ (A) Medial lemniscus
○ (B) Temporopontine fibers
○ (C) Anterolateral system
○ (D) Parietopontine fibers
○ (E) Frontopontine fibers

19. Which of the following structures of the midbrain is derived from the alar plate?

○ (A) Oculomotor nucleus
○ (B) Crus cerebri
○ (C) Edinger-Westphal nucleus
○ (D) Medial longitudinal fasciculus
○ (E) Inferior colliculus

20. During the routine neurologic examination of a 39-year-old woman the physician discovers that a light shown in the right eye does not elicit a pupillary light reflex in that eye. The patient has no other findings. Which of the following structures is the most likely synaptic center for the pupillary light reflex?

○ (A) Posterior (dorsal) raphe nucleus
○ (B) Cuneiform nucleus
○ (C) Periaqueductal gray matter
○ (D) Pretectal nuclei
○ (E) Interpeduncular nucleus

21. A 67-year-old woman presents with loss of pain and thermal sensation on the right side of the body and loss of vibratory sense and discriminative touch affecting the right lower extremity only. Which of the following labeled areas, each representing a lesion, contains tracts that, if damaged, would most likely give rise to the deficits experienced by this patient? (   )

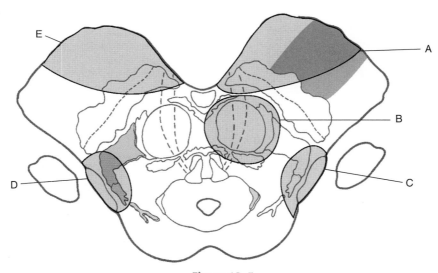

Figure 13–5

22. A 61-year-old homeless man is brought to the emergency department by paramedics after being found stumbling along a highway. He complains of headache and nausea and has an ataxic gait. A blood test reveals that he is not intoxicated. MRI reveals a hemorrhagic lesion in the tegmentum of the midbrain at a cross-sectional level of the inferior colliculus. Which of the following

structures is especially prominent in this part of the midbrain tegmentum?

○ (A) Red nucleus
○ (B) Superior colliculus
○ (C) Decussation of the superior cerebellar peduncle
○ (D) Rubrospinal tract
○ (E) Oculomotor nucleus

23. Which of the following structures of the midbrain contains fibers that convey auditory information?

○ (A) Brachium of the superior colliculus
○ (B) Medial longitudinal fasciculus
○ (C) Central tegmental tract
○ (D) Brachium of the inferior colliculus
○ (E) Medial lemniscus

24. Which of the following structures is most specifically related to the visual system and visuomotor function? (   )

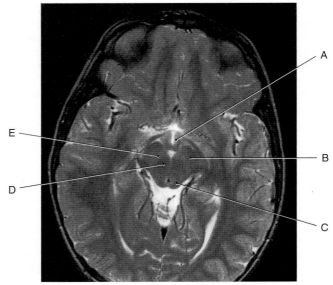

Figure 13–7

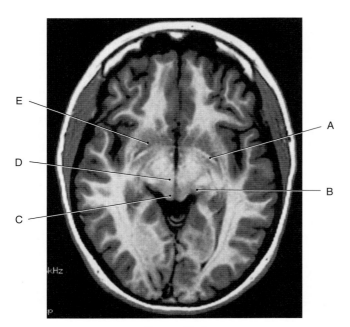

Figure 13–6

25. A 71-year-old man is referred to a neurologist for evaluation of a resting tremor, hunched posture and shuffling gait. The neurologist tells the man's family that he has Parkinson disease. The loss of dopamine-containing cells in this patient would most likely be greatest in which of the following structures? See Figure 13–7. (   )

26. Which of the following structures contains a high level of opiate receptor binding activity indicating an important role in the modulation of pain?

○ (A) Substantia nigra
○ (B) Periaqueductal gray matter
○ (C) Red nucleus
○ (D) Cuneiform nucleus
○ (E) Posterior raphe nucleus

Questions 27 and 28 are based on the following patient:

A 27-year-old man presents to the emergency department after an altercation during which he was stabbed through the left orbit with an ice pick. Remarkably, his vision is unaffected, although he complains "I can't hear right. . . ." The neurologic examination reveals an altered perception of sound, but the patient is not deaf in either ear. He also has a loss of pain and thermal sensation on the right side of his body. CT shows the tip of the ice pick has penetrated the midbrain and caused a small hemorrhage.

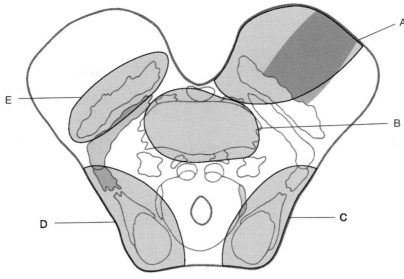

Figure 13–8

27.   Which of the labeled areas, shown above, each representing a lesion, contains the tracts or nuclei that, if damaged, would result in the deficits experienced by this patient? (   )

28.   Assuming the lesion in this patient to be the result of a hemorrhage into the brainstem, which of the following vessels is the most likely source of this hemorrhage?

○ (A) Posterior medial choroidal artery
○ (B) Posterior lateral choroidal artery
○ (C) Penetrating branches of P_1 into the midbrain
○ (D) Thalamoperforating artery
○ (E) Quadrigeminal artery

ANSWERS

1.   **(A)** The deviation of the left eye and dilated (and nonreactive) pupil indicated damage to the left eye. The oculomotor nerve contains GSE fibers to striated extraocular muscles and GVE preganglionic parasympathetic fibers that will terminate in the ciliary ganglion. An aneurysm just distal to the optic chiasm would impinge on the root of the oculomotor nerve.
FN2e 189, 195

2.   **(B)** The quadrigeminal (superior) cistern is located posterior to the superior and inferior colliculi (hence its name). It contains the great cerebral vein (vein of Galen), some branches of the posterior cerebral artery, and the exit of the trochlear. Tumors in this area, in addition to involving the trochlear root, may compress the colliculi and obstruct the cerebral aqueduct.
FN2e 189

3.   **(C)** Fibers in the optic tract traverse the brachium of the superior colliculus (located in the groove between the pulvinar and medial geniculate body) to reach the pretectal nuclei. These nuclei are located laterally adjacent to the posterior commissure at the general area of the midbrain-diencephalon junction.
FN2e 189, 195–196

4.   **(D)** The periaqueductal gray matter receives spinal input via the anterolateral system and projects to the nucleus raphe magnus located in the rostral medulla and pons-medulla junction. This nucleus, in turn, projects to the spinal trigeminal nucleus and the posterior horn of the spinal cord, where, through inhibitory interneurons, it presynaptically inhibits primary sensory fibers conveying pain and thermal sensations.
FN2e 191

5.   **(C)** The nuclei of the inferior colliculi receive ascending auditory information from the lateral lemniscus and project to the medial geniculate nucleus of the diencephalon via the brachium of the inferior colliculus. There is a tonotopic map in the inferior colliculus.
FN2e 191

6.   **(E)** The quadrigeminal artery is usually a branch of P_1, although it may be a branch of proximal P_2. This vessel is a major source of blood supply to the superior and inferior colliculi. The medial posterior choroidal artery may send a few small branches into the vicinity of the superior colliculus, and the superior cerebellar artery may send small branches into the area of the inferior colliculus. However, these vessels are not the main source of blood supply to the colliculi.
FN2e 126, 197–198

7.   **(B)** Preganglionic GVE parasympathetic fibers arise in the nucleus of Edinger-Westphal, course through the oculomotor nerve close to the surface (hence their

susceptibility to compression by external lesions), and terminate on postganglionic cell bodies of the ciliary ganglion. A mass in the subarachnoid space compressing the oculomotor nerve would affect the preganglionic fibers between the nucleus and the ciliary ganglion.
FN2e 195

8.   **(E)** The dopamine-containing cells of the compact part of the substantia nigra project to the caudate nucleus and putamen, as nigrostriatal fibers. A progressive loss of these nigral neurons and their terminals in the neostriatum (caudate + putamen) results in findings characteristic of Parkinson disease.
FN2e 197

9.   **(B)** Rubrospinal fibers originate in the red nucleus, cross the midline of the midbrain in the anterior (ventral) tegmental decussation, and descend as the rubrospinal tract to terminate in primarily cervical levels of the spinal cord.
FN2e 196

10.   **(A)** Corticospinal fibers in the crus cerebri on the patient's left side originate from the somatomotor cortex of the left cerebral hemisphere, descend through the brainstem, cross in the motor (pyramidal) decussation, and form the lateral corticospinal tract on the right side. These fibers innervate motor neurons on the right side of the spinal cord.
FN2e 191, 193–195

11.   **(D)** Pain and thermal sensations from the left side of the body are conveyed by fibers in the anterolateral system on the right side of the brainstem. These fibers originate in the posterior horn on the left side and cross in the anterior white commissure. Discriminative touch and vibratory sense are conveyed in fibers that originate from the left side of the body, ascend in the posterior columns, synapse in the posterior column nuclei, and cross the midline to form the contralateral (right) medial lemniscus. Consequently, a lesion in the midbrain on the patient's right will result in a loss of these sensations on the left side of the patient's body.
FN2e 191, 193, 197

12.   **(C)** Corticospinal fibers originate in the somatomotor cortex and descend through the brainstem (including the crus cerebri) on the left to cross the midline in the motor (pyramidal) decussation. Consequently, a lesion in the left crus cerebri (containing corticospinal fibers) results in weakness on the right.
FN2e 191, 193–195

13.   **(D)** The eye movements that are intact, abduction and looking down and out, indicate that the abducens and trochlear nerves are not damaged. Because the remaining eye movements are controlled by means of the oculomotor nerve, this lesion includes the exiting root of the oculomotor nerve.
FN2e 189, 195

14.   **(A)** A lesion of the root of the oculomotor nerve will also damage the GVE preganglionic parasympathetic fibers in this nerve. Damage to these fibers will result in dilation of the ipsilateral pupil owing to the unopposed action of the sympathetic postganglionic fibers.
FN2e 195

15.   **(B)** The superficial layers of the superior colliculus receive input from the retina and visual cortex. The deeper layers of the superior colliculus project to motor areas, some of which subserve gaze changes.
FN2e 189, 195

16.   **(D)** The substantia nigra and the crus cerebri collectively form the basis pedunculi of the midbrain.
FN2e 191–191, 193

17.   **(B)** The differential diagnosis of coma includes structural, metabolic, and psychogenic causes. Anatomically, a sudden lesion resulting in coma is clinically localizable to one of three brain regions: first, bilateral destruction of large cortical areas; second, the diencephalon; third, the ascending reticular activating system. The midbrain reticular formation contains the cuneiform and subcuneiform nuclei. This area of the midbrain receives input from lower levels of the neuraxis and projects to thalamic and hypothalamic centers that participate in maintaining an alert wakeful state. The midbrain part of the reticular formation is a portion of the reticular activating system.
FN2e 197

18.   **(E)** A vascular lesion in anteromedial medial areas of the midbrain involves the exiting roots of the oculomotor nerve, the corticospinal fibers located in the middle third of the crus cerebri, and the frontopontine fibers located in the medial third of the crus cerebri.
FN2e 193–195, 197–198

19.   **(E)** The alar plate of the developing midbrain gives rise to the superior and inferior colliculi. Some alar plate neuroblasts also migrate into anterior regions to form the red nucleus and substantia nigra.
FN2e 188

20.   **(D)** The pretectal nuclei are a collection of small nuclei located at the midbrain-diencephalon junction just rostral to the tectum (hence their name "pretectal") just lateral to the posterior commissure. This synaptic center receives input from the optic tract by means of the brachium of the superior colliculus and projects bilaterally to the Edinger-Westphal nucleus.
FN2e 195–196

21.   **(C)** Pain and thermal sensations from the body are conveyed by fibers in the anterolateral system; in the midbrain the anterolateral system on the left contains information from the right side of the body. Proprioceptive information from the right lower extremity is conveyed in lateral portions of the medial lemniscus adjacent to the anterolateral system. The upper extremity is represented in the medial portion of the medial lemniscus.
FN2e 191, 193

22.   **(C)** The tegmental area of the caudal midbrain is occupied by the decussating fibers of the superior cerebellar peduncle (brachium conjunctivum). Damage to these fibers will result in an ataxic gait.
FN2e 191–193

23.   **(D)** The brachium of the inferior colliculus is located on the lateral aspect of the midbrain and extends from the inferior colliculus to the medial geniculate

nucleus of the diencephalon. Auditory input to the inferior colliculus arrives by means of the lateral lemniscus and is relayed to the medial geniculate and, from here, to the auditory cortex in the temporal lobe.
FN2e 191

24.   **(C)** The superior colliculus receives input from the retina and visual cortex and projects to brainstem and spinal motor centers, including those that subserve eye movement.
FN2e 195

25.   **(E)** The loss of dopamine-containing cells, and their nigrostriatal terminals in the caudate and putamen, is characteristic of Parkinson disease. These cells are most concentrated in the pars compacta of the substantia nigra.
FN2e 197

26.   **(B)** The periaqueductal gray matter receives ascending inputs by means of the anterolateral system and sends descending projections to the nucleus raphe magnus. This nucleus, in turn, projects to the spinal trigeminal nucleus and to the posterior horn of the spinal cord where, through interneurons, these descending raphe fibers presynaptically inhibit primary sensory fibers.
FN2e 191

27.   **(C)** The inferior colliculus is an important relay center in the midbrain for auditory information. The lateral lemniscus conveys auditory signals from brainstem nuclei located on both sides to the inferior colliculus, which, in turn, projects to the medial geniculate nucleus. The anterolateral system is located adjacent to the lateral lemniscus. This tract conveys pain and thermal information from the contralateral side of the body; a right-sided loss is indicative of a lesion on the patient's left side.
FN2e 191–193

28.   **(E)** The primary blood supply to the superior and inferior colliculi is through branches of the quadrigeminal artery, which is usually a branch of P_1. Branches of the quadrigeminal also penetrate the lateral aspect of the midbrain to serve the area in which the anterolateral system is located.
FN2e 191–198

CHAPTER 14

A Synopsis of Cranial Nerves of the Brainstem

Questions 1 to 3 are based on the following patient:

A 26-year-old man is brought to the emergency department after a motorcycle collision. The neurologic examination reveals a confused, combative patient who is deaf in the right ear. He also has paralysis of facial muscles on the right, and, when he talks, he slurs his words. Suspecting a head injury, the physician orders CT, which reveals a basilar skull fracture that extends through a foramen. There is also a collection of blood in the immediate vicinity of the foramen.

1. The weakness of facial muscles on this patient would most likely suggest damage to the facial nerve. Which of the following deficits is also most likely being experienced by this patient?

- ○ (A) Loss of taste from the left side of the tongue
- ○ (B) Loss of sensation from the lining of the oral cavity
- ○ (C) Inability to chew
- ○ (D) Loss of the blink in response to corneal stimulation on the right (efferent limb of corneal reflex)
- ○ (E) Loss of the motor response to a gentle tap on the mandible (efferent limb of the jerk reflex)

2. The CT reveals a fracture of the petrous portion of the temporal bone. This fracture likely traverses which of the following foramina?

- ○ (A) Jugular foramen
- ○ (B) Foramen lacerum
- ○ (C) Internal acoustic meatus
- ○ (D) Foramen spinosum
- ○ (E) Hypoglossal canal

3. The neuroradiologist believes that the blood at the level of this fracture is caused by damage to a venous sinus. Which of the following sinuses is located closest to the exiting roots of the facial and vestibulocochlear nerves?

- ○ (A) Inferior petrosal sinus
- ○ (B) Superior petrosal sinus
- ○ (C) Sigmoid sinus
- ○ (D) Cavernous sinus
- ○ (E) Transverse sinus

4. The attending neonatologist notices within a few hours of birth that a male newborn is not able to move his facial muscles or suckle effectively. This newborn's cry is not appropriately loud, suggesting a weakness of the vocalis muscle. The physician suspects that the muscles

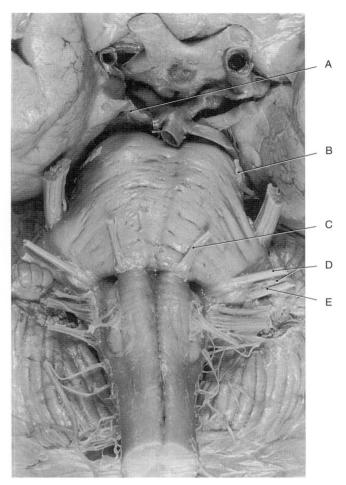

Figure 14–1

derived from the pharyngeal arches have failed to develop properly. Which of the cranial nerves above, contains special visceral efferent motor fibers that innervate muscles arising from a pharyngeal arch? (   )

5.   A 37-year-old woman presents with a lesion of the root of the hypoglossal nerve. The neurologist asks the patient to "stick your tongue out" (actually the muscles that protrude the tongue "pull" it out of the mouth) and it deviates to the left. Paralysis of which of the following muscles would most likely explain this deviation of the tongue?

○ (A) Styloglossus
○ (B) Genioglossus
○ (C) Intrinsic tongue musculature
○ (D) Hypoglossus
○ (E) Palatoglossus

6.   A 33-year-old woman is brought to the emergency department after striking her head during a fall at an ice skating rink. The neurologic examination reveals difficulty opening and closing the mouth. The jaw deviates to the right on closing, and there is a sensory loss over

the mandibular part of the face. Which of the following represents the most likely location of the lesion in this patient?

○ (A) Stylomastoid foramen
○ (B) Orbital fissure
○ (C) Foramen rotundum
○ (D) Foramen ovale
○ (E) Internal acoustic meatus

7.   A 17-year-old girl is having a neurologic examination as part of the process to be certified to play senior soccer. The physician notices that her jaw-jerk reflex is absent. Which of the following contains the motor neurons that form the efferent (motor) limb of this reflex?

○ (A) Facial motor nucleus
○ (B) Spinal trigeminal nucleus
○ (C) Trigeminal motor nucleus
○ (D) Hypoglossal nucleus
○ (E) Dorsal motor nucleus of the vagus

8.   A 21-year-old man presents with peripheral neuropathy of unknown origin. Among the various deficits seen in this patient is the absence of the corneal reflex. Which

of the following structures contains the motor cell bodies whose axons form the efferent limb of this reflex?

- ○ (A) Hypoglossal nucleus
- ○ (B) Trigeminal motor nucleus
- ○ (C) Oculomotor nucleus
- ○ (D) Trochlear nucleus
- ○ (E) Facial motor nucleus

9. Which of the following structures is the source of GVE preganglionic parasympathetic fibers to the otic ganglion?

- ○ (A) Edinger-Westphal nucleus
- ○ (B) Superior salivatory nucleus
- ○ (C) Inferior salivatory nucleus
- ○ (D) Dorsal motor nucleus of the vagus
- ○ (E) Nucleus ambiguus

10. A 71-year-old man presents with inability to abduct his right eye and has a weakness of facial muscles on the same side of his face. MRI reveals a small infarction in the brainstem. Which of the following labeled areas, each representing a lesion, contains structures that, if damaged, would most likely result in the deficits seen in this patient? (   )

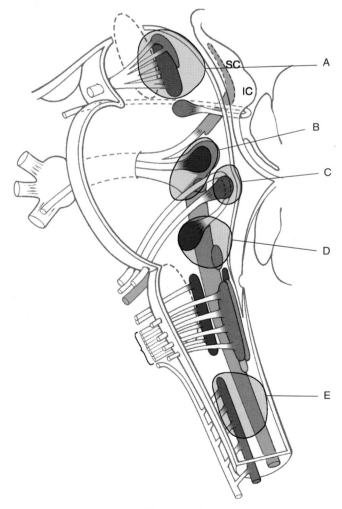

Figure 14–2

11. A 57-year-old woman presents with deviation of the tongue to the right on attempted protrusion and weakness of her left upper and lower extremities. MRI reveals a tumor, probably a meningioma, pressing on the surface of the brainstem. Which of the following labeled areas, each representing the location of a potential lesion, is the most likely site of maximal compression of the brainstem by this tumor? (   )

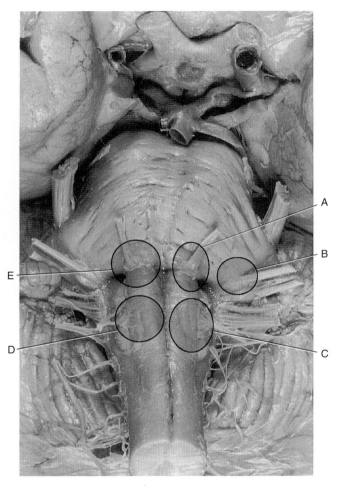

Figure 14–3

12. A 29-year-old man complains to his family physician of dizziness and diminished hearing in his left ear. He notes that the dizziness makes him nauseated almost all of the time and that his symptoms are getting worse. MRI reveals a tumor around the root of the vestibulocochlear nerve, which is filling the internal acoustic meatus. Based on the location of this tumor, which of the following additional deficits might this patient experience?

- ○ (A) Weakness of facial muscles on the right
- ○ (B) Weakness of masticatory muscles on the right
- ○ (C) Weakness of masticatory muscles on the left
- ○ (D) Weakness of facial muscles on the left
- ○ (E) Weakness in vocal muscles

13.   A 47-year-old woman presents with diplopia. The neurologic examination reveals normal vision, although her left eye is deviated slightly inward and will not abduct on attempted gaze to the left. There are no other findings. Which of the following is the most likely location of this lesion in this patient?

○ (A) Abducens root on the left
○ (B) Abducens nucleus on the left
○ (C) Abducens root within the basilar pons at caudal level on the left
○ (D) Abducens root within the basilar pons at caudal level on the right
○ (E) Abducens root on the right

14.   A 12-year-old girl presents with diplopia and signs of increased intracranial pressure. Although she can see objects clearly, she has difficulty with eye movements. On attempted gaze to the right, the right eye will not abduct and the left eye will not adduct. On attempted gaze to the left, the left eye will abduct and the right eye will adduct. Based on these observations, which of the following represents the most likely location of the lesion in this patient?

○ (A) Abducens nucleus on the left
○ (B) Abducens root on the left
○ (C) Abducens nucleus on the right

○ (D) Abducens root on the right
○ (E) Oculomotor nerve on the right

15.   A 24-year-old woman presents with waxing and waning neurologic findings that localize to multiple functional systems at different levels of the neuraxis. MRI reveals multiple lesions in the brain and spinal cord; a presumptive diagnosis of multiple sclerosis is made. The examining physician notes that on attempted gaze to the left the right eye will not adduct but on attempted gaze to the right the left eye will adduct. All other eye movements appear normal. Based on these observations, which of the following represents the most likely location of the lesion in this patient?

○ (A) Abducens nucleus on the right
○ (B) Medial longitudinal fasciculus on the right
○ (C) Abducens nucleus on the left
○ (D) Medial longitudinal fasciculus on the left
○ (E) Oculomotor nerve on the right

16.   Which of the following cranial nerves innervate muscles that originate from the first pharyngeal arch?
(   )

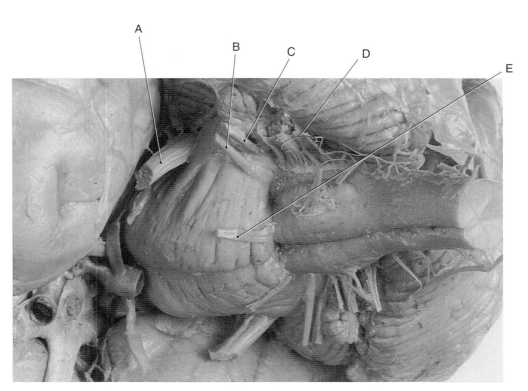

Figure 14–4

17. A 38-year-old woman complains to her family physician about intermittent pain on her face. She wonders if it might be coming from her maxillary teeth because the pain is especially acute when she attempts to brush her teeth or to put on makeup. In fact, the pain is easily triggered by anything touching the corner of her mouth. A complete neurologic examination and MRI reveals no organic disease or lesion. It is likely that this patient is suffering from which of the following?

○ (A) Bell palsy
○ (B) Wallenberg syndrome
○ (C) Central seven lesion
○ (D) Glossopharyngeal neuralgia
○ (E) Trigeminal neuralgia

18. A 43-year-old man presents with deviation of his jaw to the left, on attempted closure, and numbness over the mandibular part of his face. A contrast medium–enhanced MRI reveals a skull base tumor invading a foramen at the base of the skull. Which of the following labeled areas, each representing a lesion of cranial nerve roots, is the most likely site of this tumor? (   )

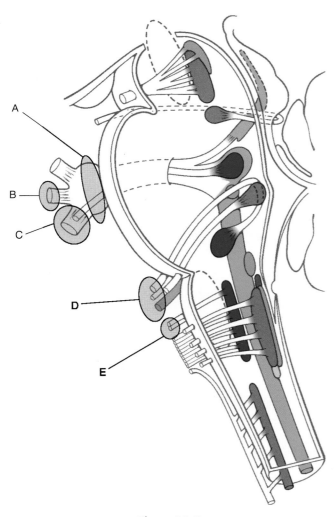

Figure 14–5

Questions 19 through 22 are based on the following patient:

A 47-year-old farmer was working on the roof of his chicken house and fell, striking his head on a concrete walk. He is brought to the emergency department unconscious. The emergency department physician orders a CT, which reveals blood in the subarachnoid space of the posterior fossa and a fracture extending through an opening in the base of the skull. On examination about 6 hours later, the patient has become lucid. He is unable to elevate the right shoulder or to turn his head to the left against resistance. The gag reflex is absent.

19. The inability to elevate the right shoulder or to look to the left against resistance most likely indicates damage to which of the following cranial nerves?

○ (A) Vagus (X)
○ (B) Glossopharyngeal (IX)
○ (C) Accessory (spinal accessory) (XI)
○ (D) Facial (VII)
○ (E) Trigeminal (V)

20. The lack of the gag reflex may result from damage to its sensory limb. Which of the following cranial nerves conveys the fibers comprising the sensory limb of the gag reflex?

○ (A) Glossopharyngeal (IX)
○ (B) Vagus (X)
○ (C) Accessory (spinal accessory) (XI)
○ (D) Facial (VII)
○ (E) Trigeminal (V)

21. Based on the deficits experienced by this patient, the basilar skull fracture has most likely damaged cranial nerves located in which of the following openings in the skull?

○ (A) Internal acoustic meatus
○ (B) Hypoglossal canal
○ (C) Orbital fissure
○ (D) Condylar canal
○ (E) Jugular foramen

22. The blood in the subarachnoid space of the posterior fossa may be the result of a tear in a venous structure. Which of the following venous structures, if damaged in the immediate area of the jugular foramen, would most likely result in blood within the subarachnoid space?

○ (A) Superior petrosal sinus
○ (B) Transverse sinus
○ (C) Inferior sagittal sinus
○ (D) Sigmoid sinus
○ (E) Confluence of sinuses

23. Branches of the recurrent laryngeal nerves serve the vocalis muscles. Which of the following brainstem nuclei

contain neuron cell bodies whose axons innervate these muscles?

○ (A) Dorsal motor nucleus of the vagus
○ (B) Accessory (spinal accessory) nucleus
○ (C) Trigeminal motor nucleus
○ (D) Nucleus ambiguus
○ (E) Superior and inferior salivatory nuclei

24. A healthy 61-year-old man develops diplopia. The neurologic examination reveals that the left eye can look down and laterally but not up or medially. MRI reveals a lesion in the brainstem. Damage to which of the following labeled areas, each representing the potential site of a lesion, would explain the findings in this patient? (   )

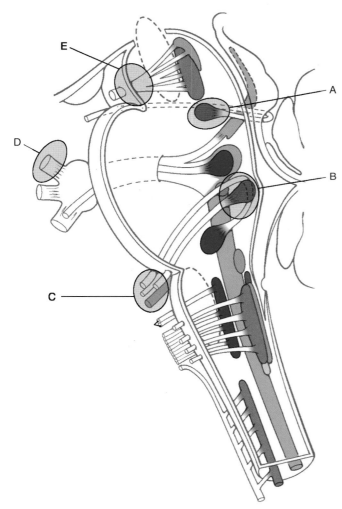

Figure 14–6

25. During the routine neurologic examination of a 29-year-old woman, the physician notices that her left pupil does not react when he flashes a light in her eye. In fact, her left pupil is larger than the right. The patient appears in good health and has no other findings. In the absence of further information, which of the following might explain this deficit in this patient?

○ (A) The patient has diabetes.
○ (B) The patient has hypertension.
○ (C) The patient has subarachnoid hemorrhage.
○ (D) The patient has a mass compressing the root of the oculomotor nerve.
○ (E) The patient has meningitis.

26. Cortical control of eye movement is mediated through relay nuclei located in the brainstem; the cerebral cortex does not project directly to brainstem nuclei controlling eye movement. Which of the following nuclei receive eye movement signals from the rostral interstitial nucleus of the medial longitudinal fasciculus (also called the vertical gaze center)?

○ (A) Abducens and trochlear nuclei
○ (B) Abducens nucleus only
○ (C) Trochlear nucleus only
○ (D) Oculomotor nucleus only
○ (E) Trochlear and oculomotor nuclei

Questions 27 through 29 are based on the following patient:

A 47-year-old woman is brought to the emergency department after a motorcycle collision. She is unconscious and has multiple soft tissue injuries to the head and face and a broken femur. CT reveals a skull fracture that passes through the superior orbital fissure. After she regains consciousness, a neurologic examination suggests that all structures traversing the superior orbital fissure are damaged.

27. Based on the extent and location of the injury, which of the following is the most obvious sensory deficit seen in this patient on the side of the skull fracture?

○ (A) Loss of pain and thermal sensations in the maxillary area of the face
○ (B) Loss of taste sensation over the anterior two thirds of the tongue
○ (C) Blindness in one eye
○ (D) Loss of pain and thermal sensation on the forehead
○ (E) Loss of pain sensations from the mandibular teeth

28. Recognizing the location of this skull fracture, which of the following represents the most obvious somatomotor deficit seen in this patient on the side of the lesion?

○ (A) Paralysis of muscles of mastication
○ (B) Paralysis of muscles of facial expression
○ (C) Paralysis of gaze laterally and inferiorly
○ (D) Paralysis of gaze medially and superiorly
○ (E) Paralysis of all eye movement

29. In addition to characteristic deficits of eye movement, which of the following visceromotor signs is seen in this patient on the injured side?

○ (A) Constriction of the pupil
○ (B) Dilation of the pupil
○ (C) Excessive salivation
○ (D) Excessive sweating
○ (E) Lack of salivation

30.   A lesion of which of the following motor nuclei will result in paralysis of a skeletal (striated) muscle or muscles on the opposite side of the midline? (   )

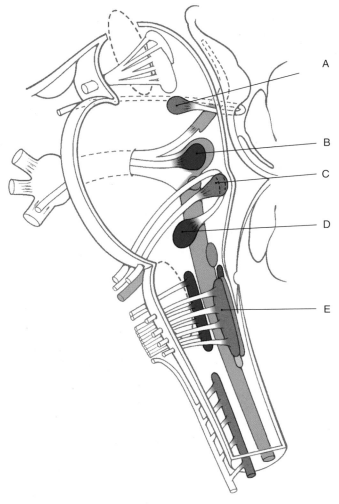

A

B

C

D

E

Figure 14–7

31.   A 38-year-old man presents to an otolaryngologist for evaluation of throat pain. He describes sudden attacks of lancinating pain that seem to coincide with swallowing with, or without, food or drink. A thorough evaluation, which includes MRI, reveals no obvious pathologic process in the throat or neck. The physician suspects that this patient is suffering from what?

○ (A) Wallenberg syndrome
○ (B) Alternating hemianesthesia
○ (C) Trigeminal neuralgia
○ (D) Glossopharyngeal neuralgia
○ (E) Polyps of the vocal folds

ANSWERS

1. **(D)** The motor nucleus of the facial nerve receives collaterals of ascending trigeminothalamic fibers and, in turn, sends axons to innervate the facial muscles around the orbit. Stimulation of the right cornea results in a blinking response, primarily of the right eye. The lesion in this patient interrupts the efferent (motor) limb of the corneal reflex.
FN2e 211–212

2. **(C)** The paralysis of facial muscles and the deafness, both on the same side, indicate a skull fracture traversing the internal acoustic meatus. In addition to the facial and vestibulocochlear nerves, this foramen also contains the labyrinthine artery.
FN2e 210–212

3. **(B)** The superior petrosal sinus lies along the upper edge of the petrous part of the temporal bone immediately above the internal acoustic meatus. In this position, it is the closest sinus to this foramen.
FN2e 131–132, 210–212

4. **(D)** The facial nerve (CN VII) contains SVE fibers that innervate the muscles of facial expression; these arise from mesenchyme of the second pharyngeal arch. The other cranial nerves that contain fibers with SVE functional components are cranial nerves V, IX, and X.
FN2e 200–201

5. **(B)** The genioglossus muscle has its origin from the inner surface of the mandible adjacent to the midline. The fibers of this muscle fan out slightly as they insert into the base of the tongue. Consequently, as these muscles contract, the tongue is pulled out of the mouth. Weakness on one side will result in deviation of the tongue to the weak side when protruded.
FN2e 202–204, 396–399

6. **(D)** The difficulty chewing, the deviation of the jaw, and the sensory loss over the mandibular area of the face is indicative of a lesion of the mandibular portion of the trigeminal (V) nerve. The motor fibers of V and the sensory fibers serving the mandibular teeth, skin over the mandible, and lining of the oral cavity pass through the foramen ovale. The deviation of the jaw is due to the action of pterygoid muscles on the intact side.
FN2e 214–215

7. **(C)** The efferent limb of jaw-jerk reflex originates from SVE cells of the trigeminal motor nucleus. The afferent limb arises from muscle spindles in the muscles of mastication, enters the brain on V_3, and has its cell bodies in the mesencephalic nucleus; the central processes of these fibers distribute bilaterally to the trigeminal motor nucleus.
FN2e 215

8. **(E)** Sensory fibers from the cornea enter the spinal trigeminal tract and terminate on cells of the medially adjacent spinal trigeminal nucleus. Second-order neurons from the spinal trigeminal nucleus send their axons across the midline to form the anterior (ventral) trigeminotha-

lamic tract. As these fibers ascend, they send collaterals to the facial motor nucleus.
FN2e 215

9. **(C)** The optic ganglion receives GVE preganglionic axons from the inferior salivatory nucleus. In turn, the neurons of the otic ganglion send postganglionic axons to the parotid gland. This central nucleus and peripheral fibers are associated with the glossopharyngeal nerve (cranial nerve IX).
FN2e 207–208

10. **(C)** The deficits in this patient result from damage to fibers of the facial nerve that innervate the facial muscles and to either the nucleus or root of the abducens nerve. Both of these structures are together in the floor of the fourth ventricle internal to the facial colliculus. Although injury to the abducens nucleus may also result in internuclear ophthalmoplegia, this is not seen in this patient.
FN2e 201, 210–213

11. **(D)** The deviation of the patient's tongue to the right accompanied by the weakness on the left side of the body places this tumor on the right side of the medulla. The deviation of the tongue is the best localizing sign in this patient. This tumor is compromising the exiting roots of the hypoglossal nerve and the corticospinal fibers in the pyramid.
FN2e 202–204

12. **(D)** A tumor located in the internal auditory meatus will potentially damage not only the root of the vestibulocochlear nerve but also the root of the facial nerve, which enters the same foramen. The most notable symptom experienced by this patient would be a facial weakness followed, possibly, by a partial loss of taste. The labyrinthine artery also passes through this foramen; compression of this vessel may also contribute to deafness in that ear.
FN2e 208–210

13. **(A)** The only complaint this patient has is diplopia resulting from a lesion of the abducens root; the left lateral rectus muscle is paralyzed. A lesion of the root of the abducens nerve results in a flaccid paralysis of this muscle on the same side; this is a good localizing sign.
FN2e 212–213

14. **(C)** The right abducens nucleus contains motor neurons that project to the lateral rectus muscle on that side and interneurons that project, via the medial longitudinal fasciculus, to motor neurons in the contralateral (left) oculomotor nucleus that innervate the medial rectus muscle on that side. Consequently, a lesion of the right abducens nucleus will result in a paralysis of the right lateral rectus muscle and an inability of the left medial rectus to contract on attempted gaze to the right.
FN2e 212–213

15. **(B)** The failure of the right medial rectus muscle to adduct the right eye on attempted gaze to the left indicates damage to interneurons of the abducens nucleus. These interneurons leave the nucleus, cross the midline, and ascend in the medial longitudinal fasciculus (MLF) to synapse on oculomotor neurons innervating the medial rectus muscle. Because the axons of these interneurons cross very close to their origin (in this case interneurons in the left abducens send axons into the right MLF), the lesion is on the right side.
FN2e 212–213

16. **(A)** The muscles of mastication arise from mesenchyme of the first pharyngeal arch and are innervated by SVE motor neurons located in the trigeminal motor nucleus. Muscles innervated by SVE motor neurons located in cranial nerves VII, IX, and X arise from pharyngeal arches 2, 3, and 4, respectively.
FN2e 200–201

17. **(E)** Idiopathic pain originating from the distribution of the peripheral branches of the trigeminal nerve is tic douloureux or trigeminal neuralgia. This pain can be severe and disabling and originates most frequently from the maxillary region of the face. While the causes of trigeminal neuralgia are unknown, this condition is seen in patients with a variety of neurologic conditions and may be related to small aberrant vascular loops compressing the root of the trigeminal nerve.
FN2e 215

18. **(C)** The maxillary division of the trigeminal nerve (V₃) and the motor root of the trigeminal nerve transverse the foramen ovale. A lesion of the ganglion of V plus the motor root of V (A) would also result in motor and sensory deficits. However, the sensory losses would be over the entire ipsilateral side of the face, not just the mandibular division.
FN2e 213–215

19. **(C)** The accessory nerve innervates the ipsilateral trapezius and sternocleidomastoid muscles. The inability to elevate the shoulder on the right indicates that the right accessory nerve is damaged. The sternocleidomastoid muscle turns the head to the opposite side when it contracts. Consequently, a paralysis of the right sternocleidomastoid muscle would result in an inability to turn the head to the left.
FN2e 205–206, 208

20. **(A)** The afferent limb of the gag reflex is conveyed by the glossopharyngeal nerve. Cell bodies of the afferent limb are in the sensory ganglia of IX, and the motor cell bodies are located in the nucleus ambiguus. The stylopharyngeus muscle originates from the third pharyngeal arch and is, therefore, innervated by SVE motor neurons.
FN2e 207–208

21. **(E)** The basilar skull fracture in this patient has transversed the jugular foramen and damaged the roots of the glossopharyngeal and accessory nerves. The vagus nerve as well as several vascular structures also pass through this space.
FN2e 205, 207–208

22. **(D)** The sigmoid sinus is continuous with the internal jugular vein at the jugular foramen. In addition, the inferior petrosal sinus empties into the internal jugular vein via the jugular foramen.
FN2e 205, 208

23. **(D)** The nucleus ambiguus provides motor innervation to muscles that originate from the third and fourth pharyngeal arches. The functional component of these fibers is SVE. The recurrent laryngeal nerves are branches of the vagus nerve that contain fibers that innervate the vocalis muscles.
FN2e 206–207

24. **(E)** The fact that the patient can rotate his left eye down and out indicates that the trochlear nerve and the abducens nerve are intact. The failure of movement in other directions indicates a lesion involving the oculomotor nerve. Because this lesion involves the nerve root, it is likely that the pupil of the affected eye would also be dilated.
FN2e 216–217

25. **(D)** In general, the GVE preganglionic parasympathetic axons in the oculomotor nerve travel at the surface of the nerve. Pressure on the nerve (as in a tumor or aneurysm) may compromise these fibers (nonreactive pupil) without affecting the larger diameter fibers innervating the extraocular muscles.
FN2e 216–217

26. **(E)** The frontal eye field, that part of the frontal lobe located in caudal parts of the middle frontal gyrus immediately rostral to the precentral gyrus, projects to the riMLF. In turn, this center projects to the oculomotor and trochlear nuclei. Cortical lesions in this part of the frontal lobe may result in conjugate deviation of the eyes toward the side of the lesion.
FN2e 215–217

27. **(D)** The ophthalmic branch of the trigeminal nerve traverses the superior orbital fissure. Damage to this nerve at the level of the superior orbital fissure will result in a loss of thermal and pain sensations and crude touch over the forehead and up to about the vertex of the skull and over the eyebrow and upper eyelid.
FN2e 213–215

28. **(E)** This patient will experience paralysis of all eye movement on the side of the injury because cranial nerves III, IV, and VI all enter the orbit via the superior orbital fissure. Because all structures traversing this fissure are damaged, there is a total loss of eye movement on this side.
FN2e 212–217

29. **(B)** The lesion to the root of the oculomotor nerve will also damage the GVE preganglionic parasympathetic fibers of the oculomotor nerve. Consequently, the pupil will be dilated, owing to the unopposed action of the sympathetic input to the iris.
FN2e 212, 216–217

30. **(A)** The trochlear nucleus is the only cranial motor nucleus in the brainstem to exclusively innervate a muscle on the contralateral side. Axons arise from the motor cells in the nucleus, arch around the periaqueductal gray matter, decussate just caudal to the inferior colliculus, and then exit the brainstem to innervate the superior oblique muscle. Consequently, a lesion of the trochlear nucleus results in paralysis of the contralateral superior oblique muscle.
FN2e 215–216

31. **(D)** Glossopharyngeal neuralgia is a sudden severe pain originating from the distribution of the cranial nerve IX. It may be initiated by any stimulus to the back of the oral cavity, including touch, chewing, talking, or swallowing.
FN2e 208

CHAPTER 15

The Diencephalon

1.   A 29-year-old woman presents with confusion. MRI reveals an enlarged right lateral ventricle resulting from a nickel-sized tumor located in the right interventricular foramen. Based on its location, this tumor is most likely to be impinging on which of the following diencephalic structures?

○ (A) Pulvinar
○ (B) Dorsomedial nucleus
○ (C) Anterior nucleus
○ (D) Ventral lateral nucleus
○ (E) Ventral anterior nucleus

Questions 2 and 3 are based on the following patient:

A 72-year-old man is brought to the emergency department by his wife. He is confused and complains of a severe headache. The neurologic examination reveals loss of the temporal visual field in the left eye and of the nasal visual field in the right eye (homonymous hemianopia) and some difficulty in localizing sound, but he is not deaf. This patient does not have motor or sensory deficits indicative of damage to long tracts, and he has no trouble walking.

2.   Based on the deficits experienced by this patient, which of the following thalamic nuclei is most likely involved in this lesion?

○ (A) Centromedian and ventral posterolateral
○ (B) Anterior and ventral anterior
○ (C) Ventral posteromedial and ventral posterolateral
○ (D) Pulvinar
○ (E) Lateral and medial geniculate

3.   The MRI of this patient reveals a lesion resulting from vascular occlusion. Which of the following vessels is most likely occluded in this patient?

○ (A) Thalamoperforating artery
○ (B) Thalamogeniculate artery
○ (C) Medial striate artery

○ (D) Medial posterior choroidal artery
○ (E) Anterior choroidal artery

4.   A 49-year-old morbidly obese man with uncontrolled diabetes presents to the emergency department complaining of headache and feeling nauseated. The examination reveals a stuporous patient with involuntary forceful movements of his left upper extremity. MRI reveals a small diencephalic infarct. Which of the following thalamic nuclei is most likely involved in a lesion that results in the deficits experienced by this patient?

○ (A) Ventral posterolateral
○ (B) Ventral lateral
○ (C) Subthalamic
○ (D) Ventral anterior
○ (E) Ventral posteromedial

5.   A 69-year-old woman presents to the emergency department complaining of severe headache and frequent vomiting. The neurologic examination reveals normal cranial nerve function but motor deficits on the left side of the body. MRI reveals a lesion in the ventral lateral thalamic nucleus. Which of the following areas is the most likely site of this lesion? (   )

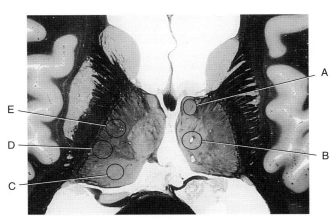

Figure 15–1

6. A 73-year-old woman presents to the emergency department with severe headache and lethargy. The examination reveals motor deficits that suggest a disconnection between the ventral lateral nucleus of the thalamus and its cortical target. Which of the following areas of the cortex receives input from the caudal part of the ventral lateral nucleus of the thalamus? (   )

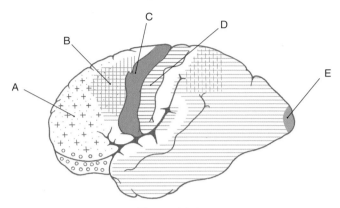

Figure 15–2

7. The MRI of a 57-year-old woman reveals diffuse degenerative changes throughout the cingulate gyrus. Which of the following thalamic nuclei project most specifically to the cingulate gyrus? (   )

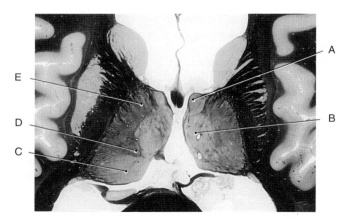

Figure 15–3

8. The circumventricular organs are specialized areas in the perimeter of the third ventricle that contain fenestrated capillaries. Which of the following structures represent a circumventricular organ?

○ (A) Habenula
○ (B) Infundibulum
○ (C) Massa intermedia
○ (D) Subcommissural organ
○ (E) Anterior thalamic nucleus

9. A 60-year-old man has a sudden severe headache and passes out. The examination at the emergency depart-

ment reveals sudden unexpected rapid movements of the left upper extremity. The neurologist describes these as hemiballistic movements and concludes that the lesion is probably in the ventral thalamus. Which of the following structures is also a portion of the ventral thalamus?

○ (A) Red nucleus
○ (B) Prerubral area (field of Forel)
○ (C) Infundibulum
○ (D) Mammillary body
○ (E) Centromedian nucleus

10. The MRI of a 57-year-old obese man with uncontrolled hypertension reveals an infarct of the primary visual cortex on the medial aspect of the occipital lobe. Which of the following thalamic nuclei relays visual information to the occipital lobe?

○ (A) Medial geniculate nucleus
○ (B) Superior colliculus
○ (C) Ventral posterolateral nucleus
○ (D) Lateral geniculate nucleus
○ (E) Lateral posterior nucleus

11. An 81-year-old woman suffering from dementia experiences a sudden loss of sensation (pain, thermal sense, proprioception) on the right side of her body. CT reveals a hemorrhage into the thalamus on the patient's left side. This hemorrhage is most likely located in which of the following thalamic nuclei?

○ (A) Ventral posteromedial nucleus
○ (B) Ventral lateral nucleus
○ (C) Pulvinar
○ (D) Centromedian
○ (E) Ventral posterolateral nucleus

12. A 27-year-old woman presents with a neurodegenerative disease affecting large portions of the frontal lobe. As a result she is suffering from dementia and personality changes. Because of its extensive connection with the frontal lobe, which of the following thalamic nuclei would most likely be adversely affected by this disease? (   )

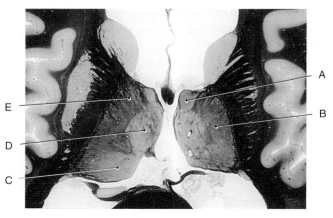

Figure 15–4

13.   The MRI of a 72-year-old man reveals a lesion that involves the thalamic nucleus that relays auditory information to the temporal lobe. Which of the following labeled structures is most likely involved in this lesion? (   )

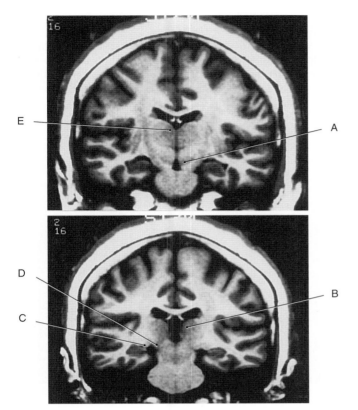

Figure 15–5

14.   A 68-year-old diabetic man with hypertension complains to his family physician of a loss of sensation on the right side of his face. MRI reveals a small lesion in the thalamus on the left side. Which of the following thalamic nuclei is most likely involved in this lesion?

○ (A) Ventral posteromedial
○ (B) Centromedian
○ (C) Ventral lateral
○ (D) Ventral anterior
○ (E) Ventral posterolateral

15.   An association nucleus of the thalamus is one that receives input from several different areas and projects to widespread areas of the cortex that may be neither specifically sensory nor motor in function. Which of the following is an association nucleus of the dorsal thalamus?

○ (A) Lateral geniculate
○ (B) Ventral lateral
○ (C) Dorsomedial nucleus
○ (D) Ventral posteromedial
○ (E) Ventral anterior

16.   Which of the following nuclei of the hypothalamus is located in the chiasmatic region of the hypothalamus?

○ (A) Posterior
○ (B) Dorsomedial
○ (C) Anterior
○ (D) Arcuate
○ (E) Mammillary

17.   Which of the following areas of the diencephalon contain a rostrocaudally oriented bundle of fibers called the medial forebrain bundle?

○ (A) Medial hypothalamic zone
○ (B) Dorsomedial nucleus
○ (C) Lateral hypothalamic zone
○ (D) Lateral thalamic nuclei
○ (E) Internal medullary lamina

18.   A 81-year-old woman complaining of severe headache and nausea is brought to the emergency department by her son. An examination reveals normal cranial nerve function but a loss of sensation on the left side of her body. Which of the following labeled areas, each representing a potential lesion, is the most likely site of a lesion that would result in the deficits seen in this patient? (   )

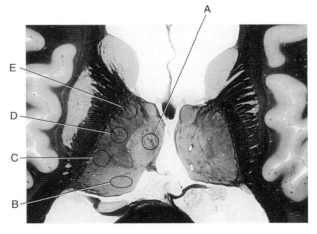

Figure 15–6

19.   A 54-year-old obese man with uncontrolled hypertension is brought to the emergency department after collapsing at a soccer game. He is breathing, has a regular heart rate, and is unresponsive. After several hours he is still unconscious. CT reveals an extensive hemorrhagic lesion in the right thalamus involving the anterior, ventral anterior, and much of the dorsomedial nuclei. The midline is shifted about 12 mm to the left by the mass effect of the hemorrhage. Which of the following vessels is most likely involved in this stroke?

○ (A) Lateral striate arteries
○ (B) Medial striate arteries
○ (C) Thalamogeniculate artery
○ (D) Posterior medial choroidal artery
○ (E) Thalamoperforating artery

20.   A 29-year-old previously athletic woman visits her family physician. She complains that her eating habits have gradually changed over the past several months to the point where she is eating constantly (hyperphagia), has gained a significant amount of weight, and is no longer able to participate in sports. Enhanced MRI reveals bilateral lesions in the hypothalamus. Which of the following labeled areas, each representative of a lesion, contains the structures that, if damaged, would result in the deficits experienced by this patient? (   )

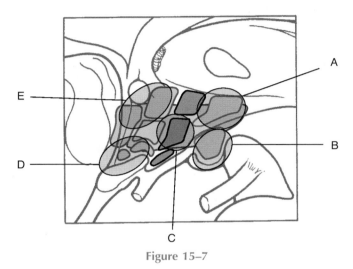

Figure 15–7

21.   A 78-year-old man is brought to the emergency department after collapsing at his grandson's birthday party. CT reveals a hemorrhagic lesion in the area outlined below.

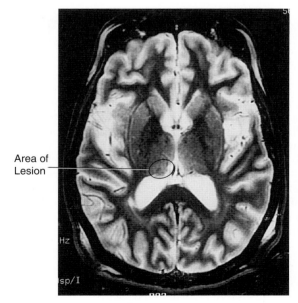

Figure 15–8

Hemorrhage from which of the following vessels is most likely responsible for this lesion?

○ (A)   Left thalamoperforating artery
○ (B)   Right thalamoperforating artery
○ (C)   Left thalamogeniculate artery
○ (D)   Right thalamogeniculate artery
○ (E)   Right lenticulostriate arteries

22.   The MRI of a 74-year-old man reveals a lesion in the area outlined below. The vessel serving this area also serves a part of the choroid plexus. Which of the following vessels is most likely involved to result in this lesion in this man?

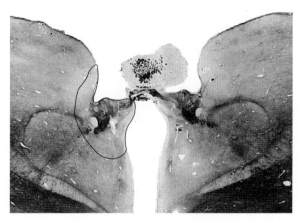

Figure 15–9

○ (A)   Posterior inferior cerebellar artery
○ (B)   Anterior inferior cerebellar artery
○ (C)   Anterior choroidal artery
○ (D)   Lateral posterior choroidal artery
○ (E)   Medial posterior choroidal artery

23.   A relay nucleus receives input from a specific source, processes the information, and sends it on to a particular region of the cerebral cortex. Which of the following is a relay nucleus in the dorsal thalamus?

○ (A)   Ventral lateral
○ (B)   Dorsomedial
○ (C)   Lateral dorsal
○ (D)   Pulvinar
○ (E)   Lateral posterior

24.   Which of the following hypothalamic nuclei receives a large input from the hippocampal formation via the fornix? (   )

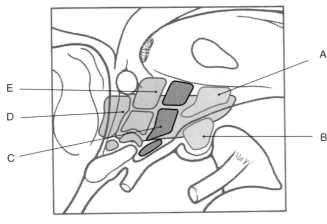

Figure 15–10

25.   A 7-year-old boy presents with visual disturbances. His evaluation, which includes an MRI, reveals a cranio-pharyngioma (Rathke pouch tumor). Under normal conditions, the Rathke pouch, an outpocketing of the stomodeum, forms which of the following structures?

○ (A) Neurohypophysis
○ (B) Adenohypophysis
○ (C) Optic chiasm
○ (D) Stalk of the pituitary
○ (E) Ventromedial hypothalamic nucleus

26.   Which of the following thalamic nuclei is an essential synaptic station in those circuits traveling through the dorsal thalamus that are related to the limbic system?

○ (A) Ventral lateral
○ (B) Centromedian
○ (C) Anterior
○ (D) Dorsomedial
○ (E) Ventral posteromedial

27.   A 74-year-old woman presents to her ophthalmologist with a variety of eye movement disturbances. The examination reveals that the extraocular muscles are not paralyzed but that eye movements are abnormal (as in ocular dysmetria). Which of the following thalamic nuclei is especially concerned with the visual system and eye movement?

○ (A) Ventral lateral
○ (B) Ventral posterolateral
○ (C) Pulvinar
○ (D) Ventral posteromedial
○ (E) Medial geniculate

28.   Which of the following thalamic nuclei is located within the internal medullary lamina?

○ (A) Ventral posterolateral
○ (B) Pulvinar
○ (C) Dorsomedial
○ (D) Centromedian
○ (E) Ventral anterior

29.   Which of the following parts of the internal capsule is located immediately lateral to the rostral aspect of the anterior nucleus of the thalamus and lateral to the position of the interventricular foramen in either axial or coronal planes?

○ (A) Anterior limb
○ (B) Genu
○ (C) Posterior limb
○ (D) External capsule
○ (E) Retrolenticular limb

Questions 30 to 31 are based on the following patient:

A 71-year-old man is brought to the emergency department by his son. The family states that his symptoms appeared suddenly and were accompanied by a severe headache. The examination reveals normal cranial nerve motor function, although there is a loss of sensation (pain, thermal sensation, proprioception) on the right side of the face. In addition, this man has a loss of the same sensations on the right side of the body. MRI reveals a hemorrhagic lesion.

30.   The sensory deficits in this man are both located on the same side of the body. In general this is indicative of a lesion located where?

○ (A) Cerebral hemisphere
○ (B) Midbrain
○ (C) Pons
○ (D) Medulla
○ (E) Cervical spinal cord

31.   Assuming the deficits experienced by this man to be the result of a thalamic lesion, which of the following nuclei is most likely involved?

○ (A) Ventral posterolateral only
○ (B) Ventral posteromedial only
○ (C) Ventral lateral only
○ (D) Ventral posterolateral and posteromedial
○ (E) Ventral lateral and ventral anterior

ANSWERS

1. **(C)** The interventricular foramen is bordered rostromedially by the column of the fornix and caudolaterally by the anterior thalamic tubercle. The anterior nucleus of the thalamus is located immediately internal to this tubercle.
FN2e 223

2. **(E)** The lateral and medial geniculate nuclei are those portions of the diencephalon that relay, respectively, visual and auditory information to the cerebral cortex. These nuclei are located in caudal portions of the diencephalon immediately inferior to the pulvinar.
FN2e 227–228

3. **(B)** This patient has visual and auditory deficits; visual information is coming from the eye, auditory information is ascending through the brainstem. The fiber bundles conveying this information converge at the level of the geniculate bodies. These structures and immediately adjacent areas of the diencephalon such as the pulvinar receive their blood supply from the thalamogeniculate artery. This vessel is usually a branch of P_2.
FN2e 233–234

4. **(C)** The subthalamic nucleus is the largest portion of the ventral thalamus. In fact, it is common to use the terms *ventral thalamus* and *subthalamus* interchangeably. The subthalamus is an important synaptic station in the motor system. It influences motor activity primarily through the basal nuclei. Subthalamic lesions result in hemiballismus.
FN2e 230–232

5. **(E)** In this axial view the lateral thalamic nucleus is located medially adjacent to the internal capsule. The ventral lateral nucleus is one of the lateral thalamic nuclei and is located in about the middle third of the rostrocaudal axis of these nuclei. This nucleus receives input from the cerebellum and basal nuclei and projects to the motor cortex.
FN2e 227–228

6. **(C)** The ventral lateral nucleus (VL) of the thalamus receives input from the cerebellum and basal nuclei and projects primarily to the somatomotor cortex. Some portions of the VL project to the area of cortex located immediately rostral to the precentral gyrus, this being the frontal eye field.
FN2e 227

7. **(A)** The anterior nucleus of the thalamus projects to the overlying cortex of the cingulate gyrus. This connection is an important part of the Papez circuit, which is a series of connections that includes the hippocampus, mammillary nuclei, anterior thalamic nucleus, and cingulate gyrus.
FN2e 223, 227, 499

8. **(D)** The subcommissural organ is located in the wall of the third ventricle adjacent to the posterior commissure at the point where the third ventricle transitions into the cerebral aqueduct.
FN2e 221

9. **(B)** The major part of the ventral thalamus is the subthalamic nucleus; sometimes these terms are used interchangeably. Smaller, but important, portions of the ventral thalamus include the zona incerta and the prerubral field. The latter consists of a small population of fiber bundles connecting the basal nuclei (and to a certain extent the cerebellum) to the thalamus.
FN2e 230–231, 409

10. **(D)** The lateral geniculate nucleus is located at the caudal aspect of the dorsal thalamus just inferior to the large bulge of the pulvinar. This thalamic nucleus receives visual input via the optic tract and, in turn, projects to the primary visual cortex.
FN2e 227–228

11. **(E)** Somatosensory information (pain, thermal sense, and proprioception) from the contralateral side of the body terminates in the ventral posterolateral nucleus. This nucleus, in turn, projects to the somatosensory cortex.
FN2e 227–228

12. **(D)** The dorsomedial nucleus of the dorsal thalamus projects extensively to the frontal cortex rostral to the somatomotor cortex. These connections are an important element in activation of the cortex. For example, infarcts in this thalamic nucleus may result in depression of consciousness.
FN2e 223–227

13. **(D)** The medial geniculate nucleus is located at the caudal level of the dorsal thalamus, inferior to the pulvinar and immediately medial to the lateral geniculate nucleus. This diencephalic nucleus receives ascending auditory input via the lateral lemniscus and projects to the temporal lobe.
FN2e 226–228

14. **(A)** The ventral posteromedial nucleus of the thalamus receives sensory input from the trigeminal nerve and, in turn, projects to the overlying somatosensory cortex, specifically the postcentral gyrus.
FN2e 226–228

15. **(C)** The dorsomedial nucleus receives input from diffuse areas of the brainstem and projects to most of the frontal lobe rostral to the somatomotor cortex. In this respect this thalamic nucleus projects to several named gyri (a widespread cortical target), none of which are specifically motor or sensory in function.
FN2e 228

16. **(C)** The anterior nucleus of the hypothalamus is found in the chiasmatic region inferior to the periventricular nucleus and caudal to the preoptic nuclei. This hypothalamic nucleus is concerned with cardiovascular function.
FN2e 230–231

17. **(C)** The medial forebrain bundle is an important fascicle of fibers that traverses the lateral hypothalamic zone. This bundle contains important projections that originate in septal areas and in the lateral hypothalamic zone and descend to brainstem nuclei. It also contains important ascending projections.
FN2e 229–230, 480, 486

18. **(C)** The ventral posterolateral nucleus of the dorsal thalamus receives sensory input via the anterolateral system (pain and thermal sense) and medial lemniscus (proprioception) and projects to the somatosensory cortex.
FN2e 227–228

19. **(E)** The rostral portions of the dorsal thalamus receive blood supply via the thalamoperforating artery, which is usually a branch of P_1. This artery serves those parts of the diencephalon that are part of the ascending reticular activating system. Injury along this pathway, such as a thalamic stroke, may result in coma. The CT finding of midline shift is an important indicator of the

severity of mass lesion affect on the entire diencephalon. In general, shift of the midline by greater than 10 mm is associated with the development of coma regardless of the cause of the shift.
FN2e 233

20. **(C)** The ventromedial nucleus, located in the tuberal region, is regarded as a satiety center. Normally, this nucleus signals a sense of fullness when adequate food is consumed. Bilateral lesions result in excessive food intake and obesity.
FN2e 230

21. **(D)** This lesion is in the territory of the thalamo-geniculate artery. The principal nuclei affected are the pulvinar, medial and lateral geniculate, centromedian, ventral posteromedial, and posterolateral. This lesion is on the patient's right side; therefore, the right artery is involved.
FN2e 226, 233–234

22. **(E)** The area of the lesion is centered on the habenular nuclei but also includes small adjacent portions of the pulvinar and dorsomedial nucleus of the thalamus. In addition to these areas/nuclei, the medial posterior choroidal artery also serves a part of the stria medullaris thalami, a portion of the habenulointerpeduncular tract and, of course, the choroid plexus of the third ventricle.
FN2e 233–234

23. **(A)** The ventral lateral nucleus receives input from the basal nuclei and the cerebellum and projects to the somatomotor cortex (motor function). This nucleus receives input from two specific sources and projects to the somatomotor cortex, which consists of the precentral and anterior paracentral gyri.
FN2e 228

24. **(B)** The mammillary nuclei receive a large input via what is commonly called the postcommissural fornix. These fibers originate mainly from the hippocampal formation.
FN2e 230

25. **(B)** The outpocketing of the stomodeum (the future oral cavity) known as the Rathke pouch opposes the neurohypophysis, an outpocketing of the floor of the diencephalon, to form the pituitary. The anterior lobe of the pituitary gland and the pars intermedia arise from the Rathke pouch.
FN2e 221

26. **(C)** The anterior nucleus of the thalamus receives input from the mammillary nuclei and, to a lesser degree, from the hippocampal formation. The mammillary bodies receive a large projection from the hippocampus. The anterior nucleus is an important relay nucleus for the limbic system and the Papez circuit.
FN2e 223

27. **(C)** The pulvinar receives input from visual-related areas of the cortex and the superior colliculus. It projects to the visual association cortex and to areas of the temporal, parietal, and frontal lobes that function in the visual sphere.
FN2e 227

28. **(D)** The internal medullary lamina is a rostrocaudally running bundle of fibers separating medial and lateral portions of the diencephalon. Particularly prominent structures located within the internal medullary lamina include the anterior nucleus of the thalamus (rostrally) and the centromedian nucleus located at more caudal levels. This delicate lamina of fibers is sometimes visible on MRI.
FN2e 228

29. **(B)** The genu of the internal capsule is located at the intersection of the anterior and posterior limbs. This is laterally adjacent to the position of the interventricular foramen, to the rostral aspect of the anterior nucleus of the thalamus (the location of the anterior tubercle), and to the position of the column of the fornix.
FN2e 229, 244–245

30. **(A)** Lesions in the cerebral hemispheres may involve thalamic nuclei, the internal capsule, or the cerebral cortex or various combinations of these. At the level of the brainstem, most testable deficits are crossed. Sensory deficits or sensory plus motor deficits are seen on the same side of the head and body resultant to lesions of the cerebral hemispheres.
FN2e 227–228

31. **(D)** This patient experiences sensory loss on the body as well as the face. For a thalamic lesion to result in these deficits, the infarct would have to encompass the ventral posterolateral as well as the ventral posteromedial nuclei. The blood supply to these nuclei is via the thalamogeniculate artery, usually a branch of P_2.
FN2e 227–228, 233–234

CHAPTER 16

The Telencephalon

1. A 67-year-old man is brought to the emergency department by his daughter. He is lethargic and complains of a headache. The examination reveals a left-sided hemiparesis and a loss of sensation on the same side of the body. MRI reveals a hemorrhagic lesion in the internal capsule. Which of the following represents the most likely location of this lesion?

○ (A) Anterior limb
○ (B) Genu
○ (C) Posterior limb
○ (D) Sublenticular limb
○ (E) Retrolenticular limb

2. The MRI of an 81-year-old woman reveals a hemorrhagic lesion (a stroke) in the posterior limb of the internal capsule. This woman presents with motor and sensory losses on the same side of the body. Which of the following vessels is the most likely source of this hemorrhage in this patient?

○ (A) Medial striate artery(ies)
○ (B) Thalamoperforating artery(ies)
○ (C) Lateral posterior choroidal artery(ies)
○ (D) Lenticulostriate arteries
○ (E) Thalamogeniculate artery(ies)

3. A 49-year-old man presents to the neurologist's office complaining that his "arm" is weak. The examination reveals normal cranial nerve function and weakness of the left upper extremity. Sensation on the weak extremity is normal. After examining the MRI, the physician concludes that a meningioma is impinging on the upper extremity area of the somatomotor cortex. Which of the following structures is most likely damaged by this tumor?

○ (A) Postcentral gyrus
○ (B) Precentral gyrus

○ (C) Anterior paracentral gyrus
○ (D) Middle frontal gyrus
○ (E) Superior frontal gyrus

4. A 39-year-old woman visits her family physician complaining of a headache. MRI reveals that this patient has agenesis of the corpus callosum. Which of the following is the first of the major commissures of the brain to form?

○ (A) Anterior commissure
○ (B) Corpus callosum
○ (C) Hippocampal commissure
○ (D) Decussation of the brachium conjunctivum
○ (E) Posterior commissure

5. The CT of a 92-year-old woman with amyloid angiopathy (deposition of amyloid in brain vessels) reveals a hemorrhagic lesion in the pars opercularis and pars triangularis. This lesion is located where?

○ (A) Occipital lobe
○ (B) Limbic lobe
○ (C) Parietal lobe
○ (D) Temporal lobe
○ (E) Frontal lobe

6. An 81-year-old woman presents with a sudden loss of vision in the nasal visual field of one eye and the temporal visual field of the other eye (homonymous hemianopsia). She tells the emergency department physician that she had a dull headache first, then noticed that she "couldn't see good afterwards." Which of the following labeled areas, each representing the location of a cortical lesion, is the most likely site of this hemorrhagic event? See Figure 16–1. (   )

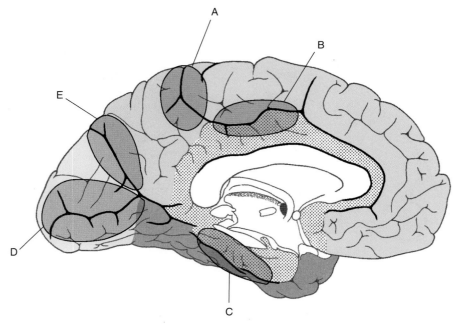

Figure 16–1

7.   Branches of which of the following vessels represent an important blood supply to the primary visual cortex?

○ (A) P$_4$
○ (B) P$_3$
○ (C) M$_4$
○ (D) M$_3$
○ (E) A$_2$

8.   A 79-year-old man has a sudden severe headache and becomes unconscious. After regaining consciousness, he is aphasic and only able to respond to questions with "yes" and "no." CT reveals a hemorrhagic stroke that involves the pars triangularis and immediately adjacent areas. Which of the following labeled areas, each representing a potential lesion, is the most likely location of this hemorrhage? (   )

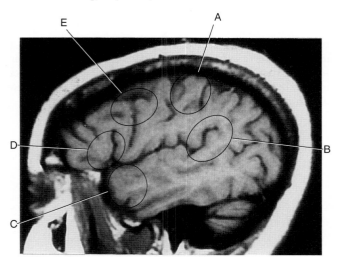

Figure 16–2

9.   A 27-year-old man is transported to the emergency department after an automobile collision in which he sustained head injuries consequent to striking the windshield and dashboard. After several weeks in the hospital he is transferred to a rehabilitation facility. The nurses in this care facility notice that he has unusual eating patterns and inappropriate sexual behavior. He also has trouble with his memory and seems unable to learn new tasks. Which of the following structures is most likely damaged in this patient to result in these deficits?

○ (A) Caudate nucleus and putamen
○ (B) Subthalamic nucleus and substantia nigra
○ (C) Amygdaloid complex and hippocampus
○ (D) Substantia nigra only
○ (E) Zona incerta and globus pallidus

10.   A 67-year-old man presents to the internist's office complaining of trouble walking, standing, and manipulating objects with his hands. The physician indicates to the man's family that the patient may have a degenerative disease of the neostriatum. Which of the following structures is most likely involved in this patient's disease?

○ (A) Globus pallidus
○ (B) Caudate nucleus and globus pallidus
○ (C) Caudate nucleus and putamen
○ (D) Putamen and globus pallidus
○ (E) Putamen

11.   A 69-year-old woman presents to the emergency department with weakness of the right lower extremity. CT reveals a small hemorrhagic lesion in the part of the primary somatomotor cortex where the lower extremity is represented (the anterior paracentral gyrus). Which of the following outlined areas represents the most likely location of this lesion? See Figure 16–3. (   )

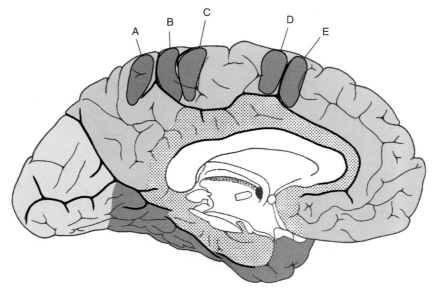

Figure 16–3

12. A 79-year-old man complains to his family physician of motor disturbances. The examination reveals normal cranial nerve function but motor dysfunction that suggests a lesion in the basal nuclei. MRI shows a hemorrhagic lesion in the territory served by the medial striate artery. Which of the following structures would be most directly affected by this stroke?

○ (A) Globus pallidus
○ (B) Putamen
○ (C) Subthalamic nucleus
○ (D) Body and tail of caudate nucleus
○ (E) Head of caudate nucleus

13. A 49-year-old woman is brought to the emergency department by her husband. The husband states that his wife became disoriented after working in her garden. Suspecting a stroke, the physician orders a CT, which reveals a large infarct in the retrolenticular limb of the internal capsule. As this patient recovers, which of the following deficits will most likely be the most obvious?

○ (A) Hearing
○ (B) Somatosensory input from the body
○ (C) Paralysis of facial and tongue movements due to infarct of corticonuclear fibers
○ (D) Vision
○ (E) Somatosensory input from the face

14. A 77-year-old man is being followed by a neurologist for dementia, which has progressively worsened over the past 6 months. The physician believes, based on a thorough examination, that this is a probable case of Alzheimer disease. In addition to the cerebral cortex, which of the following structures (see Figure 16–4), would have a significant loss of large neurons resultant to this disease? (   )

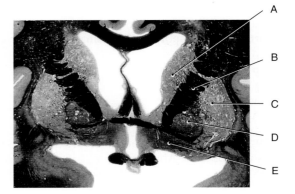

Figure 16–4

15. A 62-year-old woman presents to the emergency department with difficulty speaking. The examination reveals a partial paralysis of the facial muscles, especially around the mouth on the left side and a deviation of the tongue to the same side on protrusion. CT reveals a lesion in the internal capsule damaging corticonuclear fibers as they pass from the cortex to cranial nerve nuclei in the brainstem. This infarct is most likely located in which of the following parts of the internal capsule?

○ (A) Anterior limb
○ (B) Genu
○ (C) Posterior limb
○ (D) Sublenticular limb
○ (E) Retrolenticular limb

16. The efferent fibers of the basal nuclei that collectively form the lenticular fasciculus originate from where?

○ (A) Head of the caudate nucleus
○ (B) Putamen

○ (C) Subthalamic nucleus
○ (D) Globus pallidus
○ (E) Substantia nigra

17.   A 29-year-old woman presents to the neurologist's office complaining of recurring headaches. The examination reveals no specific motor or sensory deficits, so the physician orders an MRI. This reveals an arteriovenous malformation located in the cortex of the precuneus. Which of the following labeled areas represents the most likely location of this malformation? (   )

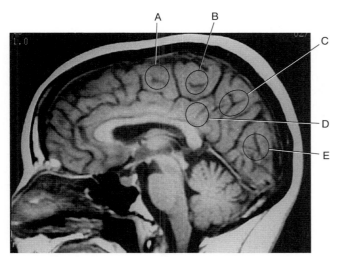

Figure 16–5

18.   A 59-year-old woman is brought to the family physician's office by her daughter. The daughter states that her mother complained of a headache and took an aspirin and then a long nap. When the mother awoke the daughter noted that, when her mother talked, her sentences made no sense (Wernicke aphasia). The physician suspects a cortical lesion and orders MRI, which reveals a lesion in the inferior parietal lobule. Which of the following structures is most likely involved in this lesion?

○ (A) Pars orbitalis and pars triangularis
○ (B) Pars triangularis and pars opercularis
○ (C) Post central gyrus and supramarginal gyrus
○ (D) Supramarginal gyrus and angular gyrus
○ (E) Angular gyrus and lateral occipital gyri

19.   A 49-year-old man with uncontrolled hypertension presents with sudden right-sided weakness and a loss of sensation on the body. MRI reveals a hemorrhagic lesion in the paracentral lobule (anterior and posterior paracentral gyri). Which of the following vessels is the most likely source of this hemorrhage?

○ (A) P_4, parieto-occipital artery
○ (B) M_4, parietal and angular branches
○ (C) A_2, frontopolar branches
○ (D) P_3, posterior temporal branches
○ (E) A_2, callosomarginal branches

20.   The frontal eye field is located in the middle frontal gyrus. This area of the cortex influences eye movement through connections to the midbrain and pontine centers. Which of the following labeled areas represents the most likely location of the frontal eye field? (   )

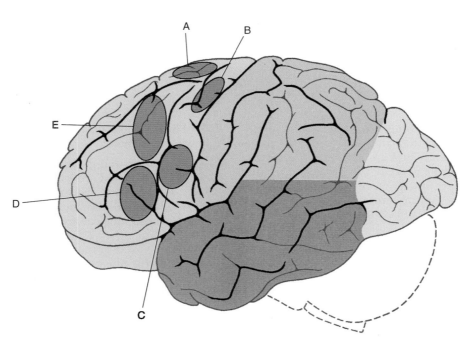

Figure 16–6

21. The MRI of a 54-year-old woman reveals a large aneurysm compromising the long (gyri longi) and short (gyri breves) gyri. These gyri are located where?

- ○ (A) Frontal lobe
- ○ (B) Limbic lobe
- ○ (C) Insular lobe
- ○ (D) Parietal lobe
- ○ (E) Temporal lobe

22. The MRI of a developmentally delayed 19-year-old man reveals a number of structural malformations of the brain. In this sagittal image, the cingulate sulcus and gyrus are not properly formed. Which of the following important structures is also most likely affected by the developmental failure in this patient?

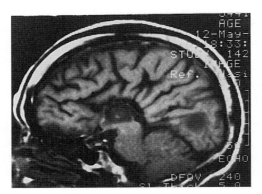

Figure 16–7

- ○ (A) Basilar pons
- ○ (B) Cerebellum
- ○ (C) Midbrain
- ○ (D) Corpus callosum
- ○ (E) Superior frontal gyrus

23. A 29-year-old man complains to his family physician of headaches that, over the past 6 months, have recurred more frequently and are getting more severe. The man is referred to a neurologist. Suspecting a brain tumor, the neurologist orders an MRI, which reveals a mass in the primary auditory cortex. Which of the following represents the most likely location of this tumor?

- ○ (A) Superior temporal gyrus
- ○ (B) Parietal operculum
- ○ (C) Pars opercularis
- ○ (D) Angular gyrus
- ○ (E) Transverse temporal gyrus

24. An 81-year-old woman is brought to the emergency department by her son. The examination reveals a con-fused and lethargic woman who has sensory loss on the left side of her face and on the upper extremity and trunk on the same side. There are no motor deficits. Suspecting a stroke, the physician orders CT, which shows a hemorrhagic lesion in the somatosensory cortex. Which of the following vessels is most likely involved to result in these deficits in this patient?

- ○ (A) Branches of A_2
- ○ (B) Branches of M_3
- ○ (C) Branches of P_4
- ○ (D) Branches of M_4
- ○ (E) Branches of P_3

25. A 49-year-old obese man with uncontrolled hypertension presents to the emergency department. The examination reveals a motor deficit that leads the physician to suspect a hemorrhage into the paleo-striatum; this was confirmed by a CT. Which of the following structures is the most likely site of his hemorrhage? (   )

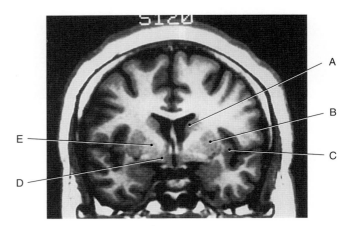

Figure 16–8

26. The lenticular nucleus is composed of which of the following structures?

- ○ (A) Putamen and globus pallidus
- ○ (B) Putamen and caudate nucleus
- ○ (C) Putamen and claustrum
- ○ (D) Globus pallidus and amygdaloid complex
- ○ (E) Caudate nucleus and amygdaloid complex

27. A 21-year-old man is brought to the emergency department after an automobile collision. He is stuporous. Suspecting injury to the brain, the physician orders a CT, which reveals a small contusion in the parahippocampal gyrus on the left side. Which of the following labeled areas represents the most likely location of the brain injury in this patient? (   )

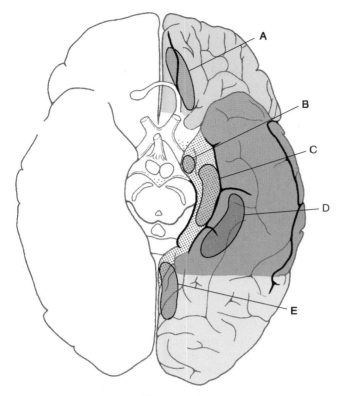

Figure 16–9

28. The MRI of an 81-year-old woman reveals hemorrhage into the lenticular nucleus and immediately adjacent portions of the internal capsule. Which of the following is the source of the lenticulostriate arteries (also called lateral striate arteries) that serve this portion of the basal nuclei?

○ (A) A_1
○ (B) M_1
○ (C) M_2
○ (D) P_1
○ (E) P_2

Questions 29 to 30 are based on the following patient:

A 19-year-old man is brought to the neurologist's office by his mother. The examination reveals a combative patient who cannot seem to follow simple instructions. His mother states that he has been getting worse over the past several months. MRI reveals a large tumor originating from the choroid plexus in the temporal (inferior) horn of the lateral ventricle. This tumor fills this portion of the ventricular space and impinges on structures located in the walls of the temporal horn.

29. Which of the following structures is located in the medial and anteromedial wall of the temporal horn of the lateral ventricle?

○ (A) Stria terminalis
○ (B) Stria medullaris thalami

○ (C) Tail of the caudate nucleus
○ (D) Hippocampal formation
○ (E) Amygdaloid complex

30. Which of the following structures is located in the rostral wall of the temporal horn of the lateral ventricle?

○ (A) Tail of the caudate nucleus
○ (B) Amygdaloid complex
○ (C) Claustrum
○ (D) Hippocampal formation
○ (E) Substantia innominata

ANSWERS

1. **(C)** The posterior limb of the internal capsule contains corticospinal fibers that serve the contralateral side of the body (hence the hemiparesis) and thalamocortical projections. These latter fibers convey somatosensory input from the thalamus to the cortex; this information has initially crossed in either the spinal cord (pain/thermal sense) or in the medulla (proprioception).
FN2e 244–245

2. **(D)** The lenticulostriate arteries (also called the lateral striate arteries) originate from M_1 and serve much of the lenticular nuclei and adjacent portions of the posterior limb of the internal capsule. The anterior choroidal artery also serves the portions of the internal capsule adjacent to the optic tract, portions of the genu, and the anterior (ventral) part of the lenticular nuclei.
FN2e 245–246, 250

3. **(B)** The somatomotor cortex (also called the primary motor cortex, Brodmann's area 4) consists of the precentral gyrus and the anterior paracentral gyrus. The face, upper extremity, and trunk are represented in the former and the lower extremity in the latter. The primary motor cortex (somatomotor cortex) is part of the frontal lobe.
FN2e 238–239, 389–390

4. **(A)** The anterior commissure, the first to form, originates from the lamina terminalis. The corpus callosum, the third to appear, originates from the general area of the anterior commissure and enlarges in a caudal direction to assume its characteristic position in the adult.
FN2e 237

5. **(E)** The inferior frontal gyrus (of the frontal lobe) consists of the pars orbitalis, pars triangularis, and pars opercularis. Lesions in this area of the frontal lobe result in Broca (expressive or nonfluent) aphasia.
FN2e 238–239, 516–517

6. **(D)** The primary visual cortex is located on the banks of the calcarine sulcus on the medial aspect of the occipital lobe. Portions of the cuneus form the upper bank, and parts of the lingual gyrus form the lower bank.
FN2e 241

7. **(A)** The calcarine artery (so named because it is located in the immediate area of the calcarine sulcus) and

the parieto-occipital artery are branches of P$_4$. The primary visual cortex receives its primary blood supply from the calcarine artery, a branch of P$_4$.
FN2e 242

8. **(D)** The inferior frontal gyrus consists of the pars opercularis, pars triangularis, and pars orbitalis. Lesions to this area of the frontal lobe result in Broca aphasia (expressive aphasia).
FN2e 238–239

9. **(C)** The amygdaloid nucleus is located in the rostromedial aspect of the temporal lobe, internal to the uncus. The hippocampus is located in the medial aspect of the temporal lobe, internal to the parahippocampal gyrus. Injury to these structures may result in a variety of behavioral changes (amygdaloid complex) or memory deficits (hippocampus). One or both of these structures may be damaged by severe impact to the head.
FN2e 250

10. **(C)** The neostriatum is composed of the caudate nucleus and the putamen. These structures have a common embryologic origin and have many structural/functional characteristics in common.
FN2e 246

11. **(C)** The paracentral lobule consists of an anterior paracentral gyrus (the medial portion—lower extremity part—of the somatomotor cortex) and the posterior paracentral gyrus (the medial portion of the somatosensory cortex). The anterior paracentral gyrus is immediately rostral to the medial continuation of the central sulcus and generally caudad to the paracentral sulcus.
FN2e 238–239

12. **(E)** The medial striate artery is a branch of the anterior cerebral artery at, or just distal to, its intersection with the anterior communicating artery. This artery, also called the artery of Heubner, is the prime blood supply to the head of the caudate nucleus and adjacent portions of the anterior limb of the internal capsule.
FN2e 246, 250

13. **(D)** The retrolenticular limb of the internal capsule contains interconnections between the occipital lobe and the diencephalon and midbrain. An especially prominent component of this part of the internal capsule is the optic radiation (geniculocalcarine radiation). These fibers convey visual information from the lateral geniculate nucleus of the diencephalon to the cortex bordering on the edges of the calcarine sulcus (the primary visual cortex).
FN2e 244–245

14. **(E)** The substantia innominata is located anterior (ventral) to the anterior commissure in the rostral and basal aspects of the cerebral hemisphere. A significant loss of neurons is seen in this brain area, as well as in the nucleus accumbens and in the parietal, temporal and frontal cortices in patients with Alzheimer disease. In addition to cell loss, there is plaque and neurofibrillary tangle formation in many areas of the affected parts of the nervous system.
FN2e 246–249

15. **(B)** Corticonuclear fibers to the brainstem are located in the genu of the internal capsule. These fibers originate from the face area of the somatomotor cortex, descend through the genu, and terminate in motor nuclei of the cranial nerves.
FN2e 244–245

16. **(D)** The efferent pathway from the basal nuclei originates from cells of the globus pallidus. These axons form the lenticular fasciculus and the ansa lenticularis and are commonly referred to as pallidothalamic fibers.
FN2e 249–250

17. **(C)** The precuneus is located on the medial surface of the hemispheres between the parieto-occipital sulcus and the marginal sulcus. This latter sulcus is sometimes called the marginal branch (or ramus) of the cingulate sulcus. The precuneus forms the medial aspect of most of the parietal lobe.
FN2e 239–240

18. **(D)** The inferior parietal lobule is composed of the supramarginal gyrus (located around the upper extreme of the lateral sulcus) and the angular gyrus (located around the upper extreme of the superior temporal gyrus). Lesions of the inferior parietal lobule result in Wernicke aphasia (fluent or receptive aphasia).
FN2e 238–239, 517

19. **(E)** The anterior paracentral gyrus (somatomotor cortex for the lower extremity) and the posterior paracentral gyrus (somatosensory cortex for the lower extremity) collectively form the paracentral lobule. The callosomarginal branch of A$_2$ courses in the general area of the cingulate sulcus; its branches serve the medial aspect of the hemisphere to the level of the parieto-occipital sulcus; this includes the paracentral gyri.
FN2e 123–124, 242

20. **(E)** The frontal eye field is located in the caudal part of the middle frontal gyrus immediately rostral to the precentral sulcus and, thus, the precentral gyrus. In general, this area is also between the superior and inferior frontal sulci.
FN2e 238–239

21. **(C)** The long and short gyri form most of the surface of the insular lobe. These gyri are separated from each other by the central sulcus of the insula, and the insula itself is separated from the surrounding frontal, parietal, and temporal opercula by the circular sulcus.
FN2e 239–241

22. **(D)** In addition to a number of developmental malformations of gyri and sulci on the medial aspect of the hemisphere, the corpus callosum is missing in this patient (agenesis of the corpus callosum). The failure of the corpus callosum to form most likely results from changes in the pattern of the adjacent cortex during the development of gyri and sulci.
FN2e 237

23. **(E)** The transverse temporal gyri are located on the upper aspect of the temporal lobe in the depth of the lateral sulcus. The primary auditory cortex is located in

these gyri. Lesions in the primary auditory cortex will not result in deafness in one ear.
FN2e 239, 241

24. **(D)** The precentral gyrus is the somatosensory cortex for the face, upper extremity, and trunk. Branches of the middle cerebral artery that issue from the lateral sulcus become the M_4 segment, the individually named branches of which serve the lateral aspect of the hemisphere including most of the precentral gyrus.
FN2e 126, 242

25. **(E)** The paleostriatum is the globus pallidus. This is the source of efferent fibers from the basal nuclei (pallidothalamic fibers) that travel via the lenticular fasciculus and the ansa lenticularis. The caudate plus the putamen represent the neostriatum.
FN2e 246, 249

26. **(A)** The putamen and globus pallidus collectively form the lenticular nucleus. This important cell group lies within the hemisphere, medial to the external capsule, and lateral to the anterior limb, genu and posterior limb of the internal capsule.
FN2e 246

27. **(C)** The parahippocampal gyrus is located in the most medial aspect of the temporal lobe; it is separated from the adjacent occipitotemporal gyri by the collateral sulcus. Internal to the parahippocampal gyrus is the hippocampal formation.
FN2e 239, 241–242

28. **(B)** The lenticulostriate arteries are branches of the M_1 segment of the middle cerebral artery. Anterior (ventral) portions of the lenticular nucleus are also served by penetrating branches of the anterior choroidal artery.
FN2e 243, 250

29. **(D)** The hippocampal complex and the small fiber bundle running along its lateral surface (the fimbria of the hippocampus) is located in the medial and anteromedial aspect of the temporal horn. The hippocampus ends before reaching the rostral wall of the ventricle and is caudally continuous as the fiber bundle comprising the fornix.
FN2e 248, 250–251

30. **(B)** The amygdaloid complex is located in the rostral aspect of the temporal horn of the lateral ventricle. In this position it is also immediately internal to the uncus, a small elevation on the rostromedial aspect of the temporal lobe. Damage to the amygdaloid complex may result in profound behavioral problems.
FN2e 248, 250–251

Systems Neurobiology

The Somatosensory System: Tactile Discrimination and Position Sense and Touch, Thermal Sense, and Pain

Questions 1 through 5 are based on the following patient:

A 59-year-old woman is referred to a neurologist by her family physician. She complains of recurring severe headaches. The examination reveals (1) normal cranial nerve function, (2) normal motor examination, and (3) bilateral loss of pain and thermal sensations and of two-point discrimination, vibratory sense, and proprioception affecting both lower extremities. When questioned, the woman states that these "funny feelings" have progressed from mild to severe over time; she is not sure but says "it has happened over a long time, maybe a couple of years." MRI reveals a single elliptical lesion measuring about 5 × 6 cm.

1. Based on this history, the deficits experienced by this patient are most likely the result of which of the following?

- ○ (A) Extrusion of an intervertebral disc
- ○ (B) Trauma
- ○ (C) Rupture of a spinal or intracranial vessel
- ○ (D) A tumor
- ○ (E) Watershed infarct

2. The loss of pain and thermal sensations in the lower extremities of this patient reflect damage, at some point, along which of the following pathways?

- ○ (A) Anterior (ventral) trigeminothalamic tract
- ○ (B) Anterolateral system
- ○ (C) Posterior column—medial lemniscus system
- ○ (D) Posterior (dorsal) trigeminothalamic tract
- ○ (E) Medial longitudinal fasciculus

3. It is highly unlikely that the loss of two-point discrimination, proprioception, and vibratory sense in this patient would reflect damage to which of the following structures?

- ○ (A) Posterior columns in the spinal cord
- ○ (B) Medial lemnisci
- ○ (C) Ventral posterolateral nuclei
- ○ (D) Posterior limbs of the internal capsules
- ○ (E) Postcentral gyrus

4. The MRI of this patient reveals a single lesion, about 5 × 6 cm, elliptical, and centered in the falx cerebri. This finding would suggest that this is what kind of lesion?

- ○ (A) Arteriovenous malformation
- ○ (B) Astrocytoma
- ○ (C) Oligodendroglioma

○ (D) Meningioma
○ (E) Glioblastoma multiforme

5.   Based on the deficits experienced by this patient, and the location of the lesion, which of the following represents the most likely structures affected by this lesion?

○ (A) Postcentral gyri
○ (B) Ventral posterolateral and posteromedial thalamic nuclei
○ (C) Posterior limb of the internal capsules
○ (D) Anterior paracentral gyri
○ (E) Posterior paracentral gyri

6.   A 53-year-old morbidly obese diabetic man presents to his family physician complaining of "numbness." The examination reveals loss of proprioception and vibratory sense on the left upper extremity and loss of pain and thermal sense on the left side of the face. Which of the following labeled areas represents the most likely location of the lesion resulting in the deficits experienced by this patient? (   )

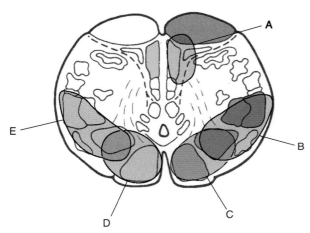

Figure 17–1

7.   A 63-year-old man presents with a loss of discriminative touch, vibratory sense, and proprioception on the right lower extremity. The cell bodies of origin for the second-order neurons in the pathway conveying this information from the periphery to the cerebral cortex are located in which of the following?

○ (A) Cuneate nucleus
○ (B) Gracile nucleus
○ (C) Ventral posterolateral nucleus
○ (D) Posterior root ganglion
○ (E) Posterior horn

8.   During a surgical procedure to remove a tumor from the posterolateral aspect of the spinal cord of a 22-year-old woman, the fibers of the medial division of the posterior root were damaged. Which of the following are characteristic of the fibers entering the medial division of the posterior root?

○ (A) Finely myelinated, slowly conducting, subserve vibratory sense and proprioception
○ (B) Finely myelinated, rapidly conducting, subserve pain and thermal sensations
○ (C) Heavily myelinated, slowly conducting, subserve vibratory sense and proprioception
○ (D) Heavily myelinated, rapidly conducting, subserve pain and thermal sensations
○ (E) Heavily myelinated, rapidly conducting, subserve vibratory sense, two-point discrimination and proprioception

9.   A 79-year-old healthy, active man complains to his family physician of "numbness" on his "arm" and of a "funny feeling" in his "leg." He is referred to a neurologist. The examination reveals a loss of pain and thermal sense on the left side of the body and a loss of proprioception and vibratory sense on the left lower extremity. CT reveals a small hemorrhagic lesion. Which of the following labeled areas represents the most likely location of the lesion in this patient? (   )

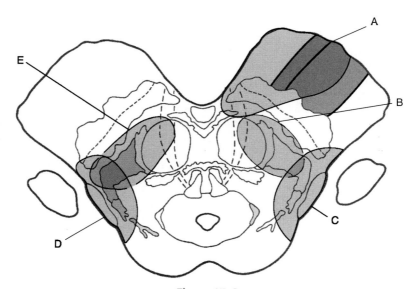

Figure 17–2

10. A small receptive field, such as that on the finger-tips or on the lips and around the oral cavity, is characterized by which of the following?

○ (A) A high receptor density and a correspondingly small area of representation in the somatosensory cortex
○ (B) Low receptor density and a correspondingly small area of representation in the somatosensory cortex
○ (C) A high receptor density and a correspondingly large area of representation in the somatosensory cortex
○ (D) A low receptor density and a correspondingly large area of representation in the somatosensory cortex

11. During the neurologic examination of a 12-year-old boy, the physician notices that the right patellar reflex is absent (areflexia). One possible explanation is that the A-alpha fibers that arise from the nuclear bag fibers of the muscle spindle may be damaged by a peripheral neuropathy. Which of the following represents the conduction velocity of A-alpha fibers?

○ (A) 80 to 120 m/sec
○ (B) 35 to 75 m/sec
○ (C) 30 to 50 m/sec
○ (D) 5 to 30 m/sec
○ (E) 0.5 to 3 m/sec

12. Slowly adapting receptors, such as Merkel cells, some hair follicles, and Ruffini endings generate action potentials

○ (A) Only at the initiation of stimulus (skin indentation) but not at its removal
○ (B) Only at the removal of a stimulus but not at its initiation
○ (C) At the initiation of a stimulus, during the time the stimulus is present (but at a lower rate), and at the removal of the stimulus
○ (D) At the initiation and removal of a stimulus, but these are absolutely silent during the time a stimulus is present
○ (E) That fire at a constant rate at all times

13. A 37-year-old woman presents with a loss of proprioception, two-point discrimination, and vibratory sense from the upper extremity. In addition to these deficits the examination reveals pigmented spots on her trunk, suggesting neurofibromatosis. MRI reveals multiple dumbbell-shaped tumors at the C4 to T3 intervertebral foramina on the left. The cell bodies for proprioceptive fibers originating from the upper extremity are located in which of the following?

○ (A) Ipsilateral posterior horn
○ (B) Ipsilateral posterior root ganglia above T6
○ (C) Ipsilateral posterior root ganglia below T6
○ (D) Ipsilateral intermediate zone of the spinal cord
○ (E) Contralateral posterior root ganglia above T6

14. A 27-year old man is brought to the emergency department from the site of a motorcycle collision. The neurologic examination reveals a normal motor examination but a loss of pain and thermal sensation over both lower extremities. Proprioception is intact. Which of the following labeled areas represents the most likely location of a lesion in this patient that would result in this deficit? (   )

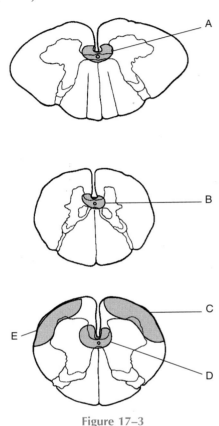

Figure 17–3

Questions 15 and 16 are based on the following patient:

A 43-year-old breast cancer survivor is being evaluated by a neurologist. She has complained, over the past several months, of a variety of motor and sensory symptoms. A peripheral neuropathy is considered in her differential diagnosis. During the examination, the physician discovers that the woman does not perceive vibration when a tuning fork is applied to bony prominences (excluding the face). The physician suspects that peripheral sensory endings or fibers may be selectively involved in the disease process.

15. Which of the following peripheral receptors are most specifically responsible for the transduction of vibratory sensations?

○ (A) Free endings
○ (B) Ruffini corpuscles
○ (C) Hair follicle receptors
○ (D) Meissner corpuscles
○ (E) Pacinian corpuscles

16. The conduction velocity of heavily myelinated fibers that conduct vibratory sensations (group II fibers) fall in the range of

○ (A) 80 to 120 m/sec
○ (B) 35 to 75 m/sec
○ (C) 5 to 30 m/sec
○ (D) 0.5 to 2 m/sec

17. A 34-year-old woman is suffering from peripheral neuropathy of undetermined etiology. An electrophysiologic evaluation suggests that group II Aβ sensory fibers are most affected. The neuropathologist confirms this finding by examining the diameters of the most severely affected fibers. Which of the following represents the fiber diameter of group II, Aβ sensory fibers?

○ (A) 13 to 20 μm
○ (B) 6 to 12 μm
○ (C) 1 to 5 μm
○ (D) 0.2 to 1.5 μm

18. An 81-year-old man is brought to the emergency department by his wife. She reports that he complained of a headache, went to lie down, and then "got real sick." The examination reveals normal motor function of the head and body and also reveals loss of pain and thermal sensation on the right side of the face and on the left side of the body. MRI reveals a small hemorrhagic lesion. Which of the following labeled areas represents the most likely location of the lesion in this patient? (   )

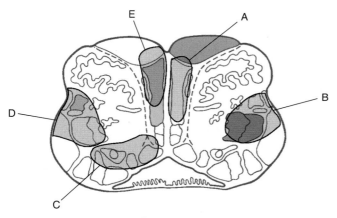

Figure 17–4

19. The somatotopic organization of the body in the medial lemniscus of the medulla oblongata is most correctly described as

○ (A) Upper extremity most anterior (ventral), lower extremity most posterior (dorsal)
○ (B) Lower extremity most anterior (ventral), upper extremity most posterior (dorsal)
○ (C) Lower extremity most anterior (ventral), upper extremity in the middle, face and head most posterior (dorsal)
○ (D) Trunk most anterior (ventral), upper extremity in the middle, lower extremity most dorsal
○ (E) Lower extremity most lateral, upper extremity most medial

20. A 61-year-old man complains to his family physician that his "face is numb." An examination reveals a loss of pain and thermal sensation on the left side of the face. MRI reveal a small hemorrhagic lesion in the area outlined below.

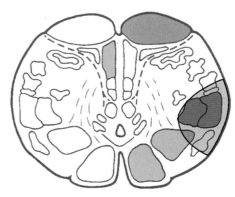

Figure 17–5

Which of the following parts of the trigeminal nuclear complex is most directly affected by this lesion?

○ (A) Pars caudalis
○ (B) Pars interpolaris
○ (C) Pars oralis
○ (D) Principal sensory nucleus
○ (E) Mesencephalic nucleus

21. A 73-year-old woman is brought to the emergency department by her housekeeper after losing consciousness. Suspecting a stroke, the physician orders CT, which reveals an infarct in the medulla. The area of the lesion includes a pyramid, medial lemniscus, and exiting hypoglossal root fibers. Which of the following fiber bundles lies immediately lateral to the medial lemniscus in the medulla, conveys pain and thermal sensations from the face and oral cavity to the thalamus, and would possibly be involved in this lesion?

○ (A) Anterolateral system
○ (B) Posterior (dorsal) trigeminothalamic tract
○ (C) Central tegmental tract
○ (D) Anterior (ventral) trigeminothalamic tract
○ (E) Spinal trigeminal tract

Questions 22 and 23 are based on the following patient:

A 77-year-old man is brought to the emergency department by his son, who found him on the floor of the garage. He is stuporous and complains of feeling sick and of a headache. The examination reveals a weakness of facial muscles on the left and loss of pain and thermal sense on the left side of the face and right side of the body. CT shows a hemorrhagic lesion in the pons.

22.   Which of the following labeled areas represents the most likely position of this hemorrhagic lesion? (   )

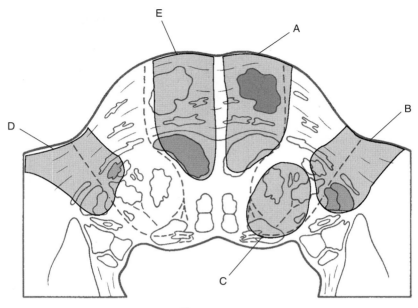

Figure 17–6

23.   Which of the following is the best localizing sign in this patient?

○ (A) Headache
○ (B) Loss of pain and thermal sensation on the body
○ (C) Loss of pain and thermal sensation on the face
○ (D) Stupor
○ (E) Weakness of facial muscles

○ (A) Left spinal laminae I and II only
○ (B) Left spinal laminae I, II, and V
○ (C) Right spinal laminae I and II only
○ (D) Right spinal laminae I, II, and V
○ (E) Right spinal laminae II, III, and IV

24.   A 4-year-old child is brought to the emergency department by her mother. The examination reveals burns on the girl's right hand that resulted from her touching a burner on the stove. Which of the following fiber types maintains a high-frequency firing rate in response to tissue damage?

○ (A) C only
○ (B) Aα
○ (C) Aβ
○ (D) Aδ only
○ (E) Aδ and C

26.   An 86-year old man presents with a loss of proprioception and vibratory sense on the left side of his body. CT reveals a small hemorrhagic lesion in the tegmentum of the midbrain. Which of the following thalamic nuclei receives input from the tract damaged by the lesion in this patient?

○ (A) Left ventral posterolateral nucleus
○ (B) Right ventral posterolateral nucleus
○ (C) Left ventral posteromedial nucleus
○ (D) Right ventral posteromedial nucleus
○ (E) Right ventral lateral nucleus

25.   A 51-year-old woman presents with a loss of pain and thermal sensation on her right foot and leg. MRI reveals an elongated tumor of the posterolateral aspect of the spinal cord suggesting damage to the primary sensory fibers conveying nociceptive (pain and thermal) input. These fibers terminate primarily in which of the following?

27.   An 87-year-old healthy man is brought to the emergency department after passing out at home. He is lethargic and has a headache. The examination reveals the loss of pain, thermal, proprioception, and vibratory sensations over his lower extremity. CT shows a hemorrhagic lesion in the somatosensory cortex. Which of the following labeled areas represent the most likely location of this lesion in this patient? See Figure 17–7. (   )

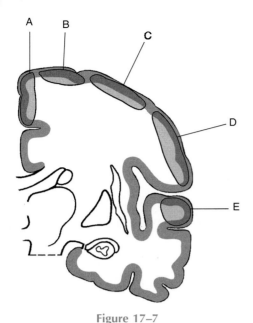

Figure 17–7

Questions 28 through 32 are based on the following patient:

A 59-year-old man with uncontrolled hypertension is brought to the emergency department by his wife. He is stuporous but is able to cooperate in the examination. His tongue deviates to the left on protrusion, but there are no other motor deficits. He has a loss of proprioception, discriminative touch, and vibratory sense over the right upper and lower extremities. The response to pain and thermal stimulation on the face or body is normal. The wife reports that these symptoms appeared suddenly while her husband was splitting firewood.

28.   Which of the following represents the best localizing sign in this patient?

○ (A) Loss of discriminative touch in the right lower extremity
○ (B) Loss of discriminative touch in the right upper extremity
○ (C) Deviation of the tongue to the left on protrusion
○ (D) Loss of proprioception on the right upper extremity
○ (E) Deviation of the tongue to the right on protrusion

29.   The combination of deficits in this patient would most likely place this lesion in which of the following areas?

○ (A) Posterior columns of cervical spinal cord
○ (B) Medial medulla
○ (C) Tegmentum of the pons

○ (D) Posterior medulla including the posterior column nuclei
○ (E) Lateral medulla

30.   The sensory deficit in this patient would suggest that the damage is specifically located where?

○ (A) Posterior column nuclei bilaterally
○ (B) Medial lemniscus of the left
○ (C) Anterior (ventral) parts of the medial lemniscus bilaterally
○ (D) Medial lemniscus on the right
○ (E) Posterior (dorsal) parts of the medial lemniscus bilaterally

31.   Based on the patient's history, which of the following is the most likely cause of this lesion?

○ (A) A small glial tumor
○ (B) An aneurysm compressing on the medulla
○ (C) A meningioma of the base of the skull
○ (D) An infarction
○ (E) Minor trauma

32.   Assuming this to be a vascular lesion, an occlusion of which of the following vessels would most likely result in the deficits experienced by this patient?

○ (A) Posterior spinal artery
○ (B) Posterior inferior cerebellar artery
○ (C) Anterior inferior cerebellar artery
○ (D) Paramedian pontine arteries
○ (E) Anterior spinal artery

33.   C-fibers conveying information from the body have their cell bodies of origin in ipsilateral posterior root ganglia, convey pain and thermal sensations, and have a conduction velocity of

○ (A) 80 to 120 m/sec
○ (B) 35 to 75 m/sec
○ (C) 30 to 50 m/sec
○ (D) 5 to 30 m/sec
○ (E) 0.5 to 3 m/sec

34.   A 27-year-old woman is referred to a neurologist by her family physician. She complains of "funny feelings" in her left "leg." The examination reveals a loss of position and vibratory sense over the left lower extremity. Suspecting multiple sclerosis, the physician orders an MRI, which shows a patch of demyelination in the pons involving the medial lemniscus. Which of the following represents the most likely location of the cell bodies of origin for these damaged fibers?

○ (A) Left gracile nucleus
○ (B) Right gracile nucleus
○ (C) Left cuneate nucleus
○ (D) Posterior root ganglia on the left below T6
○ (E) Ventral posteromedial nucleus

35.   The CT of a 62-year-old man reveals a hemorrhagic lesion in the area of the somatosensory cortex shown below. See Figure 17–8.

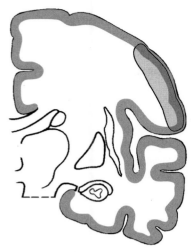

Figure 17–8

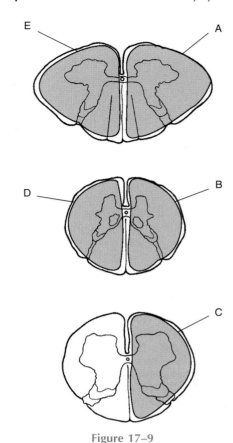

Figure 17–9

Which of the following thalamic nuclei project to this particular area of the primary somatosensory cortex?

- ○ (A) Ventral posterolateral
- ○ (B) Ventral lateral
- ○ (C) Ventral posteromedial
- ○ (D) Ventral anterior
- ○ (E) Centromedian

36. A 61-year-old man presents to the emergency department with a severe headache. He complains that his headache came on suddenly, nothing he took helped, and it made him sick to his stomach. CT reveals an infarct in the medulla on the right side within the territory served by the posterior spinal artery. Which of the following deficits would most likely be seen in this patient?

- ○ (A) Loss of pain and thermal sensation on the right side of the body
- ○ (B) Loss of pain and thermal sensation on the left side of the body
- ○ (C) Loss of proprioception, discriminative touch, and vibratory sense on the left side of the body
- ○ (D) Loss of proprioception, discriminative touch, and vibratory sense on the right side of the body
- ○ (E) Loss of pain and thermal sensation on the right side of the face

37. A 47-year-old man is brought to the emergency department after an accident at a construction site. He has sustained a severe back injury; CT reveals a fracture of two vertebrae. The examination reveals a loss of pain and thermal sensations beginning just above the umbilicus and extending caudad on the left side of the body and a loss of proprioception and vibratory sense on the right lower extremity. These are the principal sensory deficits seen in the Brown-Séquard syndrome. Which of the following labeled areas would most likely represent the location of the lesion in this patient? (   )

38. Rapidly and slowly adapting receptors are activated by skin indentations or joint movements. Rapidly adapting receptors, such as Pacinian corpuscles, generate action potentials where?

- ○ (A) At the initiation of a stimulus, during the time the stimulus is present (but at a lower rate), and at the removal of the stimulus
- ○ (B) At the removal of a stimulus but not at its initiation
- ○ (C) At the initiation of the stimulus and at the removal of the stimulus; but no action potentials are generated during maintained stimulation
- ○ (D) At the initiation of a stimulus but not at its removal
- ○ (E) At the initiation of a stimulus, during the time the stimulus is present (but at a higher rate) and at the removal of the stimulus

39. During a routine neurologic examination of a healthy 21-year-old woman, the physician purposefully stimulates receptors that code direction and velocity of movement. Which of the following receptors may function as both a rapidly adapting and a slowly adapting receptor and may code direction and velocity?

- ○ (A) Merkel cell receptor
- ○ (B) Meissner corpuscle
- ○ (C) Pacinian corpuscle
- ○ (D) Free nerve ending
- ○ (E) Hair follicle receptor

40. The posterior (dorsal) trigeminothalamic tract originates from cells located in which of the following brainstem nuclei?

○ (A) Mesencephalic nucleus
○ (B) Anterolateral region of the principal sensory nucleus
○ (C) Spinal trigeminal nucleus
○ (D) Posteromedial region of the principal sensory nucleus
○ (E) Motor nucleus of the trigeminal nerve

41. A 61-year-old morbidly obese man with uncontrolled hypertension presents with a loss of discriminative touch and pain and thermal sensations from the face and oral cavity. Which of the following represents the most likely location of the primary sensory cell bodies that relay this information into the brainstem?

○ (A) Spinal trigeminal nucleus
○ (B) Trigeminal ganglion
○ (C) Geniculate ganglion
○ (D) Superior ganglia of IX and X
○ (E) Principal (chief) sensory nucleus

42. During a routine neurologic examination of a healthy 29-year-old athlete the physician tests the jaw jerk reflex. The physician gently taps the area of the mental protuberance of the mandible, stretching muscle spindles of the masticatory muscles, and these same muscles contract. The cell bodies of origin for the primary sensory fibers forming the afferent limb of the jaw jerk reflex are located in which of the following structures?

○ (A) Spinal trigeminal nucleus, pars caudalis
○ (B) Trigeminal (semilunar) ganglion
○ (C) Geniculate ganglion
○ (D) Principal sensory nucleus
○ (E) Mesencephalic nucleus

43. A 21-year-old anorexic woman presents to her family physician complaining of sensory disturbances on her face. During the ensuing neurologic examination the physician gently touches a wisp of cotton to the woman's cornea and observes there is no response. The corneal (blink) reflex is absent. Which of the following structures contains the cell bodies of origin for the primary sensory fibers forming the afferent limb of the corneal reflex?

○ (A) Mesencephalic nucleus
○ (B) Geniculate ganglion
○ (C) Trigeminal (semilunar) ganglion
○ (D) Spinal trigeminal nucleus, pars caudalis
○ (E) Principal sensory nucleus

44. Fibers originating from cell bodies in the principal (chief) sensory nucleus that project to the contralateral dorsal thalamus travel where?

○ (A) In the anterolateral system
○ (B) In the posterior (dorsal) trigeminothalamic tract
○ (C) In the anterior (ventral) trigeminothalamic tract
○ (D) In the medial lemniscus
○ (E) In the mesencephalic tract

45. A 77-year-old morbidly obese woman is brought to the emergency department by paramedics. She is unconscious and unresponsive. Suspecting a stroke, the physician orders CT, which reveals a hemorrhagic lesion in the caudal thalamus including the centromedian, ventral posteromedial, and posterolateral nuclei. This hemorrhage has most likely originated from which of the following vessels?

○ (A) Lenticulostriate arteries
○ (B) Thalamoperforating artery(ies)
○ (C) Medial posterior choroidal artery
○ (D) Thalamogeniculate artery(ies)
○ (E) Anterior choroidal artery

Questions 46 through 50 are based on the following patient:

A 20-year-old man is brought to the emergency department by paramedics and accompanied by a policeman. The emergency department physician learns that the man's injuries are the result of an altercation at a bar. The man is alert but in pain. The examination reveals that the man has been stabbed in the back. He has profound weakness of the left lower extremity, loss of discriminative touch, vibratory sense, and proprioception on the left lower extremity, and loss of pain and thermal sensation on the right side of the body beginning at the level of the nipple. When the physician touches a tuning fork to the iliac crest and lower ribs on the left side, the man does not perceive vibration.

46. Based on information gathered in the examination of this patient, which of the following represents the most likely location of the lesion in the spinal cord of this man?

○ (A) T2–T3 levels on the left
○ (B) T2–T3 levels on the right
○ (C) T5–T6 levels on the left
○ (D) T7 level on the right
○ (E) T7 level on the left

47. The significant weakness of the left lower extremity in this patient correlates with damage to which of the following tracts of the spinal cord?

○ (A) Rubrospinal tract
○ (B) Reticulospinal fibers
○ (C) Vestibulospinal fibers
○ (D) Anterior corticospinal tract
○ (E) Lateral corticospinal tract

48. The loss of pain and thermal sensations in this patient reflects damage to which of the following spinal cord structures?

○ (A) Anterolateral system on the right
○ (B) Anterolateral system on the left
○ (C) Posterior column on the right

○ (D) Posterolateral tract (of Lissauer) on the left
○ (E) Posterior columns and posterolateral tract on the left

49. The loss of proprioception, discriminative touch, and vibratory sense in this patient is caused by damage to which of the following structures in the spinal cord?

○ (A) Cuneate fasciculus on the left
○ (B) Gracile and cuneate fasciculi on the right
○ (C) Gracile fasciculus on the left
○ (D) Cuneate and gracile fasciculi on the left
○ (E) Posterolateral tract (of Lissauer) on the right

50. Taking all the deficits seen in this patient into consideration, the injury has most likely resulted in what problem?

○ (A) Syringomyelia
○ (B) Brown-Séquard syndrome
○ (C) Claude syndrome
○ (D) Horner syndrome
○ (E) Central cord syndrome

51. The peripheral receptors most specifically associated with coding tissue damage that is perceived as pain are

○ (A) Naked (free) nerve endings
○ (B) Pacinian corpuscles
○ (C) Ruffini terminals
○ (D) Meissner corpuscle
○ (E) Merkel cell endings

52. A 9-year-old boy is brought to the emergency department by his parents after falling out of a treehouse. The examination reveals the loss of pain, thermal, and position sense on his right upper extremity. Plain spine radiographs show a fracture of C5. These findings (examination and spine radiographs) suggest that the cell bodies of primary sensory fibers are damaged. The cell bodies for pain, thermal, and position sense are located in which of the following structures?

○ (A) Spinal laminae I, II, and V
○ (B) Gracile and cuneate nuclei
○ (C) Posterior root ganglia
○ (D) Spinal laminae IV through VIII
○ (E) Sympathetic chain ganglia

53. A 37-year-old man presents to the neurologist with ill-defined sensory losses on the body. The examination reveals that stimulation of some dermatomes on the upper extremity and trunk are not perceived by the patient. Which of the following most accurately characterizes what constitutes a dermatome?

○ (A) A strip of skin innervated by two adjacent posterior roots
○ (B) A group of muscles innervated by a single anterior root
○ (C) A strip of skin innervated by the Aα and Aβ fibers of a single posterior root
○ (D) A strip of skin innervated by alpha and gamma motor neurons

○ (E) A strip of skin innervated by the C and A-delta fibers of a single posterior root

54. The MRI of an 81-year-old woman reveals a lesion in the territory served by penetrating branches of the anterior spinal artery. Which of the following structures is most likely damaged by this lesion?

○ (A) Solitary tract and nucleus
○ (B) Spinal trigeminal tract and nucleus
○ (C) Anterior (ventral) trigeminothalamic fibers
○ (D) Anterolateral system
○ (E) Nucleus ambiguus

55. A 22-year-old woman complains of "numbness" of her hands and "arms." The examination reveals that the woman does not perceive pain and thermal sensation on her left upper extremity; she actually has some cuts and bruises but she did not realize she had injured herself. An electrophysiologic test reveals dysfunction of those primary sensory fibers conveying pain and thermal sensations from the left upper extremity and trunk. Before terminating in laminae of the spinal cord, those fibers conveying pain and thermal sensations in this patient ascend or descend variable distances in which of the following?

○ (A) Anterolateral system on the left
○ (B) Anterolateral system on the right
○ (C) Anterior (ventral) white commissure
○ (D) Posterolateral tract on the right
○ (E) Posterolateral tract on the left

56. A 68-year-old morbidly obese man with uncontrolled hypertension presents with symptoms suggesting a neurodegenerative disease. The examination reveals a selective loss of nociceptive input from the face and oral cavity. An electrophysiologic examination suggests dysfunction of Aδ and C fibers. Which of the following represents the main central target for Aδ and C fibers traveling on the trigeminal nerve?

○ (A) Mesencephalic nucleus
○ (B) Principal (chief) sensory nucleus
○ (C) Spinal trigeminal nucleus, pars oralis
○ (D) Spinal trigeminal nucleus, pars interpolaris
○ (E) Spinal trigeminal nucleus, pars caudalis

57. Raphespinal fibers that modulate the transmission of pain information through synaptic contacts on inhibitory interneurons in the posterior horn and in the spinal trigeminal nucleus arise from what structure?

○ (A) Nucleus raphae pallidus
○ (B) Nucleus raphae obscurus
○ (C) Nucleus raphae magnus
○ (D) Nucleus raphae pontis
○ (E) Superior central nucleus

58. The CT of an 82-year-old man reveals a hemorrhagic lesion in the middle third of the postcentral gyrus. He complains of sensory deficits that are consistent with this lesion. The location of this lesion is shown in Figure 17–10.

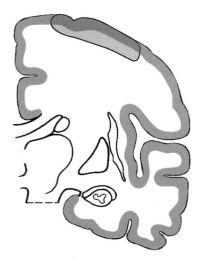

Figure 17–10

Which of the following nuclei contain the thalamic relay neurons that project to the area of the cortex involved in this lesion?

○ (A) Medial portions of the ventral posterolateral nucleus
○ (B) Ventral posteromedial nucleus
○ (C) Central lateral nucleus
○ (D) Lateral portions of the ventral posterolateral nucleus
○ (E) Ventral anterior nucleus

ANSWERS

1. **(D)** A slowly progressing deficit, especially one developing over months or even years, is highly likely to result from a tumor. This patient had no trauma; vascular lesions result in sudden deficits frequently accompanied by headache and nausea or even a loss of consciousness. Disc problems may appear slowly or quickly, but often cause back or extremity pain. It is unlikely that disc problems would result in symmetric deficits.
FN2e 8–9, 11–13, 280–282

2. **(B)** Fibers of the anterolateral system convey information that is interpreted by the nervous system as pain and thermal sensations from the body. The same sensations from the face are conveyed via the anterior (ventral) trigeminothalamic tract. The medial longitudinal fasciculus does not function in the sensory sphere.
FN2e 277–281

3. **(E)** The loss of discriminative touch, vibratory sense, and proprioception in this patient involves the lower extremities. While the postcentral gyrus is the larger portion of the primary somatosensory cortex, the lower extremity is not represented in this part (gyrus) of the cerebral cortex.
FN2e 260–263

4. **(D)** A slow-growing solid tumor located in the falx cerebri is statistically almost certainly a meningioma. Vascular lesions, such as dural arteriovenous malformations, are rarely seen. Glial cell tumors are found in the substance of the brain; some malignant astrocytomas may grow very rapidly.
FN2e 32–33, 115, 261–263, 281–283

5. **(E)** The contralateral lower extremity is somatotopically represented in the posterior paracentral gyrus; this part of the somatosensory cortex receives input interpreted as of proprioception, discriminative touch, pain, and thermal sense from this part of the body. Normally, the posterior paracentral gyri (cortex and subjacent white matter) are closely adjacent to each other at the midline, separated only by the falx cerebri and a narrow subarachnoid space; these collectively span 10 to 15 mm in width. In this patient, a large tumor in the falx cerebri has affected the posterior paracentral gyri, bilaterally resulting in the sensory losses in both lower extremities.
FN2e 261–263, 281–283

6. **(B)** The deficits in this patient indicate a lesion of the cuneate nucleus (proprioceptive loss from upper extremity) on the left and the spinal trigeminal tract and/or nucleus (pain and thermal loss from the face) on the left. These structures are adjacent to each other in the caudal medulla and are in the territories of branches of the posterior spinal artery and, in the case of the spinal trigeminal structures, the posterior inferior cerebellar artery.
FN2e 169–170, 259–261, 284–286

7. **(B)** The cell body of the first-order neuron in this pathway is located in the ipsilateral posterior root ganglion below T6 (lower extremity); the central process forms the gracile fasciculus and terminates in the ipsilateral gracile nucleus. The cell bodies of the second-order neurons are in the gracile nucleus. The axons loop toward the midline as internal arcuate fibers, cross the midline, and ascend to the ventral posterolateral nucleus as part of the medial lemniscus.
FN2e 259–262

8. **(E)** The heavily myelinated fibers conveying discriminative touch, proprioception, and vibratory sense enter the posterior root and coalesce to form the medial division of the posterior root. The lightly myelinated fibers conveying pain and thermal information collect to form the lateral division of the posterior root.
FN2e 143–144, 259–261

9. **(D)** The loss of pain and thermal sense on the left side of the body is indicative of a lesion involving anterolateral system fibers on the right. This patient also has a proprioceptive deficit of the left lower extremity. The portion of the medial lemniscus conveying this information is immediately adjacent to the anterolateral system. Because these medial lemniscus fibers originate from the gracile nucleus (leg representation) on the contralateral side of the medulla, a right-sided lesion results in a left-sided deficit. This area of the midbrain is in the territory of penetrating branches of the quadrigeminal artery.
FN2e 197–198, 261–263, 280–283

10. **(C)** There is an inverse relationship between the size of the receptive field and the representation of that body part in the somatosensory cortex. Body parts with small receptive fields (fingertips, lips) have large representations in the sensory cortex, whereas body parts with large receptive fields (proximal parts of the extremities, trunk) have correspondingly small representations in the sensory cortex.
FN2e 258

11. **(A)** Aα fibers are heavily myelinated, rapidly conducting fibers that enter the spinal cord via the medial division of the posterior root. Those that arise in the muscle spindle participate in the tendon reflex.
FN2e 143–145, 146, 258–259

12. **(C)** Slowly adapting receptors (a) respond to the initial application of the stimulus by an increase in action potentials (these receptors have a slow resting rate of action potentials); (b) continue to fire, but at a lower rate, as long as the stimulus is present; and (c) have an increased firing rate at the moment the stimulus is removed.
FN2e 257–259

13. **(B)** The central processes of primary sensory fibers conveying discriminative touch and vibratory sense arise from large unipolar cells in the posterior root ganglion and send their central processes into the posterior columns. Those inputs from the upper extremity arise from posterior root ganglia above T6 (T1–C4), whereas those inputs from the lower extremity arise from posterior root ganglia below T6.
FN2e 259–261

14. **(D)** The bilateral loss of pain and thermal sensations from the lower extremity indicates a lesion of the anterior (ventral) white commissure in lumbar and upper sacral levels of the spinal cord. This lesion damages the second-order fibers conveying pain and thermal sensations as they cross the midline. Because this lesion damages fibers coming from both sides, the deficits are bilateral and reflect those parts of the body from which the sensory input originated.
FN2e 144, 148–149, 280–281

15. **(E)** The Pacinian corpuscle is a rapidly adapting receptor that is sensitive to vibratory types of input. This encapsulated ending transduces the peripheral stimulus into a chain of action potentials that travel on heavily myelinated fibers of the posterior column–medial lemniscus system. This input is interpreted as vibration by the brain.
FN2e 256–258

16. **(B)** The Pacinian corpuscle (a mechanoreceptor) is associated with a group II fiber and has a conduction velocity in the range of 35 to 75 m/sec. This receptor, and its central fibers, conduct information interpreted by the CNS as vibratory sense.
FN2e 257, 259

17. **(B)** Group (or class) II fibers are classified as Aβ and are predominately related to skin mechanoreceptors and to some secondary muscle spindles. These fibers are in the range of 6 to 12 μm in diameter and have conduction velocities in the range of 35 to 75 m/sec.
FN2e 257–259

18. **(D)** The alternating sensory losses (crossed deficits) relating to a long tract (anterolateral system) and a cranial nerve (spinal trigeminal tract and nucleus) are characteristics of brainstem lesions. The loss of pain and thermal sense on the right side of the face is the best localizing sign because it identifies a specific cranial nerve and specifies on which side the lesion is located (in this case on the patient's right side). The lesion is within the territory served by the posterior inferior cerebellar artery (PICA), and this particular alternating sensory loss is one of the cardinal features of the PICA (Wallenberg or lateral medullary) syndrome.
FN2e 170–171, 280–282, 286–287

19. **(B)** In the medulla, the medial lemniscus (composed of second-order neurons in the posterior column–medial lemniscus system) is vertically oriented. The lower extremity is anterior, and the upper extremity is posterior within the lemniscus. An easy way to remember this is to think of one half of a headless person (the head is represented in the trigeminal system) standing on the pyramid. Located posterior to the medial lemniscus along the midline is the tectospinal tract (sometimes called the tectobulbospinal system) and the medial longitudinal fasciculus.
FN2e 260–262

20. **(A)** The pars caudalis is that portion of the spinal trigeminal nucleus located between the level of the obex of the medulla and the C2–C3 levels of the spinal cord posterior horn gray matter. This nucleus is the primary source of anterior (ventral) trigeminothalamic fibers that convey pain and thermal sensation from the medulla to the ventral posteromedial nucleus on the contralateral side.
FN2e 285–287

21. **(D)** Axons of cells of the pars caudalis of the spinal trigeminal nucleus cross the midline to form the anterior (ventral) trigeminothalamic tract on the opposite side. These fibers convey pain and thermal sense from the pars caudalis on one side to the ventral posteromedial nucleus (VPM) on the opposite side. The VPM, in turn, projects to face areas of the somatosensory cortex.
FN2e 284–287

22. **(B)** Alternating sensory deficits (alternate or crossed deficits) are generally characteristic of lesions in the brainstem. In this case the lesion involves the spinal trigeminal tract, which is composed of primary sensory fibers from the ipsilateral (left) face and fibers of the anterolateral system conveying information from the contralateral (right) side of the body. These structures are located in the lateral portion of the pontine tegmentum within the territories of long circumferential branches of the basilar artery and, to a lesser degree, penetrating branches of the anterior inferior cerebellar artery.
FN2e 178–180, 280–282

23. **(E)** The weakness of facial muscles localizes this lesion to the pons-medulla junction as likely involving

the facial nucleus and/or the root of the facial nerve. The rostral portions of the spinal trigeminal tract and the anterolateral system are located in lateral parts of the pontine tegmentum immediately adjacent to the facial nucleus and exiting facial fibers. Taking all signs and symptoms together, this lesion is at the pons-medulla junction on the patient's left and involves the lateral portion of the pontine tegmentum.
FN2e 178–180, 280–282

24.   **(E)** Aδ fibers (conduction velocity of 5 to 30 m/sec) and C fibers (conduction velocity of 0.5 to 2 m/sec) respond to tissue damage, either hot or cold, by steadily increasing their firing frequency. The pain resulting from tissue damage indicates a sustained firing rate of these fibers. C fibers are also activated by chemicals released at injury sites such as bradykinins or insect venom.
FN2e 275

25.   **(D)** Primary sensory fibers conveying nociceptive input (pain and thermal perceptions) have their cell bodies in the ipsilateral posterior root ganglion and enter through the medial division of the posterior root and terminate in laminae of the posterior horn. Aδ fibers terminate primarily in laminae I and V. C fibers terminate primarily in lamina II. Cell bodies in these laminae send their axons across the midline in the ventral (anterior) white commissure to join the contralateral anterolateral system.
FN2e 277–281

26.   **(B)** Proprioception and vibratory sense are conveyed by the posterior column–medial lemniscus system. In the midbrain, these fibers, on the right, have originated from the posterior column nuclei on the left side of the medulla and crossed at the level of the sensory decussation. Fibers within the right medial lemniscus will terminate in the ventral posterolateral nucleus on the right side.
FN2e 281–283

27.   **(A)** The primary somatosensory cortex consists of the postcentral gyrus and the posterior paracentral gyrus. The lower extremity is represented in the posterior paracentral gyrus. The postcentral gyrus can be generally divided into thirds for convenience in placing the remainder of the body in the sensory cortex. The face is represented in about the lateral third, the upper extremity and hand in about the middle third, and the trunk in about the medial third.
FN2e 263–264

28.   **(C)** The deviation of the tongue on protrusion suggests a lesion of the hypoglossal nucleus, intramedullary hypoglossal fibers, or root of the hypoglossal nerve. This clearly localizes the lesion to the medulla. Long tract signs may suggest a lesion at several different levels of the neuraxis.
FN2e 259–261, 396–398

29.   **(B)** The sensory deficit in this patient, when considered in concert with the deviation of the tongue, places this lesion in the medial regions of the medulla. This area of the medulla includes the medial lemniscus, fascicles of

the hypoglossal nerve, and ascending anterior (ventral) trigeminothalamic fibers.
FN2e 260–262

30.   **(B)** The loss of proprioceptive information on the patient's right upper and lower extremities, when considered in concert with the deviation of the tongue to the left on protrusion, puts this lesion in the medulla on the left side. Fibers of the medial lemniscus originate from the gracile and cuneate nuclei on the right side, cross in the sensory decussation, and collect to form the contralateral medial lemniscus. Consequently, a lesion of the medial lemniscus on the left will result in a loss of the corresponding sensory modalities on the right side of the body.
FN2e 260–262

31.   **(D)** The symptoms appeared suddenly while the patient was splitting firewood. Although neither the patient, nor his wife, specified an exact time frame, this type of activity requires significant exertion and these symptoms probably appeared over a few seconds. No injuries were reported. Tumors usually give rise to symptoms that appear over weeks, months or even years.
FN2e 259–261, 396–397

32.   **(E)** The nucleus and fibers of the hypoglossal nerve (deviation of the tongue), the medial lemniscus (proprioceptive and vibratory sense losses), and corticospinal fibers of the pyramid are all within the territory served by penetrating branches of the anterior spinal artery. Branches of the anterior spinal artery, in general, penetrate the medulla by alternating to the right and to the left.
FN2e 261

33.   **(E)** The central processes of these small-diameter C fibers are finely myelinated, are slowly conducting, and enter the lateral division of the posterior root. They pass into the posterolateral tract (of Lissauer), where these axons may ascend or descend and then enter the posterior horn where they synapse primarily in spinal lamina II.
FN2e 260, 275–277

34.   **(A)** The gracile nucleus on the left receives proprioceptive, discriminative touch, and vibratory sense input from the lower extremity on that side. Cell bodies in the left gracile nucleus send axons across the midline to form the contralateral medial lemniscus. In the pons, the lower extremity is represented laterally in the medial lemniscus and the upper extremity is represented in the medial part of this fiber bundle. In this patient a right-sided lesion results in left-sided deficits.
FN2e 260–263

35.   **(C)** The face area of the primary somatosensory cortex is located immediately superior to the lateral (sylvian) sulcus. This portion of the somatosensory cortex receives thalamocortical projections from the ventral posteromedial nucleus on the same side. This thalamic nucleus receives a crossed projection from the spinal trigeminal nucleus (via anterior or ventral trigeminothalamic fibers) and an uncrossed projection from the principal sensory nucleus (via the posterior or dorsal trigeminothalamic tract).
FN2e 265–267, 285–287

36. **(D)** The gracile and cuneate nuclei of the medulla are located within the territory served by branches of the posterior spinal artery. An infarct of the right gracile and cuneate nuclei would result in a loss of proprioception, vibratory sense, and discriminative touch on the same side as the lesion.
FN2e 169–170, 260–262

37. **(D)** The alternating sensory losses on the body seen in this patient are characteristic of spinal cord lesions; there are no cranial nerve motor or sensory deficits. The approximate level of the lesion is established by the pain and thermal losses beginning at about T8–T9 (the umbilicus is at T10). This would place the damage to the cord at about T9–T10. The proprioception loss is ipsilateral to the lesion, and the pain and thermal loss is contralateral to the lesion. The cord is damaged on the right side.
FN2e 278, 280–282

38. **(C)** Rapidly adapting receptors respond to the initial application of the stimulus with a burst of action potentials, are silent during a maintained stimulation, but respond with a burst of action potentials when the stimulus is removed. These receptors have little or no background activity before application of a stimulus or after its removal.
FN2e 256–258

39. **(E)** Hair follicles may function both as rapidly adapting or slowly adapting receptors. The sensory fiber (Aβ) for the hair follicle has a conduction velocity in the range of 35 to 75 m/sec. These receptors code direction of movement and can, based on the slowness or rapidity of the stimulus, code velocity.
FN2e 256–259

40. **(D)** The posterior trigeminothalamic tract is made up of second-order neurons whose cell bodies of origin are found in the principal sensory nucleus and whose axons ascend uncrossed to terminate in the ventral posteromedial nucleus (VPM). Fibers from the principal sensory nucleus that project to the contralateral VPM cross the midline and join the anterior (ventral) trigeminothalamic tract. These fibers convey discriminative tactile sensations from the face and oral cavity. The primary sensory fibers feeding this nucleus are larger-diameter Aβ axons with conduction velocities of 35 to 75 m/sec.
FN2e 265–267, 285–287

41. **(B)** The primary sensory fibers for discriminative touch, pain, and thermal sense from the face and oral cavity have their cell bodies of origin in the trigeminal (semilunar) ganglion. Whereas pain and thermal sensations from the surface of the ear, external auditory meatus, and surface of the eardrum are conveyed on cranial nerves VII, IX, and X, these are comparatively insignificant compared with the contributions of the trigeminal nerve. Centrally, these fibers terminate in the principal sensory nucleus (discriminative touch) and in the spinal trigeminal nucleus (pain and thermal sense).
FN2e 265–267, 284–287

42. **(E)** Proprioceptive input from muscle spindles in the masticatory muscles is transmitted centrally on fibers whose cell bodies are located in the mesencephalic nucleus of the trigeminal nerve. Collaterals from these primary afferent fibers distribute to the motor nuclei of the trigeminal nerve, which, in turn, activate the muscles of mastication.
FN2e 267

43. **(C)** The afferent limb of the corneal reflex travels via the nasociliary branches of the ophthalmic nerve. The cell bodies of origin for these fibers are located in the trigeminal (semilunar) ganglion on the ipsilateral side. The central processes of these afferent fibers distribute to the spinal trigeminal nucleus, pars caudalis. Collaterals of the ascending trigeminothalamic fibers distribute to the facial motor nuclei.
FN2e 285

44. **(C)** The principal sensory nucleus of the trigeminal nerve gives rise to second-order neurons, some of which ascend to the ventral posteromedial nucleus (VPM) on the ipsilateral side as the posterior (dorsal) trigeminothalamic fibers and others of which cross the midline to join the anterior (ventral) trigeminothalamic fibers to enter the contralateral VPM.
FN2e 265–266

45. **(D)** The thalamogeniculate artery usually arises from P_2 and may actually do so as several branches. These arteries, as their name implies, supply the medial and lateral geniculate nuclei as well as the ventral posteromedial and posterolateral nuclei, pulvinar, centromedian nucleus, and other structures in this immediate area.
FN2e 262–263, 283

46. **(A)** The loss of pain sensations on the right side of the body, beginning just below the nipple, points to the answer. Pain and temperature fibers (a) cross the midline in the anterior (ventral) white commissure, ascending 1 to 2 levels as they do so, and (b) the area at the level of the nipple represents the T4 dermatome. A stab wound at the T2 to T3 level on the left would damage the anterolateral system and result in the pain/temperature loss on the right (opposite to the lesion) side of the body caudad to the injury. This left-sided injury also correlates with the left-sided motor deficit and proprioception losses.
FN2e 259–261, 280–282

47. **(E)** Corticospinal fibers (as well as other descending fibers) influence the activity of lower motor neurons (alpha motor neurons). Sudden removal of the influence of corticospinal fibers will result in a loss of voluntary motor activity and a profound weakness of skeletal muscles distal to the lesion on the side of the spinal cord injury.
FN2e 280, 282

48. **(B)** Fibers conveying signals interpreted by the brain as pain and thermal sensations originate from cell bodies in the posterior horn (these are second-order neurons) and cross in the anterior white commissure to join the anterolateral system on the side contralateral to the origin of the information. The spinal lesion in this

patient resulted in a loss of pain/thermal sensations on the right side of the body; by recognizing the course of these fibers, one can determine that the lesion is on the left.
FN2e 279–280

49. **(C)** The central processes of fibers conveying signals interpreted by the nervous system as proprioception, vibratory sense, and discriminative touch arise from unipolar cell bodies in the ipsilateral posterior root ganglion, pass through the medial division of the posterior root, and turn rostrally to form the posterior columns. Consequently, these fibers are ipsilateral to their side of origin; the gracile fasciculus conveys information from the ipsilateral lower extremity and the cuneate fasciculus from the ipsilateral upper extremity.
FN2e 259–262

50. **(B)** This injury essentially resulted in a spinal cord hemisection (Brown-Séquard syndrome) at about the T2–T3 level of the spinal cord on the left. A variety of lesions can give rise to what may be called a functional hemisection of the spinal cord. For example, a tumor may compress and deform the spinal cord, impinging on one half but leaving the other half intact. Functionally, the spinal cord is "hemisected" by the tumor, although not necessarily permanently damaged.
FN2e 280, 282

51. **(A)** Group $A\delta$ and C fibers have free/naked nerve endings. These fibers respond to mechanical tissue damage (both), to heat that may result in tissue damage ($A\delta$), to cold that may result in tissue damage (both), and to substances released resultant to tissue damage, such as histamine, bradykinin, or insect venom (C-fibers). All of these events may be interpreted as pain.
FN2e 275–277

52. **(C)** The cell bodies for all primary somatosensory input from the body (except cranial nerves), including that conveyed on $A\delta$ and C fibers, are located in posterior root ganglia on the ipsilateral side. These ganglia also contain unipolar cell bodies conveying GVA information from the gut. Information conveyed on $A\delta$ and C fibers and via GVA fibers enters the spinal cord via the lateral division of the posterior root.
FN2e 275–277

53. **(E)** A dermatome is a strip of skin innervated by the cutaneous afferent fibers of a particular spinal nerve. Adjacent dermatomes partially overlap (spinal) or, in the case of the trigeminal nerve, do not overlap. In addition to some tactile/touch receptors, the dermatome contains the peripheral endings of $A\delta$ and C fibers.
FN2e 275–277

54. **(C)** The anterior trigeminothalamic tract is located laterally adjacent to the medial lemniscus as a some-what diffusely organized fiber bundle. It is in the general territory of the anterior spinal artery. This fiber bundle is composed of second-order neurons in the pathway conveying pain and thermal sensations to the thalamus from the contralateral trigeminal nucleus, pars caudalis.
FN2e 169–170, 265–266

55. **(E)** Primary sensory fibers conveying pain and thermal signals from the body are $A\delta$ and C fibers. The cell bodies of origin for these fibers are located in the posterior root ganglia and their central processes enter the cord via the posterolateral sulcus. $A\delta$ fibers bifurcate, ascend three to five levels in the posterolateral fasciculus, and terminate primarily in spinal laminae of the posterior horn. C fibers bifurcate and ascend or descend one or two levels in the posterolateral fasciculus before terminating in the posterior horn.
FN2e 279–281

56. **(E)** Pain and thermal sensations from the face, oral cavity, and external ear are carried on cranial nerve V with minor contributions from cranial nerves VII, IX, and X. These signals are carried by $A\delta$ and C fibers on each of these cranial nerves. Centrally, these primary afferent fibers join the spinal trigeminal tract and synapse in the medially adjacent caudal part (pars caudalis) of this nucleus. Each of these cranial nerves has sensory ganglia containing unipolar cell bodies.
FN2e 284–287

57. **(C)** Raphespinal fibers originate from serotonergic cells in the nucleus raphe magnus located in the rostral medulla and extending into the caudal pons. These fibers descend bilaterally in posterior parts of the lateral funiculus to terminate on interneurons primarily located in lamina II that will, in turn, presynaptically inhibit $A\delta$ and C fiber primary afferent axons. The nucleus raphe magnus also projects into the spinal trigeminal nucleus, pars caudalis.
FN2e 290–292

58. **(A)** In general, the body is somatotopically represented in the ventral posterolateral (VPL) nucleus with the lower extremity lateral and upper extremity medial. In this patient, the lesion involves the part of the somatosensory cortex in which the upper extremity and hand is represented. Cells located in medial portions of the ventral posterolateral nucleus (mVPL) receive ascending sensory input and project to about the middle third (hand and upper extremity area) of the postcentral gyrus. These thalamocortical axons traverse the posterior limb of the internal capsule. Fibers in the anterolateral system conveying input from the contralateral upper extremity arise from spinal cord levels T1 to C5 and would synapse in mVPL.
FN2e 263, 265–267, 285–287

CHAPTER 19

Viscerosensory Pathways

1. A 12-year-old girl is brought to the pediatrician's office with the complaint of severe abdominal pain. The examination suggests that she is suffering from an inflamed appendix. Her perception of pain results from impulses that are transmitted mainly by peripheral nerve fibers located where?

- ○ (A) Vagus nerve
- ○ (B) Sacral parasympathetic plexus
- ○ (C) Greater splanchnic nerve
- ○ (D) Glossopharyngeal nerve
- ○ (E) Sciatic nerve

2. A 3-year-old boy has been diagnosed with familial dysautonomia. He exhibits, as one feature typical of this disease, a reduced awareness of stimuli that normally evoke a painful sensation. Which of the following peripheral endings is characteristic of viscerosensory neurons that function as nociceptors?

- ○ (A) Pacinian corpuscles
- ○ (B) Meissner corpuscles
- ○ (C) Unencapsulated free nerve endings
- ○ (D) Ruffini endings
- ○ (E) Nuclear chain fibers

3. A 51-year-old diabetic man suffers a severe decrease in blood pressure when he rises from a supine position to a standing position. Which of the following is a potential site at which a disruption in function could lead to this condition?

- ○ (A) Solitary nucleus
- ○ (B) Superior cervical ganglion
- ○ (C) Nucleus cuneatus
- ○ (D) Hypoglossal nucleus
- ○ (E) Spinal ganglia at C5-T4 levels

4. Which of the following represents the most likely location of sensory receptors that monitor internal body temperature and serum osmolarity?

- ○ (A) Carotid bodies
- ○ (B) Hypothalamus
- ○ (C) Solitary nucleus
- ○ (D) Nucleus ambiguus
- ○ (E) Anterolateral medulla

5. A 42-year-old executive presents to his family physician with a complaint of pain in the midline of the upper abdominal wall just below the sternum. There is no evidence of trauma to the skin or musculature at the painful site. These observations suggest the possibility of a disorder involving the stomach. Why?

- ○ (A) The stomach and the skin of the painful area are innervated by the same primary afferent neurons.
- ○ (B) The stomach is innervated by vagal afferent neurons whose central processes terminate mainly in the trunk region of the ventral posterolateral nucleus of the thalamus.
- ○ (C) The stomach is innervated by sympathetic afferent neurons whose central processes terminate in the posterior horn of the spinal cord at the same levels that receive sensory input from the upper abdominal wall.
- ○ (D) The stomach is innervated by fibers of the glossopharyngeal nerve that terminate in the spinal trigeminal tract and nucleus.
- ○ (E) The stomach receives only sympathetic innervation.

6. The inability of a 29-year-old man to determine the precise origin of pain arising from inflammation in the ileum can be partially attributed to which of the following?

- ○ (A) Innervation of abdominal viscera by both vagal and sympathetic sensory neurons
- ○ (B) Large receptive fields and low density of sympathetic visceral afferent innervation of the gut
- ○ (C) Absence of a projection of viscerosensory pathways to the thalamus
- ○ (D) Absence of a projection of viscerosensory pathways to the cerebral cortex
- ○ (E) Absence of convergence in ascending viscerosensory pathways

7. Which of the following represents the most likely location of the cell bodies of primary sensory neurons that supply the carotid body and carotid sinus?

- ○ (A) Trigeminal ganglion
- ○ (B) Superior ganglion of the glossopharyngeal nerve
- ○ (C) Inferior ganglion of the glossopharyngeal nerve
- ○ (D) Superior ganglion of the vagus nerve
- ○ (E) Inferior ganglion of the vagus nerve

8. A 78-year-old man complains of increasingly frequent episodes of awakening at night to urinate. Arousal from sleep as a result of a full bladder is mediated by ascending visceral pathways that project to which of the following structures?

○ (A) Ascending reticular activating system
○ (B) Intermediolateral cell column of the lumbar spinal cord
○ (C) Solitary nucleus
○ (D) Ventral posterolateral nucleus of the thalamus
○ (E) Dorsal motor nucleus of the vagus

9. Which of the following is most characteristic of second-order sensory neurons that receive synaptic input from primary sympathetic afferent neurons?

○ (A) Have their cell bodies mainly in laminae II and III of the spinal cord posterior horn
○ (B) Project rostrally via the anterolateral system solely on the ipsilateral side
○ (C) Project rostrally primarily via the posterior columns to nucleus cuneatus and nucleus gracilis
○ (D) May project to either the ventral posterolateral nucleus or to the brainstem reticular formation
○ (E) Have no projections that contribute to perception of visceral stimuli

10. General visceral afferent (GVA) fibers of the glossopharyngeal and vagus nerves terminate mainly on second-order neurons whose cell bodies are located in which of the following structures? (   )

11. The anterolateral system conveys sympathetic, mostly nociceptive, visceral sensory signals to the ventral posterolateral (VPL) nucleus of the thalamus. Which of the following represents the main cortical target of visceral sensory signals relayed through the VPL?

○ (A) Paracentral lobule
○ (B) Parietal operculum and insula
○ (C) Cingulate gyrus
○ (D) Precentral gyrus
○ (E) Cingulate gyrus

ANSWERS

1. **(C)** The sensory fibers associated with parasympathetic nerves serve primarily physiologic functions, whereas the sensory fibers of sympathetic nerves are mainly nociceptors. Consequently, pain fibers from the appendix travel via the greater splanchnic nerve. **FN2e 295**

2. **(C)** The peripheral endings of nociceptive fibers, which may be unmyelinated (C) or thinly myelinated (Aδ), are free nerve endings. **FN2e 294**

3. **(A)** Orthostatic hypotension (an acute decrease in blood pressure when an upright position is assumed) indicates a disruption of the baroreceptor reflex. The

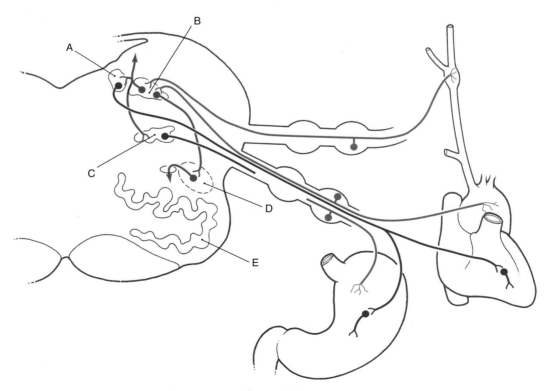

Figure 19–1

solitary nucleus, a key component of this reflex, receives signals from the baroreceptors of cranial nerves IX and X and, in turn, sends signals to vasopressor neurons of the rostral anterolateral medulla and vasodepressor cells of the dorsal vagal nucleus.
FN2e 301

4. **(B)** The hypothalamus contains neurons that directly monitor temperature and electrolyte concentrations in circulating blood. This information is used by the hypothalamus to maintain homeostasis by altering hypothalamic signals to both endocrine and visceromotor (autonomic) systems.
FN2e 295

5. **(C)** Although the mechanism of referred pain is incompletely understood, it is thought to result from convergence of visceral afferent and somatic afferent input onto second-order neurons of the spinal cord posterior horn. Signals from these second-order neurons are interpreted as originating from somatic tissues.
FN2e 297

6. **(B)** The generally imprecise localization of visceral pain is attributable to (1) the low density of nociceptor innervation of the viscera, (2) the large receptive fields of visceral nociceptors, and (3) the high degree of convergence in the visceral nociceptive pathways.
FN2e 296

7. **(C)** Cranial nerves IX (glossopharyngeal) and X (vagus) both contain baroreceptors and chemoreceptors, but the glossopharyngeal nerve conveys the axons of the baroreceptors of the carotid sinus and the chemoreceptors (sensing O_2 and CO_2 tension) of the carotid body. Cell bodies of these neurons are located in the inferior ganglion of cranial nerve IX. The superior ganglion of the glossopharyngeal nerve contains cell bodies of somatic afferent neurons.
FN2e 299–301

8. **(A)** The ascending reticular activating system is a diffuse network of brainstem neurons that promote arousal or alertness through their projections, directly and indirectly, to widespread areas of the cerebral cortex, particularly the frontal lobes. In general, the reticular activating system of the brainstem projects to thalamic nuclei, which, in turn, project to the cerebral cortex. Among the diverse inputs into the reticular activating system are visceral afferent signals arising from a full bladder.
FN2e 301–302

9. **(D)** There are two major ascending pathways that convey information from sympathetic visceral afferents. Laminae I and V and laminae VII and VIII of the spinal cord contain cell bodies of neurons that receive synaptic input from primary sympathetic visceral afferent neurons. Those second-order neurons with cell bodies in laminae I and V project rostrally mostly via the contralateral anterolateral system to the ventral posterolateral nucleus of the thalamus. Impulses conveyed by this pathway can result in perception of pain. Those second-order neurons with cell bodies in laminae VII and VIII project bilaterally as spinoreticular fibers to the brainstem reticular formation.
FN2e 295

10. **(B)** Primary visceral afferents of the glossopharyngeal and vagus nerves terminate primarily in the solitary nucleus of the medulla. Neurons of the solitary nucleus, in turn, project to the dorsal vagal nucleus (structure A), nucleus ambiguus (structure C), and the rostral ventrolateral medulla (structure D).
FN2e 300

11. **(B)** Visceral sensory signals from the VPL are conveyed to the cortex of the inferolateral postcentral gyrus (parietal operculum) and to the insula.
FN2e 296

CHAPTER 20

The Visual System

1.   A 47-year-old athletic man complains that he cannot see well out of his left eye. The results of a visual field examination suggest that the visual deficit is caused by a retinal detachment. Which of the following represents the most likely place at which this separation takes place?

○ (A) Outer plexiform layer
○ (B) Inner plexiform layer
○ (C) Junction of outer rod and cone segments with pigment epithelium
○ (D) Nerve fiber layer
○ (E) Junction of pigment epithelium with the choroid

2.   A 61-year-old woman complains of significant visual loss in one eye. The examination also reveals a loss of the pupillary light reflex in the same eye. MRI shows a lesion in the location indicated here.

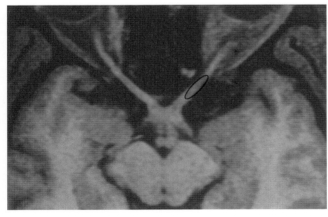

Figure 20–1A

Which of the following represents the most likely visual field deficit seen in this patient? (   )

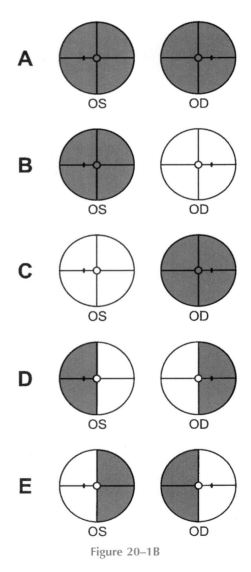

Figure 20–1B

3.   A 27-year-old woman visits her family physician with the complaint of irregular menstrual cycles. The neurologic examination reveals visual field deficits in both eyes. Further testing indicates endocrine dysfunction suggestive of a pituitary tumor. The neurologist orders an MRI, which reveals a tumor of the pituitary impinging on the structure shown here.

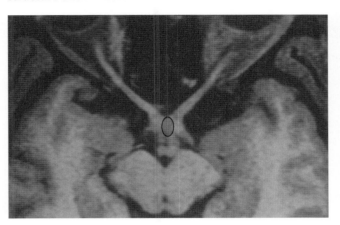

Figure 20–2A

Which of the following represents the most likely visual field deficit experienced by this patient? (   )

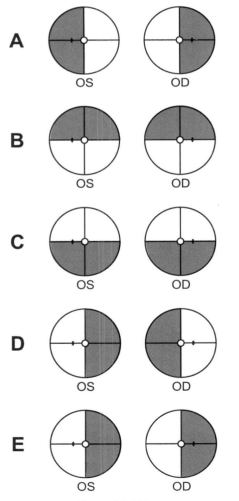

Figure 20–2B

4.   A 31-year-old woman visits her internist with complaints of headache, irregular periods, and loss of vision. The ensuing examination reveals visual deficits in both eyes and further evidence of pituitary dysfunction. MRI reveals a large dumbbell-shaped tumor of the pituitary impinging on the areas shown here.

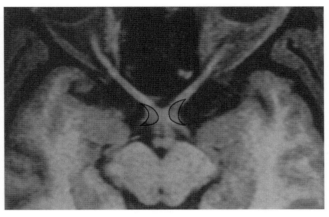

Figure 20–3A

Which of the following represents the most likely visual field deficit seen in this patient? (   )

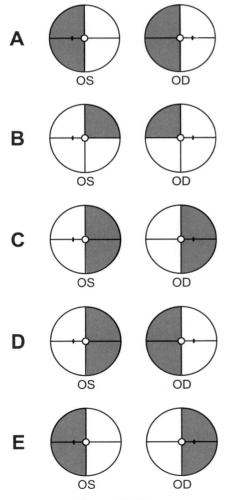

Figure 20–3B

5. A 43-year-old woman notices that she has to hold objects at arm's length to get them into focus. Which of the following most specifically characterizes this condition in this woman?

○ (A) Myopia
○ (B) Amblyopia
○ (C) Visual agnosia
○ (D) Mydriasis
○ (E) Presbyopia

Questions 6 through 9 are related to the following patient:

A 67-year-old man presents to the emergency department with headache and nausea. The examination reveals visual deficits in both eyes. The pupillary light reflex is present in both eyes, although not as brisk as in a normal patient. Suspecting a stroke, the physician orders MRI, which reveals a hemorrhagic lesion in the area outlined here.

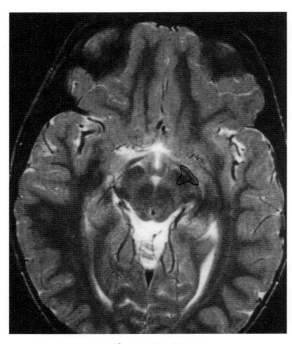

Figure 20–4A

6. Which of the following represents the most likely visual field deficit experienced by this patient? See Figure 20–4B at right. (   )

7. In addition to the visual deficits, which of the following losses related to the upper and lower extremities would most likely be seen in this patient?

○ (A) Paralysis on the right
○ (B) Paralysis on the left
○ (C) Loss of pain and thermal sensation on the left
○ (D) Loss of discriminative touch and vibratory sense on the left
○ (E) Loss of pain and thermal sense on the right

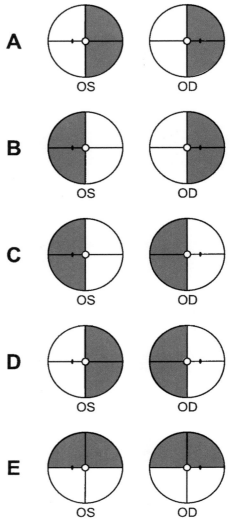

Figure 20–4B

8. Which of the following cranial nerve deficits is also most likely seen in this man?

○ (A) Bilateral paralysis of muscles of mastication
○ (B) Deviation of the tongue to left on protrusion and paralysis of lower facial muscles on right
○ (C) Deviation of the tongue to right on protrusion and paralysis of lower facial muscles on right
○ (D) Deviation of the tongue to right on protrusion and paralysis of lower facial muscles on left
○ (E) Deviation of the tongue to left on protrusion and paralysis of the lower facial muscles on left

9. Assuming this lesion to be the result of a vascular occlusion, which of the following vessels is most likely involved?

○ (A) Lenticulostriate branches of M_1
○ (B) Lateral posterior choroidal artery
○ (C) Anterior choroidal artery
○ (D) Thalamoperforating artery
○ (E) Medial striate artery

10.   A 27-year-old woman presents to the neurologist with deficits that have waxed and waned over a period of several months. Suspecting multiple sclerosis, the physician orders an MRI, which reveals demyelination in the areas outlined here.

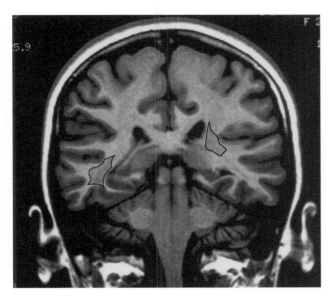

Figure 20–5A

Which of the following represents the most likely visual field deficit experienced by this patient? (   )

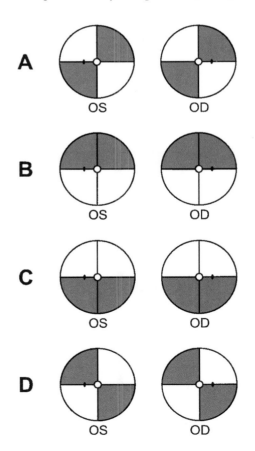

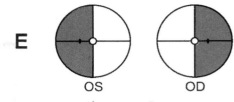

E

OS   OD

Figure 20–5B

11.   During a routine neurologic examination, the pupils of a 29-year-old man increase in diameter when the room light is turned off. Which of the following most specifically characterizes this response?

○ (A) Miosis
○ (B) Mydriasis
○ (C) Anhidrosis
○ (D) Ptosis
○ (E) Amblyopia

12.   A 54-year-old woman is diagnosed with glaucoma, an increase of pressure in the eye that, if left untreated, may result in blindness. The ophthalmologist performs a procedure to increase the egress of fluid through which of the following?

○ (A) Optic disc
○ (B) Pupil
○ (C) Canals of Schlemm
○ (D) Zonule fibers
○ (E) Optic canal

13.   An 81-year-old woman is brought to the emergency department by her son. She is confused and complains of headache and nausea. Motor and sensory function on the body are normal. Suspecting a stroke, the physician orders an MRI, which reveals a hemorrhagic lesion in the area outlined here.

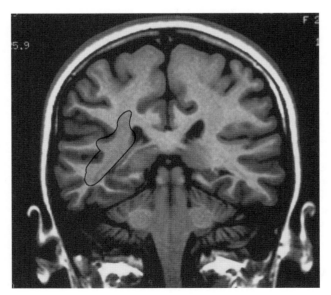

Figure 20–6A

Which of the following represents the most likely visual field deficit experienced by this patient? (   )

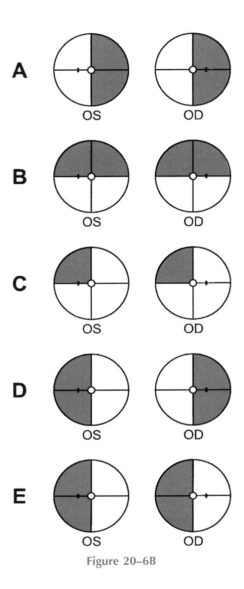

Figure 20–6B

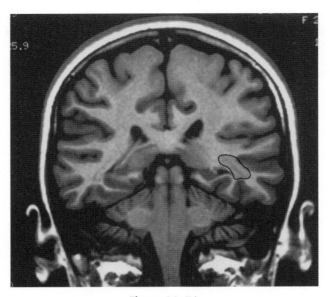

Figure 20–7A

14.   A 56-year-old morbidly obese man with untreated hypertension is brought to the emergency department from his workplace. The history reveals that the man experienced transient loss of sensation (pain and proprioception) and weakness of upper and lower extremities. He also said that he "saw flashes of light with both eyes." Subsequent MRI revealed a lesion in the area indicated in Figure 20–7A at right.

Which of the following represents the most likely visual field deficit experienced by this patient? See Figure 20–7B at right. (   )

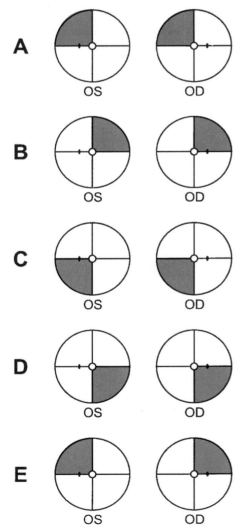

Figure 20–7B

15. Which of the following most specifically describes the physiologic events in a rod when exposed to light?

○ (A) Depolarization with corresponding increase of glutamate release
○ (B) Hyperpolarization with corresponding increase of glutamate release
○ (C) Hyperpolarization with corresponding decrease of glutamate release
○ (D) Hyperpolarization with no change in glutamate release
○ (E) Depolarization with no change in glutamate release

16. A 71-year-old right-handed man is brought to the emergency department by his wife. She explains that he complained of a sudden severe headache and then started "acting real confused." The examination reveals that the man can see objects and people but cannot name (specifically identify) the object or person. Movement and sensation on the head, face, and body is normal. CT reveals bilateral hemorrhagic lesions that are most likely located in which of the following areas?

○ (A) Temporal lobe, areas 20 and 21
○ (B) Area 17 on the left
○ (C) Lateral geniculate body on the right
○ (D) Parietal lobe, areas 6 and 8 on the left
○ (E) Temporal lobe, areas 20 and 21 on the right

17. A 26-year-old woman visits her family physician with a variety of neurologic complaints that have waxed and waned over the past several months. She complains that she stumbles when she walks and that this problem seems to be getting worse. The examination reveals normal muscle strength in the upper and lower extremities and normal sensation on the body. MRI reveals areas of demyelination, suggestive of multiple sclerosis, in the areas outlined here.

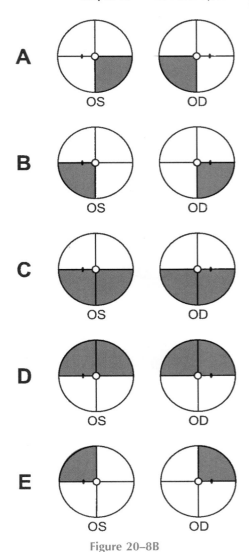

Figure 20–8B

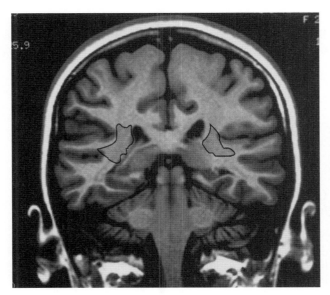

Figure 20–8A

Which of the following represents the most likely visual field deficit experienced by this patient? (   )

18. A 13-year-old boy is brought to the family physician with the main complaint of persistent headache. The physician notes that the boy is 6 feet tall and weighs 168 pounds. Suspecting a brain tumor, the physician orders an MRI, which reveals a pituitary tumor impinging on the structure indicated here.

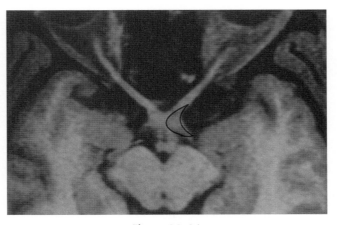

Figure 20–9A

Which of the following represents the most likely visual field deficit experienced by this boy? (   )

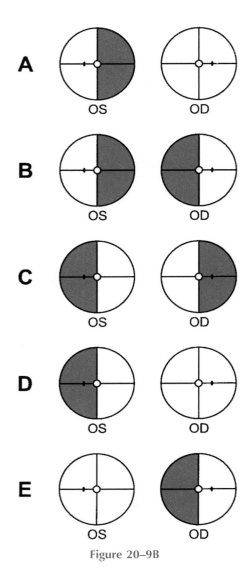

Figure 20–9B

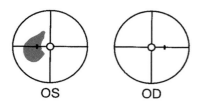

Figure 20–10

Based on these findings, what is the most likely diagnosis?

- ○ (A) Retinal detachment
- ○ (B) Scotoma from a localized infarction of branches of the left central retinal artery
- ○ (C) Pituitary tumor
- ○ (D) Infarction of the right posterior cerebral artery
- ○ (E) Infarction of the left posterior cerebral artery

21. An 89-year-old woman has an ophthalmologic examination. The ophthalmoscopic examination is normal with the exception of some drusen (yellow spots indicative of degenerative changes in the Bruch membrane) and some hazy nuclear inclusions in the lens. Intraocular pressure is normal. Her mild hypertension (140/95) is controlled by medication. The visual fields of this woman are shown here.

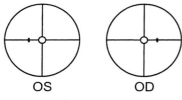

Figure 20–11

Based on these findings, what is the most likely diagnosis?

- ○ (A) Bilateral retinal detachment
- ○ (B) Bilateral retinal scotoma
- ○ (C) Normal vision
- ○ (D) Infarction of the right posterior cerebral artery
- ○ (E) Infarction of the left posterior cerebral artery

19. Which of the following most specifically represents the inability of a stroke patient to recognize faces, especially those that should be quite familiar?

- ○ (A) Achromatopsia
- ○ (B) Balint syndrome
- ○ (C) Amblyopia
- ○ (D) Prosopagnosia
- ○ (E) Presbyopia

20. A 54-year-old man has an ophthalmologic examination. The results are normal for the right eye, but the left eye shows hemorrhage and cotton wool spots in an area near the optic disc. The visual fields of this patient are shown here.

Questions 22 through 24 are based on the following patient:

A 24-year-old man is brought to the emergency department with a complaint of visual problems and headache. The man also states that he has little interest in sex and seems to be impotent. The physical examination reveals a milky discharge from both nipples. The neuro-ophthalmic examination reveals the visual field deficits shown here.

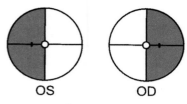

OS   OD

Figure 20–12

22. Which of the following most specifically describes the visual field loss in this man?

- ○ (A) Temporal scotoma
- ○ (B) Right homonymous hemianopia
- ○ (C) Left homonymous hemianopia
- ○ (D) Bitemporal hemianopia
- ○ (E) Binasal heteronymous hemianopia

23. Based on the visual field deficits seen in this patient, which of the following represents the most likely location of the lesion in this man?

- ○ (A) Right optic nerve or retina
- ○ (B) Left optic nerve or retina
- ○ (C) Optic chiasm
- ○ (D) Right optic radiations
- ○ (E) Left optic radiations

24. What is the most likely cause of the symptoms collectively experienced by this man?

- ○ (A) Hypertension
- ○ (B) Type II diabetes
- ○ (C) Sinusitis
- ○ (D) Prolactinoma
- ○ (E) Optic neuritis

25. A 56-year-old man presents with symptoms of increased intracranial pressure (headache, vomiting, and lethargy). Which of the following signs would most likely be caused by the increased intracranial pressure in this man?

- ○ (A) Retinal detachment
- ○ (B) Abnormal pigmentation in the neural retina
- ○ (C) Choked disc
- ○ (D) Neovascularity of the fovea
- ○ (E) Macular degeneration

26. A 3-year-old girl has congenital cataracts. Her 37-year-old mother has never been vaccinated against childhood diseases. The mother is seeking counseling regarding the genetic probability of having another child with congenital cataracts. Which of the following is the most frequent cause of congenital cataracts?

- ○ (A) Maternal exposure to rubella in the early fetal period
- ○ (B) Poor nutrition and low levels of folic acid in early pregnancy
- ○ (C) Exposure to ultraviolet light
- ○ (D) Birth trauma
- ○ (E) Elderly prima gravida

27. Which of the following cell types of the neural retina has a center-surround receptive field organization?

- ○ (A) Cone photoreceptors
- ○ (B) Rod photoreceptors
- ○ (C) Horizontal cells
- ○ (D) Amacrine cells
- ○ (E) Ganglion cells

Questions 28 through 30 are based on the following patient:

An 83-year-old woman is a resident of a convalescent home. During a routine physical examination, the physician notices the visual field deficits shown here. The ophthalmoscopic examination is normal for a person her age. Her blood pressure is 220/130 mm Hg.

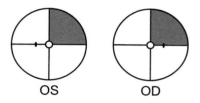

OS   OD

Figure 20–13

28. Which of the following most specifically describes the visual deficit observed in this woman?

- ○ (A) Right scotoma
- ○ (B) Right homonymous hemianopia
- ○ (C) Left homonymous hemianopia
- ○ (D) Right superior quadrantanopia
- ○ (E) Left inferior quadrantanopia

29. Which of the following represents the most likely location of the lesion in this woman?

- ○ (A) Left Meyer loop in the optic radiations
- ○ (B) Right Meyer loop in the optic radiations
- ○ (C) Right optic nerve
- ○ (D) Left lateral geniculate nucleus
- ○ (E) Right optic tract

30. The visual field deficits seen in this woman would also be consistent with a lesion in which of the following locations?

- ○ (A) Lower bank of the calcarine sulcus on the right
- ○ (B) Lower bank of the calcarine sulcus on the left
- ○ (C) Upper bank of the calcarine sulcus on the right
- ○ (D) Upper bank of the calcarine sulcus on the left
- ○ (E) Both upper and lower banks of the calcarine sulcus on the left

31. Which of the following is concerned with the circuits that allow one to discern fine detail (or form) and color?

○ (A) Medial temporal cortex
○ (B) Posterior parietal cortex
○ (C) W visual pathway
○ (D) P (or X) visual pathway
○ (E) M (or Y) visual pathway

32. Which of the following regions of the retina provides a crossed (contralateral) input to the left lateral geniculate nucleus?

○ (A) Right nasal
○ (B) Right temporal
○ (C) Right nasal and temporal
○ (D) Left nasal
○ (E) Left temporal

Questions 33 and 34 are based on the following patient:

A 16-year-old boy undergoes a visual system examination as part of a routine physical for a sports team. Visual fields, motion detection, stereoscopic vision, intraocular pressure, and pupillary light responses are all normal. However, when Ishihara test plates are used (letters or numbers printed in dot patterns in primary colors on a background of random dots of other colors), he is unable to recognize a rose-colored "6" made up of dots on a background of light green dots.

33. The most likely genetic cause of this disorder is what?

○ (A) Loss of red (L) cone opsin
○ (B) Loss of green (M) cone opsin
○ (C) Loss of blue (S) cone opsin
○ (D) Loss of rhodopsin
○ (E) Loss of both red and green (L & M) cone opsin

34. The genetic probability that this boy's sister would have a similar color vision defect is what?

○ (A) Almost 1 in 1
○ (B) About 1 in 2
○ (C) About 1 in 4
○ (D) About 1 in 8
○ (E) Almost zero

ANSWERS

1. **(C)** The junction of the outer segments of the rods and cones with the pigment epithelium is a structurally weak interface. Retinal detachment occurs at this point when the outer segments pull away from the pigment epithelium. The degree of visual loss reflects the region of the detachment.
FN2e 305

2. **(B)** The lesion in this patient is in the optic nerve on the left. Consequently, the patient is blind in her left eye and has a deficit in the corresponding visual field (OS). Also, the lesion of the optic nerve affects the afferent limb of the pupillary light reflex. A light shined in the blind eye will not result in a pupillary light reflex in either eye, but a light shined in the good (right) eye will result in a pupillary light reflex in both eyes.
FN2e 313, also 459–461

3. **(A)** The lesion in this patient involves the crossing fibers of the optic chiasm. These fibers originate from the nasal portion of both retinae. The corresponding loss is the temporal visual fields of both eyes (a bitemporal hemianopia).
FN2e 314–315

4. **(D)** The pituitary tumor in this patient has impinged on the lateral aspects of the optic chiasm. At this location the tumor impinges on the uncrossed fibers that originate from the temporal side of both retinae. Consequently, the visual deficit is in the nasal visual fields of both eyes (a binasal hemianopia).
FN2e 314–316

5. **(E)** Presbyopia, the inability to focus on near objects, is caused by the loss of lens accommodation with age. In general, this is when the near-point of focus is at a distance of about 25 cm. This condition can be resolved with corrective lenses.
FN2e 305

6. **(A)** The lesion in this patient is located in the left optic tract. This lesion interrupts optic fibers from the nasal retina of the right eye (with a loss of the temporal visual field of the right eye) and optic fibers from temporal retina of the left eye (with a loss of the nasal visual field of the left eye). This deficit in this patient represents a right homonymous hemianopia.
FN2e 316

7. **(A)** This lesion extends into the middle portion of the crus cerebri where corticospinal and corticonuclear (corticobulbar) fibers are located. Because this lesion is in the crus cerebri on the patient's left, and damages fibers therein, the upper and lower extremities on the patient's right side are paralyzed. Sensation (pain, temperature, discriminative touch, and vibratory sense) is normal on both sides of the body and face.
FN2e 316, also 393, 397

8. **(C)** The lesion in this patient damages the middle third of the crus cerebri; corticonuclear (corticobulbar) fibers are located in the medial part of this region of the crus cerebri. Corticonuclear fibers in the crus cerebri influence contralateral hypoglossal motor neurons innervating the genioglossus muscle and contralateral facial motor neurons innervating muscles of the lower portions of the face on the contralateral side. Consequently, a lesion in the crus cerebri on the left side results in a deviation of the tongue to the right on pro-

trusion and weakness of facial muscles on the lower right side of the face.
FN2e 395–396

9. **(C)** The anterior choroidal artery is usually the second major branch of the cerebral (intracranial) part of the internal carotid artery. This vessel travels along the course of the optic tract and sends branches to this tract, to immediately adjacent portions of the internal capsule, to structures of the medial temporal lobe (including the choroid plexus of the inferior horn of the lateral ventricle), and to other adjacent structures.
FN2e 316

10. **(D)** The area of demyelination on the patient's right affects axons in the lower part of the geniculocalcarine (optic) radiations on this side. This results in a left superior quadrantanopia. The area of demyelination on the patient's left affects axons in the upper (superior) part of the geniculocalcarine (optic) radiations. This results in a right inferior quadrantanopia. The overall visual deficit in this patient is a dumbbell-shaped loss involving upper left and lower right quadrants.
FN2e 318–319

11. **(B)** The pupil receives a sympathetic innervation via postganglionic fibers that arise in the superior cervical ganglion and a parasympathetic innervation via the Edinger-Westphal nucleus and the oculomotor nerve. Increase in pupil diameter, mydriasis, is mediated through the sympathetic pathway, which innervates the dilator muscle (dilator pupillae) of the iris. Dilation of the pupil is seen in conditions of fear, anger, pain, or decreased light. Drugs, both prescription and illegal, may produce pupillary dilation.
FN2e 305

12. **(C)** Fluid is continuously produced by epithelium covering the ciliary body. This fluid moves from the posterior chamber through the pupil (the opening between the anterior and posterior chambers) and into the anterior chamber. From here it drains into the canals of Schlemm. In some cases of glaucoma, the ophthalmologist may perform laser surgery to enlarge the openings between the anterior chamber and the canals with the resultant increase in the movement of fluid from the anterior chamber into the canals.
FN2e 304

13. **(E)** The lesion in this woman is located in the geniculocalcarine (optic) radiations on the right side. This represents a loss of input from the nasal visual field of the right eye and the temporal visual field of the left eye. The visual deficits experienced by this patient are essentially identical to those experienced by a patient with a lesion of the optic tract on the same side.
FN2e 318–319

14. **(B)** The history suggests that this patient may have suffered a transient ischemic attack (TIA). The lesion seen in this man is located in the inferior part of the geniculocalcarine (optic) radiation on his left side. This results in a right superior quadrantanopia.
FN2e 318

15. **(C)** Normally, there is a constant release of neurotransmitter (glutamate) at the rod spherule. When stimulated by a photon of light, the Na^+ current is blocked, the cell membrane is hyperpolarized (increasing from about $-40\,mV$ to $-60\,mV$), and the amount of neurotransmitter being released is decreased. Photoreceptors are the only sensory receptors/neurons that hyperpolarize in response to an appropriate stimulus.
FN2e 307–308

16. **(A)** Cortical lesions (in this case a hemorrhage) involving areas 20 and 21 of the temporal lobe of the dominant hemisphere may result in visual (object) agnosia. The patient can see objects or persons but is not able to identify the object or person. This leads to the impression, on the part of family members, that the patient is confused because he or she may not be able to name or identify family members.
FN2e 321

17. **(C)** The demyelinated areas in this woman's brain are located in the upper (superior) part of the geniculocalcarine (optic) radiations. These fibers are conveying information from the lower portions of the visual fields. This is basically a combined right and left inferior quadrantanopia. The motor symptoms experienced by this patient are not caused by muscle weakness or dyssynergia but because input from the lower part of the visual field is interrupted. It is especially difficult for this patient to walk down stairs.
FN2e 318

18. **(A)** This pituitary tumor is most likely one that results in the overproduction of growth hormone. It impinges on the lateral aspect of the optic chiasm on the patient's left side. This compresses fibers from the temporal side of the retina on the left, which represent the nasal visual field on the left.
FN2e 313–314

19. **(D)** Small bilateral lesions in areas of the temporal lobes associated with visual functions (areas 20, 21) may result in prosopagnosia. In this situation the patient can see the face but does not recognize the face (cannot identify the face as belonging to a particular individual). This may be the case for the patient's wife, husband, child, or close friend as well as less familiar faces.
FN2e 321

20. **(B)** Scotomas are irregular "patches" of diminished, or lost, vision that can occur anywhere in the visual field. This type of visual loss may be caused by a local detachment of the retina or infarction.
FN2e 314

21. **(C)** The visual fields are normal in this woman, with only a "blind spot" in each eye, about 12 degrees temporal to the fovea. This represents the region where the optic nerve exits the eyeball. No photoreceptors are present here, so no light can be received in this area. The changes in the lens are normal for a patient this age.
FN2e 313–314

22. **(D)** Both temporal visual fields are lost ("bitemporal"). The right visual hemifield is affected in the left eye (OS), and the left visual hemifield is affected in the right eye (OD). Therefore, the visual fields are not superimposable or congruent (they may be called "heteronymous"). Half the visual field is lost when using each eye ("hemianopia").
FN2e 315–316

23. **(C)** This pattern of visual field loss is characteristically seen resultant to a lesion of the midline portion of the optic chiasm. Typically, a lesion in this area may be related to a pituitary tumor impinging on the crossing fibers within the optic chiasm.
FN2e 315–316

24. **(D)** Based on the visual deficits identified in this patient, and the secretion of a milky substance, it is most likely this patient has a pituitary lesion. The production of a milky substance, decreased libido, and impotence in men is related to a prolactin-secreting tumor of the pituitary.
FN2e 315–316, 490

25. **(C)** Increased intracranial pressure causes the optic disc to appear to "rise" toward the ophthalmoscopic observer, a sign called a "choked disc." The increase in intracranial pressure is transmitted through the cerebrospinal fluid located within the sleeve of meninges surrounding the optic nerve. The result is a stasis of axoplasmic flow at the optic nerve head with resultant swelling (papilledema).
FN2e 314

26. **(A)** Maternal exposure to rubella may cause congenital cataracts.
FN2e 77–78

27. **(E)** Of the cells listed, only the ganglion cell has both a center and surround component of its receptive field. Ganglion cells are the efferent neurons of the retina. Their axons form the optic nerves.
FN2e 309–312

28. **(D)** Losses of only one quadrant of the visual field are called quadrantanopias. This patient has a congruent loss in the right superior visual field (i.e., a "right superior quadrantanopia"). Congruent refers to the fact that the visual loss in the visual fields of both eyes overlap if superimposed.
FN2e 318

29. **(A)** A characteristic location for lesions that result in a superior quadrantanopia is in the longer fibers wrapping around the inferior horn of the lateral ventricle. These fibers are usually termed the *Meyer loop*. This particular lesion is sometimes called a "pie-in-the-sky" lesion and is associated with either the Meyer loop or the inferior bank of the calcarine sulcus on the contralateral side. Because this patient's visual field loss is in the superior right quadrant, the lesion is on the left side of the brain.
FN2e 318

30. **(B)** The upper bank of the calcarine sulcus (i.e., cuneus) receives information from the inferior visual world. The lower bank (i.e., lingual gyrus) receives information from the superior visual world. The right visual cortex receives information from the left visual world; the left visual cortex receives information from the right visual world. The loss of the superior right quadrant of the visual field in this patient correlates with a lesion in the lower bank of the calcarine sulcus (lingual gyrus) on the patient's left side.
FN2e 318

31. **(D)** The P (or X) visual pathway encodes fine details and color information. This pathway originates from medium-sized ganglion cells (beta cells) of the retina that project to the small-celled (parvocellular) layers of the lateral geniculate nucleus. This information is processed through areas 17 and 18 and the medial temporal visual cortex.
FN2e 312, 316, 321

32. **(A)** The temporal portion of the visual field projects onto the nasal portion of the retina. The axons arising from ganglion cells located in the nasal retina cross the midline in the optic chiasm and terminate in the contralateral lateral geniculate nucleus. Consequently, the left lateral geniculate nucleus receives input from the right nasal retina.
FN2e 313–315

33. **(A)** There are several tests for color vision. The most commonly used such test, the Ishihara test, consists of different-colored dots on a background of dots. The printing is adjusted so that the luminance of the spots (the number of photons reflected off each dot) is equal; the only difference is in the wavelength of the photons, which is perceived as color. Red-green color confusion is caused by loss of red cone opsin.
FN2e 308–309

34. **(E)** The genes for red and green cone pigments are encoded on the X chromosome. Therefore, almost all colorblind individuals are men.
FN2e 309

CHAPTER 21

The Auditory System

Questions 1 and 2 are based on the following patient:

A 73-year-old man was participating in a heated discussion at the dinner table when the coffee he was drinking suddenly drooled from the right corner of his mouth and he was unable to speak. He was rushed to the emergency department where he motioned for a pen and paper. His family was relieved to know, from the note he wrote, that he was not in pain. He was admitted and underwent CT of the brain.

1. The radiologist describes mild ischemic damage, which is most likely confined to which cortical area out-lined here? (   )

2. Auditory data relayed to cortical speech centers would be processed in which sensory cortical region?

○ (A) Insular cortex
○ (B) Postcentral gyrus
○ (C) Transverse gyri of Heschl
○ (D) Inferior temporal gyrus
○ (E) Striate cortex

Questions 3 through 6 are based on the following patient:

One evening, as she applied makeup before a dinner party, a 42-year-old actress noticed that the left side of her face was "not quite normal." At the party she

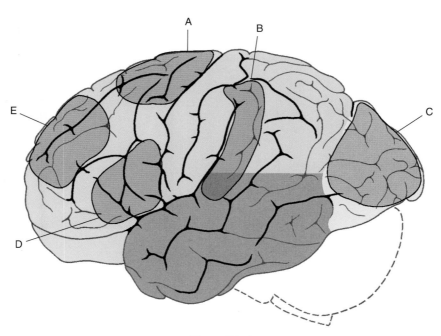

Figure 21–1

found it especially difficult to participate in conversations while the band was playing. She consulted her family physician. In a Weber test, she lateralized the tone from a vibrating tuning fork placed at the vertex of her skull to her right side. MRI revealed an acoustic neuroma on the left vestibulocochlear nerve. It was removed, and further facial paralysis was avoided. A follow-up audiogram showed normal hearing sensitivity in her right ear, but some sensorineural hearing loss in her left ear. High frequencies were lost, but frequencies below 4000 Hz were spared.

3. Peripheral branches of type I primary afferent fibers originating from which part of the spiral ganglion were spared?

- (A) Modiolus
- (B) Inner hair cells toward the apex of the cochlea
- (C) Outer hair cells toward the base of the cochlea
- (D) Helicotrema
- (E) Outer spiral bundle

4. Central branches of the primary afferent fibers from the spiral ganglion that were damaged by the tumor in this woman normally end in which of the following regions?

- (A) Anterior and posterior cochlear nuclei
- (B) Only the anterior cochlear nucleus
- (C) Only the posterior cochlear nucleus
- (D) Anterior and posterior cochlear nuclei and superior olivary nuclei
- (E) Only superior olivary nuclei

5. For speech sounds below 4000 Hz, narrowly tuned cells preserve coding of frequencies in which of the following central auditory structures?

- (A) Cochlear nuclei only
- (B) Superior olivary nuclei only
- (C) Inferior colliculus only
- (D) Auditory cortex only
- (E) Frequency coding is characteristic of all major auditory areas

6. Which of the following would most likely be more difficult for this woman?

- (A) Detection of high-frequency sounds
- (B) Localization of high-frequency sounds
- (C) Speech perception in a quiet room
- (D) Vocalization
- (E) Speaking

7. A 7-year-old child presents with bilateral otitis media. The audiology report indicates a moderate conductive hearing loss. Which one of the following is a part of the conductive hearing pathway?

- (A) Superior olive
- (B) Cochlear nucleus
- (C) Inner hair cells
- (D) Spiral ganglion
- (E) Stapes

Questions 8 through 10 are based on the following patient:

A 67-year-old war veteran with multiple sclerosis experienced abnormal auditory sensations. The audiogram showed mild high-frequency hearing loss in both ears. Recording of scalp potentials indicated that peak IV in the right auditory brainstem response (ABR) was reduced relative to the left side. Sclerotic plaques involving the lateral lemniscus and inferior colliculus on the right side were suspected as contributing to the abnormal auditory sensations. MRI confirmed these suspicions.

8. Which of the following outlined areas represents the most likely location of the lateral lemniscus? (   )

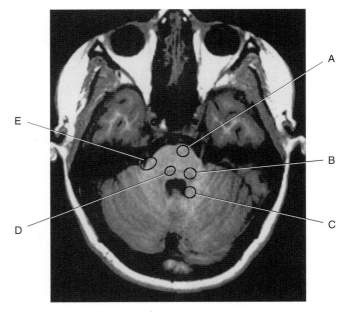

Figure 21–2

9. Which of the following labeled structures most likely represents the inferior colliculus? (   )

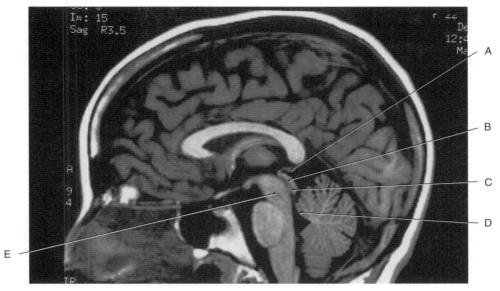

Figure 21–3

10. A reduction in activity in the fibers ascending in the lateral lemniscus to the inferior colliculus that would contribute to changes in peak IV of the auditory brain response (ABR) would not be related to damage to which of the following structures?

○ (A) Anterior cochlear nucleus
○ (B) Posterior cochlear nucleus
○ (C) Medial superior olivary nucleus
○ (D) Lateral superior olivary nucleus
○ (E) Medial geniculate nucleus

Questions 11 through 13 are based on the following patient:

A 32-year-old man returned from a Caribbean vacation where he had been scuba diving. A week later he experienced episodes of positional vertigo and nystagmus. Thinking that he simply had "water in his ears," he put off seeing his physician until he experienced sudden total hearing loss in his left ear after working out at the gym. An otologist discovered that the man had perilymphatic fluid leaking from the cochlea into the middle ear and that hair cell function was compromised.

11. Leaks of perilymphatic fluid into the middle ear cavity could occur through channels that developed around the edges of which of the following structures?

○ (A) Basilar membrane
○ (B) Spiral ligament
○ (C) Round window
○ (D) Tympanic membrane
○ (E) Tectorial membrane

12. Which of the labeled spaces in the figure below is filled with perilymphatic fluid?

Type I cell afferent
Type II cell afferent
Medial olivocochlear efferent
Lateral olivocochlear efferent

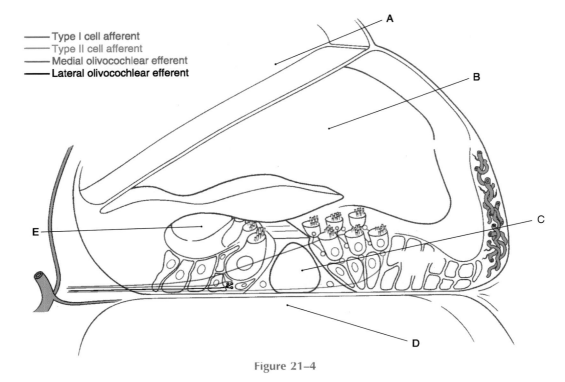

Figure 21–4

○ (A) A and B
○ (B) A and D
○ (C) A only
○ (D) B only
○ (E) B and C

13. When compared with endolymph, the fluid leaking from the cochlea in this man is

○ (A) Produced by the stria vascularis
○ (B) High in sodium concentration
○ (C) High in magnesium concentration
○ (D) High in calcium concentration
○ (E) High in chloride concentration

Questions 14 through 16 are based on the following patient:

A 39-year-old man had a normal hearing test at the beginning of his employment in a noisy factory. Ten years later he could not hear the alarm on his watch or even localize a cricket in his basement. His hearing was retested.

14. Cues about the location of a sound are unlikely to be related to which of the following?

○ (A) Differences in the time of arrival of low-frequency sounds at the left versus right ear
○ (B) Differences in the level of high-frequency sounds at the left versus right ear
○ (C) Spectral cues introduced by the outer ear

○ (D) Time differences in high frequencies introduced by the outer ear

15. Inhibitory pathways are important in the binaural circuits within the superior olivary nuclei that are important for sound localization. Which one of the following is the neurotransmitter used by interneurons in this region?

○ (A) Acetylcholine
○ (B) Glycine
○ (C) Aspartate
○ (D) Glutamate
○ (E) Serotonin

16. Feedback to the outer hair cells influencing the sensitivity of the cochlea is mediated by circuits that arise from which one of the following?

○ (A) Anterior cochlear nucleus
○ (B) Posterior cochlear nucleus
○ (C) Periolivary nuclei
○ (D) Inferior colliculus
○ (E) Facial nucleus

17. An ischemic infarction in a 46-year-old man results in total deafness in only the right ear. Which of the following arteries is most likely to be involved in this lesion?

○ (A) Middle cerebral artery
○ (B) Right anterior inferior cerebellar artery
○ (C) Right superior cerebellar artery
○ (D) Left thalamogeniculate artery
○ (E) Right thalamogeniculate artery

ANSWERS

1. **(D)** The patient is unable to speak but can write. Therefore, areas 44 and 45 (the expressive speech and language areas) must be damaged along with, perhaps, the adjacent motor cortical regions representing regions of the face. The patient is able to hear and answer questions by writing; therefore, auditory association areas (labeled B) are not involved.
FN2e 336–337

2. **(C)** The primary auditory cortex is located on the superior surface of the temporal lobe in the transverse gyri of Heschl. The arcuate fasciculus connects this area with surrounding association cortex including areas 39 and 40 (Wernicke area).
FN2e 336–337

3. **(B)** Peripheral branches of the spiral ganglion cells innervate the hair cells; type I terminals end specifically on inner hair cells. The patient has a high-frequency hearing loss. The cochlea is organized such that high frequencies are represented at the base and low frequencies more toward the apex.
FN2e 328–329

4. **(A)** Primary afferent fibers from the spiral ganglion make up the cochlear portion of the vestibulocochlear nerve. These cochlear fibers enter the cochlear nuclei where the axons divide and innervate each of the subnuclei in a tonotopic order.
FN2e 331–332

5. **(E)** Frequency tuning is a primary characteristic of all major auditory regions from the cochlear nuclei to the auditory cortex.
FN2e 329

6. **(B)** The patient has a high-frequency hearing loss in one ear. Localization of sounds depends largely on binaural cues, whereas detection of high frequencies with the intact ear is still possible. Human speech is made up of relatively low frequencies and also requires only monaural hearing, if not masked by background noise.
FN2e 324, 335

7. **(E)** The function of the outer and middle ear is to collect and conduct the vibrations of air molecules to the inner ear where transduction takes place. Disease of the middle ear (location of the stapes) results in conductive hearing loss as opposed to damage to the inner ear, which results in sensorineural hearing loss.
FN2e 324–325

8. **(B)** The lateral lemniscus is located in the anterolateral part of the pontine tegmentum. Insinuated within the lateral lemniscus are cells forming the nuclei of the lateral lemniscus. This bundle continues rostrally to enter the inferior colliculus.
FN2e 333–334, also 181–182, 191–192

9. **(C)** The inferior colliculus, shown here in a sagittal MRI, is located on the posterior aspect of the midbrain. It receives auditory input through the lateral lemniscus and projects to the medial geniculate nucleus through the brachium of the inferior colliculus. This structure is a prominent landmark in MRI in all planes.
FN2e 333, 335–336

10. **(C)** Peaks I through IV of the auditory brain response (ABR) relate to activity in the auditory nerve, cochlear nuclei, superior olive, and lateral lemniscus, respectively. A change in peaks I through IV of the ABR could relate to damage to one (or more) of these structures. A lesion in the medial geniculate nucleus (MGNu) would result in changes in peak VI or VII because these are related to activity in the MGNu and auditory cortex, respectively.
FN2e 330–331

11. **(C)** Scala vestibuli and tympani contain perilymphatic fluid. The scala tympani ends at the round window. Trauma or a pathologic process at this area could result in a fluid leak into the middle ear.
FN2e 326

12. **(B)** The scala vestibuli, located above the Reissner membrane, and the scala tympani, located below the basilar membrane, contain perilymphatic fluid.
FN2e 325–326

13. **(B)** Perilymph has a high concentration of sodium, whereas endolymph has a high concentration of potassium.
FN2e 327–328

14. **(B)** Time differences in the arrival of low-frequency sounds, introduced by the difference in the length of the path of sound to each ear, are related to the location from which the sound originates. Such differences assist in the location of sound in space.
FN2e 334–336

15. **(B)** Glycine is an important inhibitory neurotransmitter used in local circuits in the superior olivary nuclear complex.
FN2e 334

16. **(C)** Periolivary nuclei give rise to the medial and lateral olivocochlear efferent pathways that selectively influence the sensitivity and frequency selectivity of hair cells in the cochlea.
FN2e 338

17. **(B)** Lesions of the central auditory pathway seldom result in total deafness in one ear. However, deafness can occur from damage to the cochlear nuclei, vestibulocochlear nerve, or the cochlea itself. These regions receive their blood supply from branches of the anterior inferior cerebellar artery, specifically through branches of the labyrinthine artery.
FN2e 324, 329

CHAPTER 22

The Vestibular System

1. A 39-year-old man has severe vertigo, positional nystagmus, and tinnitus that are episodic. The man complains that these attacks can be severe, with nausea and vomiting. An audiogram shows low-frequency hearing loss that the man states "comes and goes." Which of the following represents the most likely diagnosis and corresponding treatment?

- ○ (A) Acoustic neuroma, surgery
- ○ (B) Temporal bone fracture, rest
- ○ (C) Meniere disease, diuretics and salt restriction
- ○ (D) Psychosomatic disorder, psychiatric consult
- ○ (E) Hypertensive cardiovascular disease, reserpine

2. The peripheral receptors of the vestibular system lie in five separate organs for each inner ear, including three semicircular canals and two otolith organs. The three semicircular canals are responsible for the transduction of what?

- ○ (A) Linear accelerations of the head in the horizontal plane
- ○ (B) Rotational head motion
- ○ (C) Tilts of the head relative to gravity
- ○ (D) Static head position
- ○ (E) Up-down head motion aligned with gravity

3. The peripheral otolith receptor organs of the vestibular system contain tiny calcium carbonate crystals, the otoconia, which lie on top of a gelatinous membrane encasing the stereocilia of the receptor hair cells. These otoconia become displaced during certain types of movement. The otolith receptors are responsible for transduction of what?

- ○ (A) Linear accelerations and tilts of the head relative to gravity
- ○ (B) Head rotations toward the ipsilateral side
- ○ (C) Displacement of the limbs relative to the body
- ○ (D) Angular accelerations of the head, left and right
- ○ (E) Hyperbaric changes

4. The vestibular receptor cells are termed *hair cells*. Stereocilia arising from the apical portion of the cell are arranged in a stereotypical manner, with a single kinocilium at one end of the cell near the largest stereocilia.

Each hair cell is physiologically responsive to directional movement by displacement of the stereocilia according to which of the following schemes?

- ○ (A) Displacement of the stereocilia toward the kinocilium produces excitatory responses.
- ○ (B) Displacement of the stereocilia away from the kinocilium produces excitatory responses.
- ○ (C) The hair cells in the semicircular canals are polarized differently relative to a central line.
- ○ (D) Compression of the stereocilia produces excitatory responses for vertical accelerations.

5. The receptor cells of the vestibular system are termed *hair cells*. Signal transduction in the hair cell results from a cascade of several events. Initially, when movement occurs, stereocilia are deflected. For excitatory signal transduction in hair cells, which of the following series of events is correct?

- ○ (A) The stereocilia are compressed toward the cell surface by acceleration forces, K^+ channels in the stereocilia close, Ca^{2+} channels in the basolateral cell membrane close, and excitatory neurotransmitter is released.
- ○ (B) The stereocilia are bent away from the kinocilium, K^+ channels in the stereocilia close, Ca^{2+} channels in the basolateral cell membrane close, and excitatory neurotransmitter is released.
- ○ (C) The stereocilia are rigid and do not move, endolymph motion forces the K^+ channels in the stereocilia open, Ca^{2+} channels in the basolateral cell membrane close, and excitatory neurotransmitter is released.
- ○ (D) The stereocilia are bent toward the kinocilium, K^+ channels in the stereocilia open, Ca^{2+} channels in the basolateral cell membrane open, and excitatory neurotransmitter is released.
- ○ (E) The stereocilia are bent perpendicular to the kinocilium, K^+ channels in the stereocilia close, Ca^{2+} channels in the basolateral membrane open, and excitatory neurotransmitter is released.

6. During surgery on a 47-year-old woman to remove a large acoustic neuroma, cranial nerve VIII on the left side of the head was inadvertently transected. Once the

woman is recumbent, the physician performs a bedside postoperative evaluation. Which of the following would be most characteristic of the symptoms experienced by this woman?

- ○ (A) A profound hearing loss on the right side with no nystagmus and paralysis of left lower extremity
- ○ (B) Nystagmus with fast phases directed toward the right ear, gait disturbance using left lower extremity, and deafness in left ear
- ○ (C) Unsteadiness in gait when standing using right lower extremity only and a right-sided hearing loss
- ○ (D) Positional nystagmus with rightward head turns and paralysis of right lower extremity

7. When the head of a 23-year-old man is tilted (rolled) toward the right, the otolith organs of the vestibular system produce a compensatory oculomotor response. The response can be observed by viewing the man's eyes during the head-tilt procedure. Which of the following represents the compensatory response observed in this man assuming he has normal vestibular system function?

- ○ (A) Counter-roll (torsion) of the eyes toward the right
- ○ (B) Counter-roll (torsion) of the eyes toward the left
- ○ (C) An upward eye deflection
- ○ (D) A leftward beating horizontal nystagmus
- ○ (E) A rightward and upward eye deflection

8. A 39-year-old woman presents to the otorhinolaryngology clinic with complaints of dizziness and blurred vision that occur when her child is playing loud music. She also complains of spinning sensations that occur during sneezing or when traveling by airplane. The examination reveals nystagmus (beating downward and rightward) that may be generated by increasing the pressure within the middle ear. Which of the following would most likely explain the symptoms experienced by this woman and would be visible in a thin-cut temporal bone CT?

- ○ (A) A small acoustic neuroma on left side
- ○ (B) Squamous cell carcinoma of middle ear
- ○ (C) Left hairline temporal bone fracture
- ○ (D) Dehiscence of the right superior semicircular canal
- ○ (E) Occlusion of the posterior inferior cerebellar artery

9. A 17-year-old boy is brought to the emergency department with head trauma after a motorcycle crash. The boy complains of being unable to detect movements of the head forward and backward (flexion and extension). The boy says that he knows when he is turning to his left or to his right. Electronystagmography shows that compensatory eye movements are normal with left and right head turns but greatly reduced with flexion and extension of the head. CT is ordered. Which of the following would most likely explain the deficits seen in this boy?

- ○ (A) Temporal fractures that include only the horizontal canals

- ○ (B) Temporal fractures that include only the vertical canals
- ○ (C) An occipital fracture over the cerebellum
- ○ (D) No fractures, but a severed left VIII cranial nerve
- ○ (E) Large subdural hematoma over left temporal lobe

10. A 42-year-old man visits the otolaryngology clinic with the complaint of dizziness and blurred vision. Caloric and posturographic tests are performed. Caloric irrigation of the right ear produces normal responses. Caloric irrigation of the left ear produces no response. The patient also has instability when standing on the left leg. MRI reveals the cause of the symptoms experienced by this man. Which of the following is most congruent with the evaluation in this patient?

- ○ (A) An acoustic neuroma of the left VIII cranial nerve
- ○ (B) A large neuroma of the cerebellar cortex
- ○ (C) A large glomus tumor of the right brainstem
- ○ (D) The left medial vestibulospinal tract only has been affected
- ○ (E) Large subdural hematoma over left temporal lobe

11. Vestibular function is tested in a 19-year-old woman using a caloric test. Which of the following most likely occurs in a normal patient when cold water is introduced into the right ear?

- ○ (A) Vertical nystagmus with the fast phase directed downward
- ○ (B) Vertical nystagmus with alternating direction fast phases
- ○ (C) Horizontal nystagmus with the fast phase directed toward the left
- ○ (D) Horizontal nystagmus with the fast phase directed toward the right
- ○ (E) Ocular counter-roll to the right

12. An interruption of the right medial vestibulospinal tract fibers originating in the right vestibular nuclei would most likely produce which of the following deficits?

- ○ (A) Muscle tremors in the left lower extremity
- ○ (B) Difficulty in moving the left upper extremity
- ○ (C) Postural instability of the head only, with no effect on the lower body
- ○ (D) Postural difficulty involving all right side muscles from the neck down
- ○ (E) Bilateral postural difficulty in the lower extremities only

13. The vestibulo-ocular reflex provides compensatory eye movements in response to head movements to stabilize images on the retina. For a leftward horizontal head movement, which of the following is correct?

- ○ (A) Left horizontal canal vestibular receptors will be inhibited.
- ○ (B) Right horizontal canal vestibular receptors will be excited.

○ (C) Left vestibular nuclei neurons will be excited, which, in turn, excite right abducens motor neurons, and the eyes will have a slow phase to the right.

○ (D) Left vestibular nuclei neurons will be excited, which, in turn, excite left abducens motor neurons, and the eyes will have a slow phase to the left.

○ (E) A fast phase reset of the eyes to the right will occur.

14. A 16-year-old boy is brought to the emergency department after a motorcycle crash. There is hemorrhage from the left ear, and the boy complains of a spinning sensation, dizziness, and blurred vision. In addition to these symptoms which of the following would also most likely be seen in this boy?

○ (A) A profound hearing loss on the right side
○ (B) Nystagmus with fast phases directed toward the right (opposite) ear
○ (C) A head tilt to the right
○ (D) Nystagmus with fast phases directed toward the left (same) ear
○ (E) Weakness in the right leg

15. A 23-year-old woman is brought to the emergency department from the site of an automobile collision. CT reveals blood in the vestibular labyrinth. Damage to branches of which of the following arteries would most likely explain this observation?

○ (A) Anterior inferior cerebellar artery
○ (B) Posteior superior cerebellar artery
○ (C) Anterior spinal artery
○ (D) Thalamogeniculate artery
○ (E) Anterior choroidal artery

16. The semicircular canals of the vestibular system are arranged in specific orientations for detection of head rotations in three-dimensional space. Which of the following best describes the relative positions of the three semicircular canals?

○ (A) The horizontal canals lie below the Earth's horizontal plane by 30 degrees.
○ (B) The vertical canals lie at right angles to each other and to the horizontal canals.
○ (C) All semicircular canals lie parallel to the cochlea in the inner ear.
○ (D) The anterior canals lie in the horizontal head plane.
○ (E) The horizontal canals of the left ear are at right angles to the horizontal canals of the right ear.

17. The vestibulocollic reflex (VCR) provides compensatory posture adjustments of the head during movement. A 14-year-old boy trips and falls forward while walking on a cobblestone street. Which of the following occurs as part of the normal VCR response in this boy during this event?

○ (A) Upward head movement (dorsiflexion–extension)

○ (B) Downward head movement (ventroflexion–flexion)
○ (C) Leftward head movement and upward eye movement
○ (D) Rightward head movement and downward eye movement
○ (E) Extension of the legs bilaterally

ANSWERS

1. **(C)** These symptoms are characteristic of Meniere disease, caused by endolymphatic hydrops in the vestibular and cochlear membranous labyrinth. Attacks are typically episodic and can be severe. Although the cause of Meniere disease is unknown, most cases respond well to diuretics, such as hydrochlorothiazide, and to salt-restricted diets.
FN2e 344–345

2. **(B)** The three semicircular canals respond to rotational motion of the head. Endolymph becomes displaced relative to the receptor stereocilia during head turns, thereby eliciting membrane polarizations that affect transmitter release. Each canal is approximately aligned in an orthogonal plane to the other canals. Neither static head position nor linear accelerations affect semicircular canal receptors.
FN2e 347–349

3. **(A)** The otolith organs respond to linear accelerations and tilts of the head relative to gravity. These receptors respond as inertial sensors and are not sensitive to rotational head motion.
FN2e 349

4. **(A)** Movement of the stereocilia toward the kinocilium depolarize the cell, whereas stereocilia movements away from the kinocilium hyperpolarize the cell. All of the hair cells are morphologically polarized in the same direction for the semicircular canals but are differentially polarized either toward or away from a central reversal line in the utricle and saccule, respectively.
FN2e 346–347

5. **(D)** Hair cell transduction relies on the potassium-rich environment of the endolymph fluid bathing the cell surface. For excitatory transduction, stereocilia are deflected toward the kinocilium, which opens the K^+ channels in the stereocilia tips. K^+ influx produces opening of the basolateral Ca^{2+} channels, which forces synaptic vesicles to fuse with the membrane, and an excitatory neurotransmitter is released.
FN2e 346

6. **(B)** A complete loss of ipsilateral nerve transduction would produce hearing loss, nystagmus with fast phases directed opposite to the lesion, unsteady gait, and vertigo.
FN2e 346–347

7. **(B)** For tilts of the head to the right or left, an ocular counter roll is produced as a compensatory eye movement. The counter roll consists of a torsional eye move-

ment toward the side of the head opposite to the tilt. If the head is tilted to the right, an ocular counter roll to the left will be observed.
FN2e 350

8. **(D)** Occasionally, a portion of the temporal bone overlaying the semicircular canals thins so as to create a bony defect adjacent to the dura. This defect exposes the ducts of either the anterior or posterior semicircular canals (membranous labyrinth) to the extradural space. In these patients, Tulio's phenomenon is often observed consisting of dizziness and oscillopsia in response to loud sounds or to changes in middle ear or intracranial pressure. Other symptoms include nystagmus evoked by these stimuli in the plane of the affected canal.
FN2e 345

9. **(B)** The reduced capacity to detect movements of the head forward and backward (flexion and extension) would be produced by insult to the vertical semicircular canals. Temporal bone fractures involving these structures would reduce proper function and lead to an inability to detect motion in the planes of the vertical canals. Horizontal head motion detection would be unaffected.
FN2e 343–344

10. **(A)** An "acoustic neuroma" is usually a benign intradural tumor that involves cranial nerve VIII. This tumor most commonly arises from the superior division of this nerve and is actually a vestibular schwannoma. The tumor often produces compression of the nerve, reducing the signals from the receptors on the ipsilateral side. Symptoms include dizziness, nausea, and blurred vision. Caloric irrigation of the left ear shows a reduced response with ipsilateral weakness on posturography.
FN2e 349, 354

11. **(C)** Caloric irrigation is an often-used diagnostic test for vestibular system function. Warm water introduced into the external ear canal produces nystagmus with a fast phase directed toward the same side. Cold water produces nystagmus to the opposite side. This relationship is easily indicated by the mnemonic COWS: cold opposite—warm same.
FN2e 354

12. **(C)** The medial vestibulospinal tract (MVST) originates from the vestibular nuclei to descend through the medial longitudinal fasciculus and terminate bilaterally in the cervical spinal cord. MVST fibers terminate on neck flexor and extensor motor neurons, as well as on propriospinal neurons. MVST neurons primarily affect neck and head posture.
FN2e 355

13. **(D)** During a leftward head turn, the following events occur to produce the compensatory VOR. Left horizontal semicircular canal receptors are excited, left vestibular nuclei neurons are excited, right abducens motor neurons are excited, right lateral rectus muscles contract, and rightward slow phase eye movements occur. With continued leftward rotation, a resetting fast phase toward the rotation (leftward) occurs after each slow phase.
FN2e 353

14. **(B)** Trauma to the left vestibular nerve or labyrinth would reduce normal signals from the affected side. Reduced nerve activity would be processed by central vestibular neurons as an inhibitory signal and result in nystagmus with a fast phase directed toward the opposite ear.
FN2e 347, 353–354

15. **(A)** Blood flow to the vestibular labyrinth is provided through the labyrinthine artery, which is a branch of the anterior inferior cerebellar artery.
FN2e 343

16. **(E)** The three semicircular canals lie in approximately orthogonal planes to each other within the inner ear. The horizontal semicircular canal lies elevated approximately 30 degrees above the naso-occipital plane, and the vertical canals lie approximately at 45 degree positions between the nose, ear, and posterior occiput.
FN2e 343–344

17. **(A)** The vestibulocollic reflex (VCR) arises primarily through activation of the medial and lateral vestibulospinal pathways as part of compensatory head movement responses. The VCR can serve as a protective response, such as occurs during falling forward, where the head extension (dorsiflexion) would occur through activation of the neck extensor musculature.
FN2e 355

CHAPTER 23

Olfaction and Taste

1. A 21-year-old woman is brought to the emergency department from the site of an automobile collision. The CT reveals bilateral contusions on the medial surface of the temporal lobes, including portions of the periamygdaloid, piriform, and entorhinal cortices. Which of the following sensory deficits is most likely to be perceived by this patient?

- ○ (A) Altered sense of smell only
- ○ (B) Visual loss (partial blindness)
- ○ (C) Altered sense of taste and smell
- ○ (D) Loss of a sense of balance and equilibrium (dizziness)
- ○ (E) Paralysis of facial musculature

2. A 27-year-old man complains to his family physician that he seems to have lost much of his sense of taste. During the examination the physician discovers that the man was in a fist fight 2 weeks ago. With the exception of the taste disorder, affecting the anterior two thirds of the tongue, the motor and sensory function of cranial nerves appears normal. These observations suggest possible damage to which of the following?

- ○ (A) Lingual nerve
- ○ (B) Root of the facial nerve
- ○ (C) Geniculate ganglion
- ○ (D) Greater superficial petrosal nerve
- ○ (E) Chorda tympani

3. Which of the following is an essential step in the generation of an action potential in a fiber conveying taste information?

- ○ (A) Closing of Ca^{2+} pores in the cell membrane of the receptor cells
- ○ (B) Soluble chemicals interacting with receptors on the membranes of receptor cells
- ○ (C) The blockage of Ca^{2+} release from intracellular Ca^{2+} stores
- ○ (D) The release of Na^+ from intracellular Na^+ stores
- ○ (E) The release of K^+ from intracellular K^+ stores

4. Vallate (circumvallate) papillae, and their corresponding taste buds, are most characteristically found at which of the following locations?

- ○ (A) Over the surface of the posterior two thirds of the tongue
- ○ (B) At the root of the tongue
- ○ (C) On the epiglottis
- ○ (D) Over the surface of the anterior two thirds of the tongue
- ○ (E) At the junction of the rostral two thirds of the tongue (oral part) with the caudal part of the tongue

5. An 81-year-old woman is brought to her family physician. Her daughter explains that her mother has stopped eating because "nothing tastes good anymore." The woman also complains that her mouth is numb. MRI reveals a clearly outlined vascular lesion in the medulla. Damage to which of the following structures would most specifically relate to the altered perception of taste?

- ○ (A) Spinal trigeminal tract and nucleus
- ○ (B) Rostral portions of the solitary tract and nucleus
- ○ (C) Inferior salivatory nucleus of the glossopharyngeal nerve
- ○ (D) Superior salivatory nucleus of the facial nerve
- ○ (E) Caudalmost portions of the solitary tract and nucleus

6. After recovering from a motorcycle crash, a 21-year-old man complains that everything he eats "tastes funny." Which of the following most specifically describes a distorted or perverted sense of taste?

- ○ (A) Hyposmia
- ○ (B) Ageusia
- ○ (C) Anosmia
- ○ (D) Dysgeusia
- ○ (E) Alexia

7. A 73-year-old man is brought to the emergency department after experiencing a loss of sensation on the left side of his body and face. CT reveals a hemorrhagic lesion in the forebrain. In addition to conveying general sensation (pain and thermal sense, touch) from face regions of the brainstem to the cerebral cortex, which of the following nuclei also conveys taste information to the sensory cortex?

- ○ (A) Ventral lateral nucleus
- ○ (B) Ventral posterolateral nucleus

○ (C) Centromedian nucleus
○ (D) Ventral anterior nucleus
○ (E) Ventral posteromedial nucleus

8. Olfactory receptor cells have a life span of 30 to 60 days and, consequently, are replaced throughout life. Which of the following is the stem cell from which olfactory receptor cells arise?

○ (A) Mitral cell
○ (B) Basal cell
○ (C) Tufted cell
○ (D) Sustentacular cell
○ (E) Periglomerular cell

9. Which of the following is a feature specifically characteristic of sensory input conveyed through the olfactory system?

○ (A) Olfactory neurons have chemical synapses.
○ (B) A generator potential in olfactory receptor cells may lead to depolarization and may initiate an action potential.
○ (C) There is a region of sensory cortex that receives olfactory input.
○ (D) Olfactory input travels directly to the cortex without a synaptic relay in a thalamic nucleus.
○ (E) The olfactory bulb, as a sensory structure, is laminated.

10. A neuropathologist examines a tumor removed from the olfactory mucosa of a 7-year-old boy. The tumor contains the sensory cell type characteristic of receptor neurons in the olfactory epithelium. Which of the following cell types is most likely seen in this tumor?

○ (A) Pseudounipolar
○ (B) Unipolar
○ (C) Multipolar
○ (D) Bipolar
○ (E) Pyramidal

11. Taste buds are located in specialized structures called papillae. Which of the following represents the most widely distributed papillae in the oral cavity?

○ (A) Fungiform
○ (B) Vallate
○ (C) Foliate
○ (D) Circumvallate
○ (E) Bowman gland

12. Which of the following neurotransmitters is associated with the synapse of the olfactory receptor neurons on the next neurons (such as mitral or tufted cells) in the olfactory pathway?

○ (A) Dopamine
○ (B) Acetylcholine
○ (C) Histamine
○ (D) GABA
○ (E) Glutamate

13. Which of the following cranial nerves (CNs) contain primary sensory taste fibers that enter the soli-

tary tract to eventually terminate in the adjacent solitary nucleus?

○ (A) CNs V, VI, and VII
○ (B) CNs IX, X, and XII
○ (C) CNs VII, IX, and X
○ (D) CNs VIII, IX, and XI
○ (E) CNs V, VII, and XI

14. Perception of salty tastes most likely requires which of the following mechanisms in the receptor cell?

○ (A) Marked decrease in intracellular Ca^{2+} stores
○ (B) Movement of H^+ out of the cell
○ (C) Movement of Na^+ into the receptor cell via apical cation channels
○ (D) Release of K^+ from intracellular stores
○ (E) Activation of extracellular G protein–mediated second-messenger pathways

ANSWERS

1. **(C)** Olfactory fibers project to the amygdaloid complex and to the adjacent periamygdaloid, piriform, and entorhinal cortices. Lesions of the medial temporal lobes may result in an altered or perverted perception of odors (parosmia). However, because smell and taste function in concert this patient would also experience an alteration in her sense of taste. Remember how a bad cold alters the sense of smell and taste. Such lesions in the medial temporal lobe(s) may also result in deficits characteristic of injury to the amygdaloid complex and/or hippocampal formation.
FN2e 363–364, 499–500, 501, 522

2. **(E)** The chorda tympani is a branch of the facial nerve that conveys taste fibers from the anterior two thirds of the tongue. Taste fibers from the anterior two thirds of the tongue first travel on the lingual nerve and then join the facial nerve via the chorda tympani. These taste fibers distribute to the brainstem on the facial nerve. The lingual nerve conveys general sensation (pain and thermal sense) from the surface of the tongue via the trigeminal nerve.
FN2e 369, 210–211, 213–215

3. **(B)** Taste transduction (the conversion of a chemical stimulus to an electrical impulse on an axon) is initiated by the interaction of soluble substances with membrane receptors on the apical microvilli of the taste receptor cells. This interaction initiates a cascade of events, both at the cell membrane and within the cell, that results in the perception of taste.
FN2e 368–369

4. **(E)** The vallate papillae form a V-shaped configuration on the surface of the tongue at about the junction of the oval area of the tongue with the pharyngeal area of the tongue. These large structures are visible when examining the surface of the tongue.
FN2e 367–368

5.   **(B)** Taste fibers (special visceral afferent, SVA) are conveyed on cranial nerves VII (from anterior two thirds of tongue), IX (from posterior one third of tongue), and X (from root of tongue). These fibers terminate primarily in rostral portions of the solitary nucleus after their central processes traverse the solitary tract.
FN2e 369–370

6.   **(D)** Dysgeusia (or parageusia) is a distorted perception of taste. Something may taste unpleasant when it should be pleasant, or vice versa. There may also be a perception of taste when no substances are present that should produce such a perception. The latter may also be called a gustatory hallucination.
FN2e 262, 265

7.   **(E)** The ventral posteromedial nucleus (VPM, specifically its parvocellular division) of the diencephalon relays taste information to the face portion of the postcentral gyrus and to parts of the adjacent operculum. Fibers conveying taste information to the VPM originate from rostral areas of the solitary nucleus (also called the gustatory nucleus) and ascend ipsilaterally to terminate in this thalamic nucleus.
FN2e 370–371

8.   **(B)** Basal cells are located on the inner aspect of the olfactory epithelium. These cells sit on a basal lamina and give rise to a new generation of olfactory receptor cells.
FN2e 361–362

9.   **(D)** The olfactory system is the only sensory system that projects directly to the cerebral cortex without first synapsing in a relay nucleus of the thalamus.
FN2e 364–365

10.   **(D)** As is the case for other neuroepithelial cells involved in special sense (retina, vestibular, and cochlear receptors), the receptor cells of the olfactory epithelium are bipolar. Olfactory receptor cells also have a knoblike structure called the olfactory vesicle from which about 10 to 30 nonmobile cilia protrude. These cilia contain the receptors for odorant molecules.
FN2e 360

11.   **(A)** Fungiform papillae are widely distributed over the anterior two thirds of the tongue. These are distributed among many filiform papillae, which have a nongustatory function.
FN2e 367–368

12.   **(E)** The synaptic contact of the olfactory receptor neuron on the mitral cell, tufted cell, and periglomerular cell is excitatory. The neurotransmitter at this synapse is glutamate.
FN2e 363

13.   **(C)** The facial, glossopharyngeal, and vagus nerves convey taste fibers centrally. These fibers have their cell bodies of origin in the geniculate ganglion (VII) and the inferior ganglia of CNs IX and X. Centrally, these taste fibers terminate in the rostral portions of the solitary tract. This part of the nucleus is also called the gustatory nucleus.
FN2e 370–371

14.   **(C)** Perception of salty tastes is a result of the direct action of Na^+ with membrane receptors located in the membrane at the apical surface of taste receptor cells. Similar pathways may also exist for potassium salts.
FN2e 368–369

The Motor System: Peripheral Sensory, Brainstem, and Spinal Influence on Anterior Horn Neurons and Corticofugal Systems and the Control of Movement

Questions 1 through 5 are based on the following patient:

A 23-year-old man is brought to the emergency department after an automobile collision. The evaluation, which includes CT, reveals a man with multiple injuries who is stuporous and responds only to deep painful stimulation. Within a few hours he exhibits the characteristics of decorticate (flexor) posturing. Within 24 hours the decorticate posturing converts to decerebrate (extensor) posturing and he no longer responds to painful stimulation.

1. The initial appearance of decorticate rigidity (decorticate posturing) would most likely indicate damage in which of the following?

- ○ (A) A supratentorial location
- ○ (B) An infratentorial location
- ○ (C) The midbrain
- ○ (D) The pons and medulla
- ○ (E) The cerebellum

2. In a patient who exhibits decorticate posturing (decorticate rigidity) the upper and lower extremities assume which of the following positions?

- ○ (A) Lower extremities flexed, upper extremities extended
- ○ (B) Lower and upper extremities flexed
- ○ (C) Lower and upper extremities extended
- ○ (D) Lower extremities extended, upper extremities flexed
- ○ (E) Upper and lower extremities flaccid

3. The fact that this patient went from being decorticate to being decerebrate suggests that the damage within the brain is what?

- ○ (A) Extending from a supratentorial location downward through the tentorial notch into an infratentorial location
- ○ (B) Extending from an infratentorial location upward through the tentorial notch into a supratentorial location
- ○ (C) Extending through the foramen magnum into the cervical spinal cord (tonsilar herniation)
- ○ (D) Extending from the pons into the cerebellum
- ○ (E) Extending from pons into the medulla

4. Which of the following would most correctly describe a patient with decerebrate rigidity (posturing)?

- ○ (A) Lower and upper extremities flexed
- ○ (B) Lower and upper extremities extended

147

○ (C) Lower and upper extremities completely flaccid
○ (D) Lower extremities flexed, upper extremities extended
○ (E) Lower extremities extended, upper extremities flexed

5. The probability that this patient will regain consciousness and any of his normal function is about

○ (A) 80%
○ (B) 60%
○ (C) 40%
○ (D) 20%
○ (E) Negligible

6. A 17-year-old boy has weakness of extrafusal muscles that has progressed from mild to severe over about a year. Which of the following is the primary source of innervation of these muscle fibers?

○ (A) Posterior horn track neurons
○ (B) Gamma motor neurons
○ (C) Interneurons
○ (D) Alpha motor neurons
○ (E) Renshaw cells

7. A 29-year-old woman is referred to a neurologist for muscle weakness. She complains that she feels weak then seems to "get better" only to feel weak again. The examination reveals a weakness in the ocular muscles, slight drooping of the eyelids, and limb weakness. The neurologist suspects a disease of the neuromuscular junction. Which of the following neurotransmitters would be most affected by a disease at this location?

○ (A) GABA
○ (B) Acetylcholine
○ (C) Glutamate
○ (D) Dopamine
○ (E) Glycine

8. A 67-year-old man presents with weakness of axial (truncal) muscles. Distal (appendicular) muscle strength is normal. Sensation and deep tendon reflexes are also normal. Which of the following is the most likely location of lower motor neurons innervating axial musculature?

○ (A) Lateral areas of the anterior horn
○ (B) Upper (more dorsal parts) of the anterior horn
○ (C) Lower (more ventral parts) of the anterior horn
○ (D) Medial areas of the anterior horn
○ (E) Intermediolateral cell column

9. A 67-year-old man with uncontrolled hypertension becomes decorticate subsequent to a stroke. The flexed posture of his upper extremities is caused primarily by action of fibers contained in which of the following tracts?

○ (A) Medial reticulospinal tract
○ (B) Medial vestibulospinal tract
○ (C) Tectospinal tract
○ (D) Rubrospinal tract
○ (E) Lateral vestibulospinal tract

10. The ultimate action of lateral vestibulospinal tract axons, after making synaptic contacts with interneurons, is to

○ (A) Inhibit motor neurons innervating distal musculature
○ (B) Excite motor neurons innervating distal musculature
○ (C) Inhibit motor neurons innervating flexor musculature
○ (D) Inhibit motor neurons innervating paravertebral (axial) and proximal limb extensor musculature
○ (E) Excite motor neurons innervating paravertebral (axial) and proximal limb extensor musculature

11. A 78-year-old woman experiences transient neurologic deficits suggestive of a partial occlusion of the internal carotid artery (stenosis). During an angiogram performed to determine the patency of the internal carotid artery, she experiences sudden weakness of her left upper extremity. CT reveals a hemorrhage in the motor cortex. Which of the following labeled areas, each indicating a potential lesion in the somatomotor cortex, represents the most likely location of this lesion? (   )

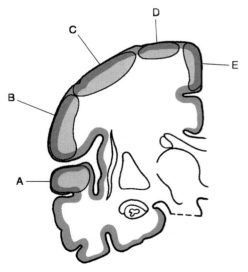

Figure 24–1

12. A 59-year-old morbidly obese man with untreated diabetes suffered from several neurologic problems before his death. The family requested an autopsy in an effort to identify some of the particulars of his neurologic disorders. A stained section of the brainstem reveals an obvious defect. Which of the following represents the most likely location of the origin of the missing fibers? See Figure 24–2.

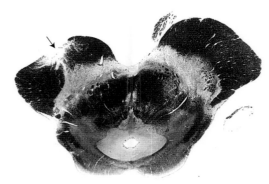

Figure 24–2

○ (A) Postcentral and posterior paracentral gyri on the right
○ (B) Precentral and anterior paracentral gyri on the right
○ (C) Postcentral and posterior paracentral gyri on the left
○ (D) Precentral and anterior paracentral gyri on the left
○ (E) Internal capsule on the left

13.   A 29-year-old construction worker is brought to the emergency department by a coworker. He states that he was lifting very heavy steel bars and felt a sudden shearing pain in his "arm." The examination reveals a tear in the biceps muscle at its junction with the flat tendon attaching to the radial tuberosity. This injury suggests a failure of the reflex known as autogenic inhibition that arises from the Golgi tendon organ. Which of the following fiber types is most specifically related to the afferent limb of this reflex?

○ (A) Ia fibers
○ (B) Ib fibers
○ (C) C fibers
○ (D) III (Aδ)
○ (E) II (Aβ)

Questions 14 through 19 are based on the following patient:

A 79-year-old man is brought to the emergency department by his son and daughter-in-law. They report that he complained of a headache, became nauseated, and then seemed to be confused. The examination reveals that the patient has a weakness of facial muscles on the left lower half of the face, especially at the corner of the mouth, and is unable to elevate his right shoulder (especially against resistance); his tongue protrudes to the left on attempted protrusion. Sensation from the face and body is normal. MRI reveals a hemorrhagic lesion.

14.   Weakness of which of the following muscles would explain a droop of the right shoulder or an inability to elevate (shrug) the right shoulder, especially against resistance?

○ (A) Deltoid
○ (B) Levator scapulae
○ (C) Sternocleidomastoid
○ (D) Trapezius
○ (E) Rhomboid muscle

15.   Weakness of which of the following muscles explains the deviation of the tongue to the left, on protrusion, in this patient?

○ (A) Superior constrictor
○ (B) Thyroglossus
○ (C) Hyoglossus
○ (D) Genioglossus
○ (E) Palatoglossus

16.   The pattern of weakness of the facial muscles in this patient suggests a lesion at which of the following locations?

○ (A) Root of the facial nerve at the brainstem
○ (B) Nucleus of the facial nerve in the brainstem
○ (C) Posterior limb of the internal capsule
○ (D) At some point between the precentral gyrus and the motor facial nucleus
○ (E) Facial nerve at the stylomastoid foramen

17.   The difficulty in elevating the shoulder, especially against resistance, as experienced by this particular patient suggests damage at which of the following locations?

○ (A) Root of the accessory nerve
○ (B) Nucleus of the accessory nerve
○ (C) Cerebral cortical input to the accessory nucleus
○ (D) Root of the phrenic nerve
○ (E) Corticospinal input to motor neurons of the cervical enlargement and phrenic motor neurons

18.   The combination of signs and symptoms experienced by this patient suggests that the lesion is most likely located in which of the following?

○ (A) Left posterior limb of the internal capsule
○ (B) Right genu of the internal capsule
○ (C) Right posterior limb of the internal capsule
○ (D) Left genu of the internal capsule
○ (E) Right anterior limb of the internal capsule

19.   In addition to being served by branches of the anterior choroidal artery, corticonuclear (corticobulbar) fibers also receive blood supply through which of the following?

○ (A) Lenticulostriate arteries
○ (B) Medial posterior choroidal artery(ies)
○ (C) Ophthalmic artery
○ (D) Precentral branch of the middle cerebral artery
○ (E) Posterior lateral choroidal artery

20.   A 47-year-old man is brought to the emergency department with decorticate rigidity. MRI reveals a

hemorrhagic lesion. The patient's upper extremities and fingers are flexed, the hands are rotated outward (extreme supination), and the lower extremities are extended. Which of the following fibers are most specifically responsible for the flexed upper extremities in this patient?

○ (A) Reticulospinal
○ (B) Vestibulospinal
○ (C) Hypothalamospinal
○ (D) Corticospinal
○ (E) Rubrospinal

21.   A neurologist sees three patients in her clinic. These are a 47-year-old man with a Brown-Séquard syndrome resulting from trauma to the spinal cord at C3-C5, a 67-year-old woman with a lateral medullary syndrome, and an 81-year-old woman with a hemorrhagic stroke into the lateral portions of the pontine tegmentum. Which of the following deficits would most likely be seen in all of these patients?

○ (A) Weakness of muscles of the extremities on one side of the body
○ (B) Loss of pain and thermal sense from one side of the face
○ (C) Loss of proprioception and discriminative touch on one side of the body
○ (D) Constriction of the pupil (miosis) on the side of the lesion
○ (E) Deviation of the tongue and weakness of the facial and masticatory muscles

22.   A 61-year-old man with uncontrolled hypertension and diabetes becomes decorticate after a large hemorrhagic stroke in the right hemisphere. The lesion has caused significant midline shift. Which of the following tracts is most specifically responsible for the extensor rigidity of the neck, trunk, and lower extremities in this patient?

○ (A) Rubrospinal only
○ (B) Vestibulospinal only
○ (C) Corticospinal and rubrospinal
○ (D) Vestibulospinal and reticulospinal
○ (E) Tectospinal

23.   A 74-year-old man is brought to the emergency department by paramedics. His family reports that he became confused and sick to his stomach. The examination reveals right-sided loss of sensation (pain, thermal sense, proprioception, and discriminative touch) on the face and body and weakness of the upper and lower extremities on the right. MRI reveals a hemorrhagic lesion in the forebrain. Which of the following labeled areas, each representing the location of a potential lesion, is the most likely site of this infarct? See Figure 24–3. (   )

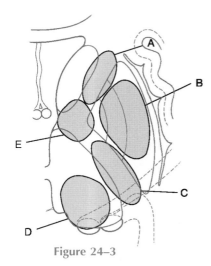

Figure 24–3

24.   An 81-year-old woman complains to her family physician that she "had a real bad headache and felt awful." The examination reveals deviation of the tongue to the left on protrusion and weakness of muscles on the lower face on the left, especially around the corner of the mouth. Motor and sensory function on the body is normal. MRI shows a lesion in the somatomotor cortex. Which of the following labeled areas, each representing the location of a potential lesion, is the most likely site of this infarct? (   )

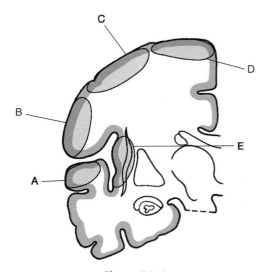

Figure 24–4

25.   An 83-year-old woman is brought to the emergency department from an assisted living facility after becoming confused. The examination reveals weakness of muscle function associated with cranial nerves. MRI reveals a hemorrhagic lesion in the genu of the left internal capsule. Which of the following deficits correlates most specifically with a lesion in the genu of the left internal capsule?

○ (A) Deviation of the tongue to the left
○ (B) Weakness of facial muscles on the left lower face

○ (C) Inability to elevate the right shoulder
○ (D) Weakness of facial muscles on the right upper face
○ (E) Deviation of the uvula to the right

26. A 27-year-old man who is a drug addict (cocaine abuse) is brought to the emergency department by the police. In addition to a drug-induced delirium, this man's tongue deviates, as shown here, on protrusion.

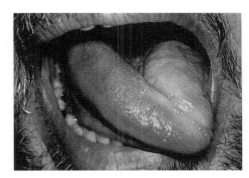

Figure 24–5

This is the only neurologic sign seen by the physician. This lesion is most likely located at which of the following locations or is a result of the occlusion of which of the following vessels?

○ (A) Right hypoglossal nucleus
○ (B) Genu of the internal capsule
○ (C) Anterior spinal artery branches on right
○ (D) Anterior spinal artery branches on left
○ (E) Left hypoglossal nucleus

27. A 29-year-old man presents with cerebellar rigidity. That is, he has an increase in extensor muscle tone as the result of a hemorrhagic lesion in the anterior lobe of the cerebellum. Which of the following is the most likely cause of this rigidity?

○ (A) Pressure on the medulla by tonsillar herniation
○ (B) Removal of Purkinje cell inhibition of vestibulospinal neurons
○ (C) Removal of Purkinje cell excitation of vestibulospinal neurons
○ (D) Damage to the corticopontocerebellar circuit
○ (E) Increase in the outflow of inhibitory signals from the fastigial nucleus

28. During the routine neurologic examination of a 42-year-old man the physician taps the patient's patellar tendon and elicits a normal knee-jerk reflex. Which of the following fiber types and corresponding conduction velocity is representative of the afferent limb of this reflex?

○ (A) C (class IV), 0.5 to 2.0 m/sec
○ (B) Aα (class Ia), 80 to 120 m/sec
○ (C) Aδ (class III), 5 to 30 m/sec
○ (D) Aγ, 12 to 48 m/sec
○ (B) B, 6 to 18 m/sec

Questions 29 through 32 are based on the following patient:

A 71-year-old man is brought to the emergency department by his wife. The physician is told that the man suddenly became nauseated, complained of a severe headache, and then became somnolent over the next hour or so. Although lethargic, the man is able to cooperate with the examination. There is deviation of the tongue to the right on protrusion, a left-sided weakness of the upper and lower extremities, and loss of proprioception and vibratory sense on the left side of the body. CT reveals a hemorrhagic lesion in the brain.

29. Which of the following is the best localizing sign in this patient?

○ (A) Upper extremity weakness on the left
○ (B) Lower extremity weakness on the left
○ (C) Proprioceptive loss on the left upper extremity
○ (D) Proprioceptive loss on the left lower extremity
○ (E) Deviation of the tongue to the right

30. Which of the following represents the location of the cell bodies of origin for those lesioned fibers that give rise to the weakness of the extremities?

○ (A) Right precentral gyrus
○ (B) Right somatomotor cortex
○ (C) Left precentral gyrus
○ (D) Left somatomotor cortex
○ (E) Right premotor cortex

31. This patient's deficits are the result of a small hemorrhagic infarction. Hemorrhage from which of the following vessels would most likely explain these deficits?

○ (A) Paramedian branches of the basilar artery on the left
○ (B) Branches of the anterior spinal artery to the right
○ (C) Branches of the anterior spinal artery to the left
○ (D) Branches of the posterior inferior cerebellar artery on the left
○ (E) Branches of the posterior inferior cerebellar artery on the right

32. The loss of proprioception and vibratory sense in this patient reflects damage to which of the following?

○ (A) Posterior columns on the left
○ (B) Posterior columns on the right
○ (C) Internal arcuate fibers bilaterally
○ (D) Medial lemniscus on the right
○ (E) Medial lemniscus on the left

33. A 71-year-old man experiences several small infarctions during the final 10 years of his life. Following his death from a myocardial infarction, his family requests an autopsy. The neuropathologist identifies a degenerated bundle of fibers in the brainstem.

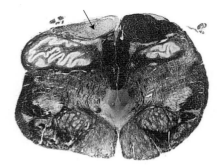

Figure 24–6

A lesion in which of the following would most likely explain the loss of fibers in this prominent fiber bundle?

○ (A) Right posterior limb of internal capsule
○ (B) Left posterior limb of internal capsule
○ (C) Right genu of internal capsule
○ (D) Left genu of internal capsule
○ (E) Left somatomotor cortex

34.   A 61-year-old man collapses at work and is transported to the emergency department by paramedics. The evaluation reveals normal motor and sensory cranial nerve function, profound weakness of both lower extremities, and normal sensation (pain, thermal sense, proprioception) from the body. Suspecting a small brain lesion, the physician orders an MRI. Which of the following represents the most likely location of this lesion?

○ (A) Caudal pons including both corticospinal tracts
○ (B) Right pyramid of medulla
○ (C) Left pyramid of medulla
○ (D) Rostral part of motor decussation
○ (E) Caudal part of motor decussation

35.   An 89-year-old woman complains to her family physician of weakness on the right side of her body and double vision. The physician writes "middle alternating hemiplegia" on the chart. Which of the following represents the most likely location of the lesion in this patient?

○ (A) Anteromedial area of the midbrain
○ (B) Anteromedial area of the pons-medulla junction
○ (C) Anteromedial area of the medulla at about mid-olivary levels
○ (D) Decussation of the superior cerebellar peduncle
○ (E) Genu of the internal capsule

36.   Which of the following sensory endings codes only the change in muscle length (the event) but does not code the rate of change in muscle length?

○ (A) Pacinian corpuscle
○ (B) Dynamic bag fibers
○ (C) Free endings
○ (D) Flower-spray endings
○ (E) Ruffini endings

37.   Descending inputs from supraspinal centers excite spinal motor neurons innervating intrafusal muscle fibers. Contraction of these fibers results in an increase in Ia fiber activity and a corresponding increase in the activity of alpha motor neurons and extrafusal muscle contraction. What is this circuit called?

○ (A) Monosynaptic myotatic reflex
○ (B) Reciprocal inhibition
○ (C) Crossed extensor reflex
○ (D) Gamma loop
○ (E) Flexor (or withdrawal) reflex

Questions 38 and 39 are based on the following patient:

A 59-year-old man with untreated diabetes presents to the emergency department complaining that he "can't walk right." The examination reveals that cranial nerve function is normal. The man's left lower extremity is paralyzed, but sensory function from the body is normal. CT reveals a hemorrhagic infarction in the motor cortex.

38.   Which of the following labeled areas, each representing the location of a potential lesion, is the most likely location of this lesion? (   )

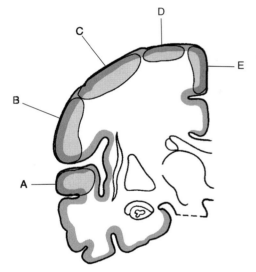

Figure 24–7

39.   Which of the following vessels is the most likely source of the hemorrhage in this patient?

○ (A) Precentral branches of M_4
○ (B) Central branches of M_4
○ (C) Branches of callosomarginal artery of A_2
○ (D) Parieto-occipital branches of P_4
○ (E) Anterior and posterior parietal branches of M_4

40.   Which of the following is seen in a patient with a lower motor neuron lesion?

○ (A) Muscle spasticity
○ (B) Muscle fasciculations
○ (C) Hyperreflexia
○ (D) Hypertonia
○ (E) Groups of muscles are adversely affected

41. A 28-year-old woman presents to her internist with neurologic symptoms that wax and wane. After referral to a neurologist, a diagnosis of multiple sclerosis is made. The MRI shows areas of demyelination at several places in her brain. Which of the following deficits would correlate most specifically with demyelination in the area shown here?

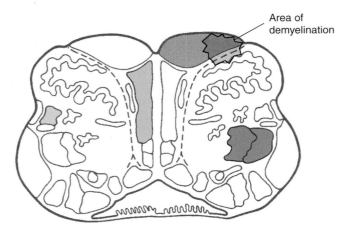

Figure 24–8

- ○ (A) Tongue deviation to the right with weakness of the left lower extremity
- ○ (B) Tongue deviation to the left with weakness of the right upper and lower extremities
- ○ (C) Tongue deviation to the left with weakness of the right lower extremity
- ○ (D) Tongue deviation to the right with weakness of left upper and lower extremities
- ○ (E) Tongue deviation to the left with weakness of the right upper extremity

42. Which of the following receptors is part of the afferent limb of the patellar tendon reflex or jaw jerk reflex?

- ○ (A) Golgi tendon organ
- ○ (B) Pacinian corpuscle
- ○ (C) Meissner corpuscle
- ○ (D) Muscle spindle
- ○ (E) Ruffini ending

Questions 43 through 46 are related to the following patient:

A 16-year-old boy is brought to the emergency department by paramedics from the site of an automobile collision. He is unconscious and has multiple injuries. CT reveals a vertebral fracture with bone displacement. After the boy regains consciousness, the examination reveals a flaccid paralysis of the left upper extremity and loss of pain and thermal sensation sense on the right side of the body beginning at the shoulder (about the C5 dermatome).

43. The flaccid paralysis of the left upper extremity in this patient most specifically correlates with damage to which of the following?

- ○ (A) Corticospinal fibers on the right
- ○ (B) Corticospinal fibers on the left
- ○ (C) Anterior (ventral) horn on the left
- ○ (D) Anterior ventral horn on the right
- ○ (E) Anterior paracentral gyrus on the right

44. After several weeks the boy develops increased muscle tone and hyperreflexia in the left lower extremity. This correlates with damage to which of the following?

- ○ (A) Posterior columns on the left
- ○ (B) Corticospinal fibers on the right
- ○ (C) Anterolateral system on the left
- ○ (D) Corticospinal fibers on the left
- ○ (E) Spinocerebellar tracts on the right

45. The loss of pain and thermal sensation on the right side of the body in this patient is most specifically related to a lesion of which of the following?

- ○ (A) Anterolateral system on the right
- ○ (B) Posterior column system on the right
- ○ (C) Posterior column system on the left
- ○ (D) Anterior spinocerebellar tract on the left
- ○ (E) Anterolateral system on the left

46. The constellation of deficits experienced by this patient would suggest that the lesion is located at about which of the following spinal cord levels?

- ○ (A) C_3-C_4 on the left
- ○ (B) C_3-T_1 on the left
- ○ (C) C_2-C_3 on the right
- ○ (D) C_3-T_1 on the right
- ○ (E) C_7-T_3 on the left

47. Lateral vestibulospinal tract fibers extend the length of the spinal cord and excite extensor motor neurons innervating paravertebral and proximal limb muscles. Which of the following is the primary source of these tract cells?

- ○ (A) Superior vestibular nucleus
- ○ (B) Medial vestibular nucleus
- ○ (C) Lateral vestibular nucleus
- ○ (D) Inferior (spinal) vestibular nucleus
- ○ (E) Medial and inferior vestibular nuclei together

48. The reticular formation receives input from the cerebral cortex as corticoreticular fibers and from the spinal cord via the anterolateral system. In turn, cells of the gigantocellular reticular nucleus give rise to what?

- ○ (A) Medial reticulospinal tract
- ○ (B) Medial vestibulospinal tract
- ○ (C) Pontine reticulospinal tract
- ○ (D) Lateral reticulospinal tract
- ○ (E) Lateral vestibulospinal tract

Questions 49 and 50 are based on the following patient:

A 70-year-old woman living in a rural area is brought to the local medical clinic by her daughter. She is confused. Suspecting an intracranial lesion, the physician refers the woman to a regional medical center. The examination reveals weakness of the muscles on the lower right face, inability to elevate the left shoulder especially against resistance, and deviation of the tongue to the right on protrusion. MRI reveals a small hemorrhagic lesion.

49.   Taking into consideration the combination of deficits experienced by this patient, which of the following represents the most likely location of her lesion?

- ○ (A) Genu of internal capsule on left
- ○ (B) Posterior limb of internal capsule on left
- ○ (C) Genu of internal capsule on right
- ○ (D) Posterior limb of internal capsule on right
- ○ (E) Precentral gyrus and frontal eye field on right

50.   In addition to the deficits just described, which of the following would also be seen in this woman when she attempts phonation (says "Ah")?

- ○ (A) Drooping of the soft palate only
- ○ (B) Deviation of the uvula to the right
- ○ (C) Deviation of the uvula to the left
- ○ (D) Drooping of the soft palate and no deviation of the tongue
- ○ (E) Elevation of the tongue

Questions 51 and 52 are based on the following patient:

A 23-year-old woman presents to her family physician with the complaint of generalized weakness. She says that her "arm feels funny." The neurologic examination reveals visual deficits, weakness of the right upper extremity, and loss of vibratory and position sense on the left upper extremity. MRI shows areas of demyelination in the brain that have sharply demarcated borders. Cerebrospinal fluid tests show elevated levels of gamma globulin in the cerebrospinal fluid. The evidence suggests a diagnosis of multiple sclerosis.

51.   Damage to which of the following labeled areas in the midbrain, each representing an area of demyelination, would account for the weakness of the upper extremity in this patient? (   )

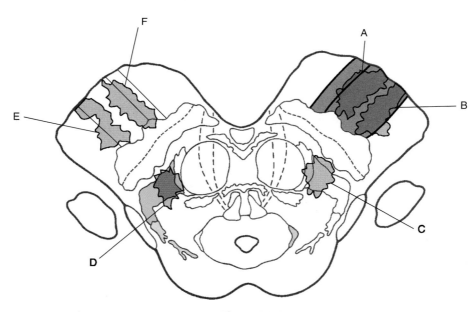

Figure 24–9

52.   Damage to fibers in which of the following labeled areas, each representing an area of demyelination, would most likely correlate with the sensory deficits experienced by this patient? See Figure 24–10. (   )

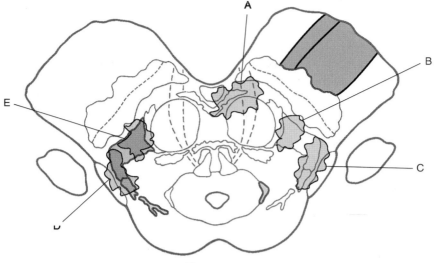

Figure 24–10

53.   A 49-year-old man with untreated hypertension is brought to the emergency department by paramedics. His wife explains that they were working in the yard when he complained of a headache and had to lie down in the grass because he felt like he was going to pass out. The examination reveals that on gaze to the right the right eye will not abduct and the left eye will not adduct. On gaze to the left, eye movement is normal. In addition, there is a weakness of facial muscles on one side of the face. MRI reveals a hemorrhagic lesion in the pons. Which of the following labeled areas below, each representing the site of a potential lesion, is the most likely site of this infarct? See Figure 24–11. (   )

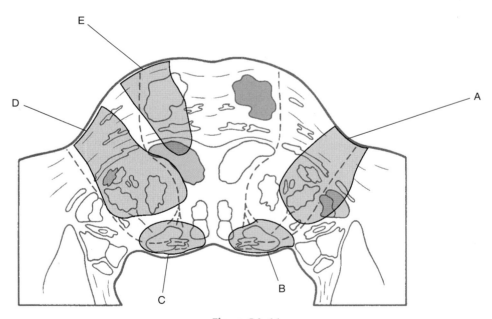

Figure 24–11

54.   A 22-year-old woman has waxing and waning muscle weakness that seems to especially affect ocular muscles. The woman complains of "seeing double" (diplopia). The administration of a cholinergic drug resolves the muscle weakness. Which of the following diseases is associated with the autoantibody destruction of nicotinic acetylcholine receptors in the neuromuscular junction?

○ (A) Huntington chorea
○ (B) Peripheral neuropathy
○ (C) Wilson disease
○ (D) Myasthenia gravis
○ (E) Muscular dystrophy

55.   Rubrospinal fibers originate from the large-celled (magnocellular) part of the red nucleus, cross in the

anterior (ventral) tegmental decussation, and descend through lateral parts of the brainstem. At spinal cord levels the primary action of rubrospinal axons is to

- (A) Excite extensor motor neurons innervating musculature of the lower extremity
- (B) Excite extensor motor neurons innervating musculature of the upper extremity
- (C) Excite flexor motor neurons innervating musculature of the lower extremity
- (D) Excite flexor motor neurons innervating musculature of the upper extremity
- (E) Excite motor neurons innervating paravertebral (axial) musculature

56.   Intrafusal muscle fibers are small striated muscles associated with the muscle spindle. These muscle fibers are innervated by

- (A) Alpha motor neurons
- (B) Interneurons of the anterior horn
- (C) Gamma motor neurons
- (D) Renshaw cells
- (E) Granule cells

57.   A 79-year-old man presents with a brainstem lesion that damages the axons of vestibulospinal and reticulospinal tracts. These tracts terminate primarily in which of the following spinal laminae?

- (A) I–III
- (B) I and II
- (C) III–V
- (D) VII and VIII
- (E) IX

Questions 58 through 62 are based on the following patient:

A 64-year-old man is transported from a rural location to a regional medical center by paramedics. The emergency department physician learns that the man was working on his chicken house roof, became dizzy and nauseated, and fell. He is conscious but complains of a bad headache and "seeing two of everything." The examination reveals a dilated right pupil and an almost complete lack of eye movement of the right eye (the eye is rotated slightly down and out and the patient can make eye movements in these directions). Sensation from the face and body is normal. In addition, the man has a profound left-sided weakness of upper and lower extremities.

58.   Based on the voluntary eye movements that this patient can perform, which of the following muscles are most likely functioning normally?

- (A) Superior oblique and lateral rectus
- (B) Superior rectus and lateral rectus
- (C) Medial rectus and inferior oblique
- (D) Superior oblique and medial rectus
- (E) Inferior rectus and inferior oblique

59.   Damage to which of the following would most likely result in the dilated pupil in this patient?

- (A) Optic nerve
- (B) GSE fibers of the oculomotor nerve
- (C) GVE postganglionic sympathetic fibers arising in the superior cervical ganglion
- (D) GVE fibers of the oculomotor nerve
- (E) GVE fibers of the abducens nerve

60.   The weakness of the extremities in this patient most likely represents injury to which of the following?

- (A) Rubrospinal fibers on the left
- (B) Rubrospinal fibers on the right
- (C) Corticospinal fibers on the left
- (D) Corticospinal fibers on the right
- (E) Medial lemniscus fibers on the right

61.   The combination of deficits seen in this patient most likely indicates a lesion in which of the following?

- (A) Telencephalon
- (B) Diencephalon
- (C) Mesencephalon
- (D) Metencephalon
- (E) Myelencephalon

62.   The particular combination of deficits seen in this patient can also be referred to as which of the following?

- (A) Weber syndrome
- (B) Foville syndrome
- (C) Wallenberg syndrome
- (D) Parinaud syndrome
- (E) Benedikt syndrome

63.   Descending cortical fibers (corticonuclear fibers) that influence the activity of lower motor neurons of the facial, spinal accessory and hypoglossal nuclei primarily traverse the

- (A) Anterior limb of the internal capsule
- (B) Genu of the internal capsule
- (C) Posterior limb of the internal capsule
- (D) Retrolenticular limb of the internal capsule
- (E) Sublenticular limb of the internal capsule

64.   A 29-year-old man is brought to the emergency department after an automobile collision. The examination reveals that the gag reflex is absent, and the man has a hoarse, gravely voice. Which of the following functional components is associated with the innervation of the vocalis and stylopharyngeus muscles?

- (A) GSE
- (B) GVE
- (C) SVE
- (D) GSE and GVE
- (E) SVE and GSE

65.   The largest axons in the corticospinal tract range from 12 to 15 μm in diameter and have a conduction velocity in the range of

- (A) 40 m/sec
- (B) 55 m/sec

○ (C) 70 m/sec
○ (D) 90 m/sec
○ (E) 110 m/sec

66. A 59-year-old man is brought to the emergency department after collapsing at his desk at a local office building. MRI reveals a massive hemorrhage. The man becomes decorticate, followed at 4 hours by decerebrate rigidity. Decerebrate rigidity results from which of the following?

○ (A) Increased excitatory activity of corticospinal axons at spinal levels on extensor motor neurons
○ (B) Increased excitatory activity of rubrospinal axons at spinal levels or extensor motor neurons
○ (C) A loss of excitatory outflow of cerebellar corticovestibular axons
○ (D) Unopposed (and overriding) excitatory activity of reticulospinal and vestibulospinal axons on flexor motor neurons at spinal levels
○ (E) Unopposed (and overriding) excitatory activity of reticulospinal and vestibulospinal axons on extensor motor neurons at spinal levels

67. A 31-year-old woman visits her internist with a headache and nausea of several weeks duration. Suspecting a brain lesion, the physician orders MRI, which reveals a large tumor occupying the anterior lobe of the cerebellum. Assuming this lesion has removed the influence of anterior lobe Purkinje cells on their targets, which of the following is most likely the cause of the resulting decerebellate (cerebellar) rigidity?

○ (A) Increased excitatory activity of rubrospinal fibers
○ (B) Decreased inhibitory activity of corticospinal fibers
○ (C) Increased excitatory activity of vestibulospinal fibers
○ (D) Increased inhibitory activity of spinoreticular fibers
○ (E) Decreased excitatory activity of rubrospinal fibers

68. Which of the following signals the rate of change in extrafusal muscle length?

○ (A) Golgi tendons organ
○ (B) Static nuclear bag fiber
○ (C) Tree nerve ending
○ (D) Dynamic nuclear bag fiber
○ (E) Pacinian corpuscle

69. Stretch of the Golgi tendon organ will, through appropriate neural circuits, ultimately result in which of the following?

○ (A) Monosynaptic excitation of alpha motor neurons innervating muscles associated with the activated tendon organ
○ (B) Excitation (through interneurons) of alpha motor neurons innervating muscles associated with the activated tendon organ
○ (C) Monosynaptic inhibition of alpha motor neurons innervating muscles associated with the activated tendon organ

○ (D) Inhibition (through interneurons) of alpha motor neurons innervating muscles associated with the activated tendon organ
○ (E) A monosynaptic myotatic reflex on the ipsilateral side of the body

70. Contraction of the intrafusal muscle fiber consequent to activation of a gamma motor neuron by descending fibers from the cortex or brainstem will result in

○ (A) Decreased firing rates in Ia fibers
○ (B) Increased firing rates in Ib fibers
○ (C) Decreased firing rates in Ib fibers
○ (D) Increased firing rates in Ia fibers
○ (E) Increased firing rates in C fibers

Questions 71 and 72 are based on the following patient:

A 22-year-old man is brought to the emergency department from the site of a motorcycle collision. He has extensive facial injuries and is stuporous. The examination reveals a paralysis of the left lower leg, a loss of proprioception and vibratory sense from the left lower extremity, and a right-sided loss of pain and thermal sensation beginning at the dermatome for T9 and extending caudally. CT reveals fractures of the facial bones and of two adjacent vertebrae.

71. Which of the following labeled areas, each representing the location of potential damage to the spinal cord, is the most likely site of the injury in this patient? (   )

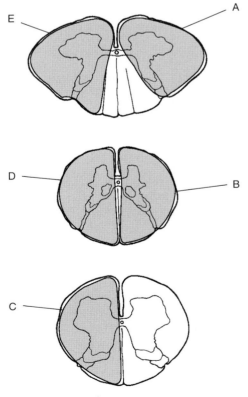

Figure 24–12

72. Which of the following most specifically includes the combination of deficits experienced by this patient?

○ (A) Weber syndrome
○ (B) Duane syndrome
○ (C) Wallenberg syndrome
○ (D) Brown-Séquard syndrome
○ (E) Foville syndrome

ANSWERS

1. **(A)** Decorticate rigidity reflects a large lesion within one hemisphere that extends into the opposite hemisphere or bilateral damage within both hemispheres. In effect this removes most of the descending influence of the cortex from the brainstem and spinal cord. The internal capsule and descending cortical fibers, including corticospinal fibers, are compromised by the injury.
FN2e 384–385

2. **(D)** In the patient with decorticate posturing, the cerebral cortex is removed from its influence on spinal motor neurons, but the rubrospinal tract and descending brainstem tracts (vestibulospinal, reticulospinal) are intact. Consequently, the upper extremities are flexed and hands rotated inward (extreme supination, rubrospinal influence) and the lower extremities are extended and rigid (vestibulospinal, reticulospinal influence). In addition, the toes are pointed slightly inward, the hand rotated slightly outward (extreme pronation), and the head extended. Collaterals of spinoreticular fibers in the anterolateral system increase the excitatory activity of reticulospinal neurons innervating extensor motor neurons.
FN2e 382–385

3. **(A)** Proceeding from decorticate to decerebrate posturing indicates that the damage has extended from a supratentorial position to an infratentorial position by passing through the tentorial notch. In doing so, the area of damage extended into the midbrain tegmentum, the red nucleus, and adjacent structures.
FN2e 382–383

4. **(B)** In the patient with decerebrate posturing, the descending cortical influence and the rubrospinal influence on spinal lower motor neurons have been removed. All that is left are descending, and predominately excitatory, brainstem projections to extensor motor neurons in the spinal cord. Consequently, the upper and lower extremities are extended and rigid, the toes pointed, and the head extended. Spinoreticular fibers in the anterolateral system add an additional excitatory input into the brainstem centers (reticular formation) projecting to spinal motor neurons.
FN2e 382–385

5. **(E)** Patients with traumatic brain injury (TBI) that proceed from decorticate to decerebrate rigidity have a poor chance of significant recovery or survival.
FN2e 383–385

6. **(D)** Large lower motor neurons (alpha motor neurons) of the anterior horn innervate skeletal muscles. Motor nuclei of cranial nerves also contain similar cells that innervate skeletal muscles of the head that are associated with cranial nerves.
FN2e 374–376

7. **(B)** In addition to the neuromuscular junction, acetylcholine is found in visceromotor preganglionic neurons (and at their synapse with postganglionic cells), in postganglionic neurons innervating sweat glands and blood vessels, and in cells of the caudate nucleus, the basal forebrain and the brainstem tegmental area. Myasthenia gravis is a neuromuscular disease caused by an antibody-mediated destruction of the nicotinic acetylcholine receptors in the neuromuscular junction.
FN2e 375–376

8. **(D)** Lower motor neurons (alpha motor neurons) are, in general, somatotopically arranged in the anterior horn. Neurons innervating proximal muscles are medial, those innervating more distal muscles are located more lateral, those innervating extensor muscles more anterior in the horn, and those innervating flexor muscles located more posteriorly in the anterior horn.
FN2e 374

9. **(D)** Rubrospinal axons originate from the magnocellular portion of the red nucleus, arch toward the midline of the midbrain, and then cross as the anterior (ventral) tegmental decussation. These fibers descend through lateral portions of the brainstem to assume a position in the lateral funiculus of the spinal cord overlapping with the lateral corticospinal tract. The action of rubrospinal fibers is to excite motor neurons innervating proximal limb flexor muscles.
FN2e 380–382

10. **(E)** Lateral vestibulospinal fibers originate from the lateral vestibular nucleus, descend ipsilaterally, and exert an excitatory influence on extensor motor neurons. This pathway is one that contributes to the extensor rigidity seen in decorticate and decerebrate patients.
FN2e 379–380

11. **(C)** The weakness of the left upper extremity correlates with an infarct located in about the middle one third of the precentral gyrus on the contralateral side. The face is represented in the lateral third, and the trunk in about the medial third of this gyrus. The blood supply to this area of the motor cortex is primarily via central and precentral branches of the middle cerebral artery (M_4).
FN2e 389–390

12. **(B)** The middle portion of the crus cerebri is atrophic on the patient's right side consequent to the missing corticospinal fibers. This is the location of corticospinal and corticonuclear (corticobulbar) fibers that originate from the somatomotor cortex (precentral and anterior paracentral gyri) on the right side. A lesion of the somatomotor cortex on the right or of the internal capsule (also on the right) would result in the loss of these fibers in the crus cerebri of the midbrain. This lesion results in a left-sided hemiparesis.
FN2e 391–393, 397

13. **(B)** The Golgi tendon organ is the peripheral receptor associated with Ib fibers. The cell bodies of these fibers are located in the posterior root ganglion and their central processes end in relation to inhibitory interneurons. These interneurons synapse on (and inhibit) motor neurons innervating the muscle from which the afferent volley originated. The result is muscle relaxation and protection from overstretch.
FN2e 146, 259, 377–378

14. **(D)** The trapezius muscle, innervated predominately by the accessory nerve, elevates the shoulder. Injury to the accessory nerve or to inputs to the accessory nuclei (e.g., corticonuclear fibers) will result in muscle weakness, especially in attempted voluntary movement. When standing, the affected shoulder may droop slightly when compared with the normal side.
FN2e 396–398

15. **(D)** The genioglossus muscle arises from the superior mental spine on the inner surface of the mandibular symphysis; the superior fibers enter the basal aspect of the full length of the tongue. Each genioglossus muscle pulls obliquely toward the midline. Consequently, weakness/paralysis of one genioglossus muscle will result in the tongue deviating toward the weak side, on attempted protrusion, owing to the pull of muscles on the unaffected side.
FN2e 396–399

16. **(D)** The fact that this patient has weakness of facial muscles on the lower half of the face excludes the root or the nucleus of the facial nerve as probable locations of the damage. Corticonuclear (corticobulbar) fibers to the motor neurons of the facial nucleus innervating muscles on about the lower half of the face are predominately crossed. Those projections to facial motor neurons innervating the muscles on the upper half of the face are mainly bilateral. Consequently, the lesion involves inputs to the facial nucleus between the nucleus and precentral gyrus.
FN2e 396–398

17. **(C)** In addition to a drooping shoulder this patient has motor deficits related to other cranial nerves. Consequently, the lesion cannot involve only the accessory root or nucleus. The lesion has to be located more rostral (at least rostral to the level of the facial motor nucleus) and most likely involves cortical fibers influencing lower motor neurons of cranial nerves (corticonuclear fibers). Corticonuclear (corticobulbar) projections to the accessory motor nucleus in upper levels of the cervical spinal cord are ipsilateral.
FN2e 396–399

18. **(B)** Taking all the signs and symptoms of this patient into consideration, the lesion is in the genu of the internal capsule on the patient's right side. Corticonuclear (corticobulbar) fibers to motor nuclei of cranial nerves primarily traverse the genu of the internal capsule. Those to the genioglossus motor neurons of the hypoglossal nucleus are crossed, those to the facial motor neurons serving the lower half of the face are predominately crossed, and those to the accessory nucleus serving the trapezius muscle are uncrossed.
FN2e 396–397

19. **(A)** Lenticulostriate branches of M_1 penetrate the hemisphere and serve much of the genu and portions of the posterior limb of the internal capsule, portions of the lenticular nucleus, and adjacent structures. In addition, the genu may also receive small blood supply from the anterior choroidal artery and medial striate artery (recurrent artery of Heubner). Occlusion of, or a hemorrhage from, lenticulostriate, medial striate, or anterior choroidal vessels may damage corticonuclear (corticobulbar) fibers in the genu of the internal capsule.
FN2e 390–392

20. **(E)** Rubrospinal fibers originate primarily from the large-celled (magnocellular) portion of the nucleus and cross in the anterior (ventral) tegmental decussation. As these axons proceed caudad they move into the lateral portion of the pontine tegmentum and descend through the lateral area of the medulla to eventually enter the lateral funiculus of the spinal cord. Rubrospinal axons terminate primarily in cervical levels, where they have an excitatory influence on flexor motor neurons, innervating flexors of the upper extremity.
FN2e 380–382

21. **(D)** Descending hypothalamospinal fibers pass through the lateral portion of the pontine tegmentum, lateral medulla, and lateral funiculus of the spinal cord en route to the intermediolateral cell column (IMLCC). These fibers provide input to the IMLCC, which, in turn, is the source of sympathetic preganglionic fibers to the superior cervical ganglion (SCG). The SCG, in turn, sends postganglionic fibers to the superior cervical ganglion. All three of these lesions will interrupt descending hypothalamospinal fibers and result in a Horner syndrome on the side of the lesion. This syndrome includes ptosis, anhidrosis, and constriction of the pupil (miosis) owing to a lesion within the sympathetic pathway.
FN2e 149, 170, 442–453, 470–471

22. **(D)** Both vestibulospinal and reticulospinal fibers influence extensor motor neurons at spinal levels. Whereas there are some small differences between the influence of medial and lateral vestibulospinal fibers and medial and lateral reticulospinal fibers, the overall affect of these descending projections is to excite extensor motor neurons. The result is contraction of extensor muscles and the characteristic (decerebrate) rigidity seen in the patient.
FN2e 379–383, 385

23. **(C)** The symptoms experienced by this patient indicate a disconnect of sensory input from the body and face going to the cerebral cortex and a disruption of descending corticospinal fibers. All of the deficits are on the same side in this patient; this is characteristic of a lesion in the cerebral hemisphere. The lesion in the posterior limb of the internal capsule interrupts descending corticospinal fibers and thalamocortical projections originating in the ventral posteromedial and ventral posterolateral nuclei and traveling to the somatosensory cortex.
FN2e 244–245, 390–391

24. **(B)** The face portions of the somatomotor cortex occupies about the lateral one third of the precentral

gyrus; this is the part immediately superior to the lateral sulcus. The cranial nerve deficits experienced by this patient (deviation of the tongue to the left, weakness of facial muscles around the mouth on the left) are consistent with a lesion in the face area of the right motor cortex.
FN2e 390, 396–397

25.   **(D)** A lesion in the left genu of the internal capsule will damage corticonuclear (corticobulbar) fibers as they exit the hemisphere. An infarct in this location will result in weakness of facial muscles on the right lower face, an inability to elevate the left shoulder, and deviation of the tongue to the right on attempted protrusion. The deviation of the tongue and the inability to elevate the shoulder are also seen resulting from lesions in other locations, such as in the medulla or at the roots of the nerves. Weakness of facial muscles on the right lower face is specifically related to the lesion in the genu.
FN2e 396–398

26.   **(E)** The patient's tongue is protruding to the left, and he exhibits no other neurologic signs. This observation indicates that the lesion is in the left hypoglossal nucleus or nerve. Lesions at other locations or in the territory of the anterior spinal artery would also produce deviation of the tongue, but there would be other signs and symptoms.
FN2e 396–399

27.   **(B)** Purkinje cells are inhibitory to their targets, including neurons in the vestibular nuclei of the brainstem that, in turn, project to the spinal cord. Removal of this inhibitory influence, due to an infarct in the anterior lobe, results in an increase in the excitatory outflow of the vestibulospinal projection to extensor motor neurons in the spinal cord. Another source of this imbalance is the fact that spinoreticular fibers in the anterolateral system are excitatory to the reticular nuclei that contribute, via reticulospinal fibers, to spinal extensor motor neurons.
FN2e 382–385

28.   **(B)** The afferent limb of the patellar tendon reflex originates from the muscle spindle as an Ia (Aα) fiber. These are heavily myelinated fibers with conduction velocities in the range of 80 to 120 m/sec. Aγ fibers arise from gamma motor neurons and innervate intrafusal muscles fibers, and B fibers are preganglionic visceromotor fibers. C fibers and Aδ fibers are concerned with pain and thermal sense and mechanoreceptors.
FN2e 259, 376–377

29.   **(E)** The weakness and proprioception/vibratory sense loss are indicative of a lesion of long tracts. The deviation of the tongue to the right is the best localizing sign. This observation, taken in concert with the long tract signs, points to a lesion in the caudal medulla of the nucleus or root of the hypoglossal nerve on the right side.
FN2e 261, 393, 395–397

30.   **(B)** This patient has weakness of upper and lower extremities, indicating damage to fibers originating from the upper extremity and trunk (precentral gyrus) areas and the lower extremity (anterior paracentral gyrus) area of the motor cortex. Both of these together are the somatomotor cortex; the precentral gyrus is only part of this cortical region. The right pyramid is damaged (rostral to the decussation); therefore, the right cortex is the source of these fibers.
FN2e 391–393

31.   **(B)** The deviation of the tongue is the best localizing sign in this patient; the root of this nerve is immediately lateral to the pyramid, which contains corticospinal fibers. The exiting roots and nucleus of the hypoglossal nerve, corticospinal fibers, and the medial lemniscus (conveying proprioception) are in the territory of penetrating branches of the anterior spinal artery. The hemorrhage originated from branches to the right; this correlates with the crossed (alternating) deficits.
FN2e 391–393

32.   **(D)** This patient has a medial medullary syndrome. He has alternating (crossed) motor deficits (tongue on right, body on left) and a contralateral sensory deficit that correlates with the position of the lesion. Sensory fibers conveying proprioception and vibratory sense ascend in the posterior column and synapse in the gracile and cuneate nuclei. The axons arising in the gracile and cuneate nuclei arch toward the midline as internal arcuate fibers, cross, and collect to form the medial lemniscus on the contralateral side. This lesion involves the right medial lemniscus.
FN2e 260–262, 393

33.   **(A)** The right pyramid of the medulla is atrophic in this patient. This reflects a loss of corticospinal fibers. These fibers originate from portions of the right somatomotor cortex (no fibers in the pyramid arise from face areas), descend through the right posterior limb of the internal capsule, and proceed through the brainstem on the right. Most corticospinal fibers cross in the motor decussation.
FN2e 391–393

34.   **(E)** The crossing of corticospinal fibers in the motor (pyramidal) decussation has a general somatotopic pattern. Fibers originating from the upper-extremity area of the somatomotor cortex generally cross in rostral portions of the decussation and terminate in the cervical enlargement. Fibers originating in the lower-extremity portion of the somatomotor cortex generally cross in the caudal portions of the decussation and descend to the lumbosacral enlargement. Consequently, a small lesion involving the caudal portions of the pyramidal decussation will result in bilateral weakness of the lower extremities with no other signs or symptoms.
FN2e 392–393

35.   **(B)** A "middle alternating hemiplegia" specifies a lesion involving corticospinal fibers and the immediately adjacent exiting roots of the abducens nerve—"middle" because it is between the superior and inferior alternating hemiplegias, "alternating" because it is a cranial nerve deficit on one side and a body deficit on the other side, and "hemiplegia" because it is a motor deficit. Alternating hemiplegias are also called crossed deficits. "Hemi-" refers to one half of the body or face.
FN2e 391–392

36. **(D)** The flower-spray ending in the muscle spindle codes the change in the length of muscle but does not code the rate at which the change is taking place. An easy way to remember this is flower-spray = event, not rate. The dynamic bag fiber is sensitive to the rate of change.
FN2e 377

37. **(D)** Gamma motor neurons receive an excitatory supraspinal input that results in the contraction of intrafusal muscle fibers. This action stretches the equatorial portion of the muscle spindle and in doing so increases the firing rate of Ia fibers (conduction velocity 80 to 120 m/sec). These Ia fibers excite alpha motor neurons, which causes the contraction of extrafusal muscle fibers. This circuit is the gamma loop.
FN2e 377–378

38. **(E)** The lower extremity is represented in the anterior paracentral gyrus. This is the most medial portion of the somatomotor cortex, is located on the medial aspect of hemisphere (adjacent to the falx cerebri), and is laterally continuous with the precentral gyrus. Neurons in this portion of the cortex influence the activity of lower motor neurons in lumbosacral levels of the spinal cord on the contralateral side.
FN2e 390, 393

39. **(C)** The callosomarginal artery is one of two large branches comprising A$_2$, the other being the pericallosal artery. It serves much of the medial surface of the hemisphere, including the paracentral lobule, through paracentral branches. The paracentral lobule consists of the anterior (motor cortex for lower extremity) and posterior (sensory cortex for lower extremity) paracentral gyri.
FN2e 390–393

40. **(B)** Muscle fibrillations and fasciculations are seen in patients with lower motor neuron disease. These involuntary contractions are caused by infrequent and irregular firing patterns of lower motor neurons as their cell bodies or axons die. Other characteristics of lower motor neuron disease include (a) muscles that are flaccid and will eventually undergo atrophy, (b) hypotonia, and (c) weak or absent reflexes (hyporeflexia, areflexia).
FN2e 388

41. **(C)** The somatotopic arrangement of corticospinal fibers in the pyramid is such that fibers to the lumbosacral spinal cord (lower extremity or "leg" fibers) are lateral and fibers to the cervical enlargement of the spinal cord (upper extremity or "arm" fibers) are medially located. This sclerotic plaque is located in the lateral portion of the patient's left pyramid (lower extremity weakness on the right) and involves the exiting root of the hypoglossal nerve (tongue deviates to the left on protrusion).
FN2e 392–393, 396, 398

42. **(D)** The muscle spindle is the afferent ending for the monosynaptic myotatic reflex. The central processes of the Ia fiber from the spindle is excitatory to alpha motor neurons innervating extrafusal muscle fibers of the muscle from which the afferent volley originated.
FN2e 376–377

43. **(C)** Flaccid paralysis is one of the cardinal signs of a lower motor neuron lesion. Other signs include mus-

cle atrophy, fasciculations/fibrillations, hypotonia, and hyporeflexia/areflexia. In this patient damage to the anterior horn on the left side is the cause of the flaccid paralysis of the left upper extremity.
FN2e 393–395

44. **(D)** Corticospinal fibers are upper motor neurons; they influence the activity of lower motor neurons (alpha motor neurons). Removing the influence of upper motor neurons, which includes corticospinal fibers and may encompass other smaller tracts, may eventually result in upper motor neuron signs. In addition to hypertonia (increased muscle tone) and hyperreflexia, the signs of upper motor neuron lesions are muscle spasticity, dorsiflexion of the great toe (Babinski sign), and the involvement of muscles groups as opposed to individual muscles.
FN2e 393–395

45. **(E)** Fibers conveying pain and thermal sensation originate from cells in the posterior horn, cross in the anterior (ventral) white commissure, and coalesce to form the anterolateral system contralateral to their origin. As these fibers cross the midline, they ascend one to two segments. In this patient a right-sided loss of pain and thermal sensations is indicative of a lesion on the left side of the spinal cord.
FN2e 277–281, 394–395

46. **(A)** The flaccid (lower motor neuron) paralysis of the patient's left upper extremity indicates damage to left anterior horn from about C3 to C4. The sensory level is about C5, indicating a lesion of fibers conveying pain and thermal sensations at about C3-C4 on the left side. These fibers ascend one to two segments as they cross the midline in the anterior (ventral) white commissure. The approximate level is established by a combination of the sensory level and the lower motor neuron paralysis of the upper extremity. This patient has certain elements of the Brown-Séquard syndrome.
FN2e 280–282, 394–395

47. **(C)** Lateral vestibulospinal fibers originate mainly from cells of the lateral vestibular nucleus and descend on the ipsilateral side in the anterior area of the spinal cord white matter. These fibers terminate mainly in spinal laminae VII and VIII on interneurons that influence lower motor neurons in the anterior horn.
FN2e 379–381

48. **(D)** The gigantocellular reticular nucleus of the medulla gives rise to a predominantly ipsilateral reticulospinal projection that terminates mainly in lamina VII (some in VI and VIII, IX). These fibers are called the medullary reticulospinal tract because of their origin from the reticular nuclei of the medulla, or the lateral reticulospinal tract because of their position (relative to other reticulospinal fibers) in the spinal cord white matter.
FN2e 380–381

49. **(A)** Corticonuclear (corticobulbar) fibers in the genu of the internal capsule to the genioglossus motor neurons in the hypoglossal nucleus and to the portion of the facial nucleus innervating the lower portion of the face are primarily crossed. The fibers to the accessory

nucleus are uncrossed. Consequently, the lesion is ipsilateral to the affected shoulder and contralateral to the tongue and facial paralysis. In this patient, the lesion is in the genu of the left internal capsule. The following is an easy way to remember the positions of lesions resulting in deviation of the tongue. When the lesion is in the genu, the tongue points to the side opposite the lesion; when the lesion is in the medulla, the tongue points to the side of the lesion.
FN2e 395–398

50.   **(C)** Corticonuclear (corticobulbar) fibers to neurons in the accessory nucleus that innervate muscles of the uvula are predominately crossed. Consequently, a lesion in the left genu results in the weakness of muscles of the uvula on the right. When the patient says "Ah," the intact muscles on the left contract and the uvula deviates to the left, toward the side of the lesion.
FN2e 397–399

51.   **(A)** Corticospinal fibers are somatotopically arranged in about the middle third of the crus cerebri. Fibers to the cervical enlargement (to influence the upper extremity) are located medially, and fibers to the lumbosacral enlargement (and influencing the lower extremity) are located laterally. Corticonuclear (corticobulbar) fibers are located medial to the corticospinal bundle. These latter fibers originate from the somatomotor cortex and descend uncrossed through the brainstem; most cross in the motor decussation. Weakness of the right upper extremity is consistent with demyelination of the crus cerebri on the patient's left.
FN2e 391–393

52.   **(E)** Fibers conveying vibratory sense, position sense (proprioception), and discriminative touch are located in the medial lemniscus in the brainstem. At midbrain levels these fibers are somatotopcially arranged; lower extremity fibers are located in the posterolateral portion of the medial lemniscus and upper extremity fibers in its anteromedial portion. Medial lemniscus fibers originate from the posterior column nuclei in medulla on the contralateral side and terminate in the ipsilateral ventral posterolateral nucleus. A proprioceptive deficit affecting the patient's left upper extremity correlates with a lesion in anteromedial portions of the medial lemniscus on the right.
FN2e 260–262, 392–394

53.   **(C)** The abducens nucleus contains large lower motor neurons that innervate the lateral rectus muscle on the same side and interneurons whose axons cross the midline, enter the medial longitudinal fasciculus, and ascend to influence oculomotor neurons that innervate the medial rectus muscle on the opposite side. A lesion of the abducens nucleus on the right side will result in the deficits experienced by this patient. The internal genu is intimately associated with (loops around) the abducens nucleus. The weakness of facial muscles indicates damage to the internal genu as it loops around the abducens muscles. Facial muscles are weak on the patient's right side.
FN2e 213, 280, 394–397, 452

54.   **(D)** The production of antibodies by plasma cells in patient's thymus or lymphoid organs results in a saturation of receptors and subsequent damage to the postsynaptic membrane at the neuromuscular junction. The membrane is reduced, receptors are lost, and the pattern of subjunctional folds profoundly altered. The resulting disease, myasthenia gravis, presents as muscle weakness that may wax and wane over a period of minutes, hours, or days and frequently affects ocular movements.
FN2e 374–375

55.   **(D)** In humans it is believed that rubrospinal fibers project primarily to cervical levels of the spinal cord. Their primary action is to excite flexor motor neurons innervating the upper extremity. This explains the flexion of the upper extremity characteristic of decorticate rigidity.
FN2e 380–382

56.   **(C)** The small intrafusal striated muscles of the muscle spindle are innervated by the small gamma motor neurons of the anterior horn. The muscle spindle is a receptor for important reflexes tested during a neurologic examination, and it provides information on stretch, rate of stretch, and tension within skeletal muscles.
FN2e 376–378

57.   **(D)** The action of vestibulospinal and reticulospinal fibers is to excite extensor motor neurons of the anterior horn that innervate axial muscles (sometimes called antigravity muscles). These descending fibers terminate primarily in spinal laminae VII and VIII on interneurons, which, in turn, excite lower motor neurons.
FN2e 379–382

58.   **(A)** The patient can move his eye down and out, indicating that the superior oblique muscle (innervated by the trochlear nerve) and the lateral rectus muscle (innervated by the abducens nerve) are functioning. The other four main extraocular muscles (innervated by the oculomotor nerve) are not functioning.
FN2e 212, 216–217, 395–397

59.   **(D)** Damage to the preganglionic parasympathetic (GVE) fibers traveling with the oculomotor nerve removes the innervation of the sphincter pupillae muscle of the iris on the side of the lesion. These fibers originate in the Edinger-Westphal nucleus on the side of the lesion and terminate in the ipsilateral ciliary ganglion. The pupil dilates owing to the unopposed influence of the sympathetic postganglionic fibers (still intact) innervating the dilator pupillae muscle. The deficits of eye movement, coupled with the dilated pupil, are the best localizing signs in this patient.
FN2e 216–217, 391

60.   **(D)** This patient has a combination of deficits that indicate damage to lower motor neurons (eye movement problems) and to the axons of upper motor neurons (weakness of extremities). The lower motor neuron deficit is on the right side and the upper motor neuron deficit affects the left side of the body. This pattern represents a crossed deficit or alternating hemiplegia that specifically localizes to the side of the cranial nerve (lower motor neuron) deficit. Consequently, the weakness of

extremities on the left side of the body reflects damage to corticospinal fibers on the right.
FN2e 216–217, 391

61. **(C)** The paralysis of most eye movement, the best localizing sign in this patient, when coupled with the weakness of upper and lower extremities on the contralateral side of the body indicates a lesion in anteromedial areas of the midbrain involving corticospinal fibers and the exiting roots of the oculomotor nerve.
FN2e 212, 216–217, 394–396

62. **(A)** The combination of a third nerve paralysis, coupled with a contralateral weakness of the extremities is a superior (the most rostral in the brainstem), alternating (cranial nerve on one side, long tract sign on the other side) hemiplegia (motor deficit/paralysis); these are the major components of the Weber syndrome. This syndrome may also include deviation of the tongue away from the side of the lesion and weakness of facial muscles on the lower half of the face opposite the lesion. These reflect damage to corticonuclear (corticobulbar) fibers descending to the hypoglossal nucleus and facial nucleus on the opposite side.
FN2e 395–398, 450

63. **(B)** Corticonuclear fibers project to the motor nuclei of cranial nerves (and to other targets) by passing primarily through the genu of the internal capsule. Some corticobulbar fibers may also descend through the anterior portion of the posterior limb of the internal capsule.
FN2e 394–398

64. **(C)** The nucleus ambiguus innervates skeletal muscles that originate from the mesoderm of the third and fourth pharyngeal arches. The functional component of these motor neurons is SVE. The muscles innervated are the stylopharyngeus (third arch–ninth nerve) and the pharyngeal and laryngeal muscles, including the fine medial part of the thyroarytenoid muscle commonly called the vocalis muscle (fourth arch–tenth nerve).
FN2e 206–208, 395–398

65. **(C)** The large pyramidal cells of the primary motor cortex give rise to larger-diameter, rapidly conducting axons that descend as part of the corticospinal tract. These axons constitute about 10% of all fibers in this tract; the majority of corticospinal fibers are in the range of 5 μm in diameter.
FN2e 391

66. **(E)** In the decerebrate patient the damage to the brain has extended from a supratentorial location through the tentorial notch and into an infratentorial location to involve the midbrain and rostral pons. The red nucleus and rubrospinal tract are compromised, and the overwhelming influence on spinal motor neurons is through reticulospinal and vestibulospinal axons. The predominant result is excessive excitation of extensor motor neurons.
FN2e 382–383

67. **(C)** Removal of the anterior lobe and its efferent neurons (the Purkinje cells) has the following effects. First, it removes the Purkinje cell inhibitory influence on the neurons of the fastigial nucleus that project to the vestibular nuclei. Second, it removes the inhibitory influence of Purkinje cells that project directly to the vestibular nuclei as cerebellar corticovestibular projections. The net effect of removing this inhibitory cerebellar influence is an increase in the excitatory outflow of the vestibular nuclei and an increased input to lower motor neurons in the spinal cord. Decerebellate (extensor) rigidity is the result.
FN2e 382, 384

68. **(D)** The dynamic nuclear bag fiber is sensitive to the rate of change of extrafusal muscle length whereas the static nuclear bag fiber responds only to a change in length but is not sensitive to the rate at which this change takes place.
FN2e 376–378

69. **(D)** The Golgi tendon organ (GTO) is a mechanoreceptor sensitive to excessive stretch. Excitation of the Ib fiber attached to the GTO, in response to an excessive stretch, results in the initiation of an action potential. The Ib fiber synapses (and excites) an inhibitory interneuron, which, in turn inhibits the alpha motor neurons innervating the stretched muscle. The muscle relaxes and is protected from the damage to the tendon, muscle, or both that may result from excessive stretch.
FN2e 377–378

70. **(D)** Descending cortical or brainstem excitation of gamma motor neurons results in a contraction of the intrafusal muscle fibers of the neuromuscular spindle. This is, in turn, interpreted by the spindle as stretch (potentially of the extrafusal fibers), and the Ia fiber of the spindle is either activated or its baseline firing rate increases.
FN2e 377–378

71. **(B)** The level of the lesion is determined by the pain and thermal sense loss. Because fibers conveying this information ascend one or two levels as they cross the midline in the anterior (ventral) white commissure, the injury is at about T7-T8 spinal cord level on the patient's left side. Corticospinal fibers cross in the motor decussation and influence spinal motor neurons on the side of the lesion. Posterior column fibers are the central processes of primary sensory fibers that ascend ipsilateral to their origin. Consequently, posterior column and motor signs are ipsilateral to the lesion; pain and thermal sensation losses are on the contralateral side.
FN2e 280–282, 394–395

72. **(D)** The combination of deficits seen in this patient (ipsilateral paralysis, ipsilateral loss of proprioception and vibratory sense, and contralateral loss of pain and thermal sensation) is characteristic of the Brown-Séquard syndrome. The level of the lesion is most specifically determined by the pain and thermal sense loss since this follows dermatomes.
FN2e 394–395

CHAPTER 26

The Basal Nuclei

1.   A 61-year-old man has a movement disorder (chorea) and dementia, both of which have become progressively worse over the past 5 years. The MRI of this patient reveals what appear to be enlarged ventricles.

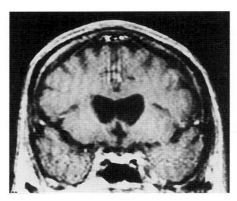

Figure 26–1

Which of the following is the most likely cause of this change in the volume of the ventricular spaces?

○ (A) Obstructive hydrocephalus
○ (B) Normal pressure hydrocephalus
○ (C) Aqueductal stenosis
○ (D) Hydrocephalus ex vacuo
○ (E) Idiopathic intracranial hypertension

2.   A 68-year-old man is brought to his family physician by his wife. The examination reveals rhythmic movements of the man's fingers and hands as he sits quietly in a chair. Which of the following most specifically describes this movement disorder?

○ (A) Titubation
○ (B) Intention tremor
○ (C) Dysdiadochokinesia
○ (D) Athetosis
○ (E) Resting tremor

Questions 3 through 5 are based on the following patient:

A 71-year-old man is brought to the emergency department by his son. According to the son, the man felt ill and went to sleep for several hours. On waking the man still felt ill and had what his son called "fits." On examination, the man is confused but able to cooperate. He has uncontrolled and unpredictable violent flinging movements of his right extremities, especially the upper.

3.   Which of the following most specifically describes the motor symptoms experienced by this man?

○ (A) Hemidysmetria
○ (B) Hemiplegia
○ (C) Hemiparesis
○ (D) Hemiballism
○ (E) Hemihypertonia

4.   Which of the following represents the most likely location of the lesion in this man?

○ (A) Right subthalamic nucleus
○ (B) Left subthalamic nucleus
○ (C) Right globus pallidus
○ (D) Left globus pallidus
○ (E) Left putamen

5.   Which of the following is the most likely cause of the lesion leading to the motor deficits in this man?

○ (A) Tumor
○ (B) A neurodegenerative disease
○ (C) Hemorrhagic lesion
○ (D) Demyelinating disease
○ (E) Trauma

6.   Which of the following structures contains GABA-ergic neurons that project to the tectum, thalamus and striatum?

○ (A) Red nucleus
○ (B) Putamen
○ (C) Substantia nigra, pars compacta
○ (D) Substantia nigra, pars reticularis
○ (E) Subthalamic nucleus

7. A 7-year-old girl is brought to the pediatrician by her mother. The mother states that the girl had a serious infection about 4 months before the onset of her motor symptoms; she was treated for this infection with antibiotics. The examination reveals a girl with rapid, flowing (choreiform) movements of her extremities and facial muscles. This girl is most likely suffering from which of the following motor disorders?

- ○ (A) Parkinson disease
- ○ (B) Wilson disease
- ○ (C) Huntington disease
- ○ (D) Tardive dyskinesia
- ○ (E) Sydenham chorea

8. Which of the following neurotransmitter substances is associated with the efferent fibers arising in the medial segment of the globus pallidus?

- ○ (A) GABA (γ-aminobutyric acid)
- ○ (B) Dopamine
- ○ (C) Acetylcholine
- ○ (D) Glycine
- ○ (E) Glutamate

Questions 9 through 12 are based on the following patient:

A 21-year-old man is referred to the neurologist by his family physician for evaluation of a movement disorder. The evaluation reveals dysarthria, tremor, and unsteady gait. The tremor is characterized by repeated dorsiflexion of the hand and spreading of the fingers and up-and-down movements of the arms. Further tests reveal abnormal levels of liver enzymes and abnormal kidney function. This patient also has a yellow-green ring at the periphery of the pigmented portion of the iris.

9. Which of the following most characteristically describes the tremor seen in this patient?

- ○ (A) Choreiform
- ○ (B) Intention
- ○ (C) Athetoid
- ○ (D) Ballistic
- ○ (E) Asterixis

10. The MRI of this patient reveals small cavities in the brain. Which of the following represents the most likely location of these cavities?

- ○ (A) Hippocampus
- ○ (B) Putamen
- ○ (C) Head of the caudate nucleus
- ○ (D) Dorsal thalamus
- ○ (E) Globus pallidus

11. The yellow-green ring in the cornea of this patient is specifically characteristic of this disease. This ring is most likely the result of which of the following?

- ○ (A) Depositions of magnesium
- ○ (B) Small hemorrhages
- ○ (C) Depositions of calcium
- ○ (D) Small arteriovenous malformations
- ○ (E) Depositions of copper

12. This man is most likely suffering from which of the following?

- ○ (A) Wilson disease
- ○ (B) Parkinson disease
- ○ (C) Sydenham chorea
- ○ (D) Huntington disease
- ○ (E) Tardive dyskinesia

13. An 81-year-old woman is diagnosed with probable Alzheimer disease. In this disease, there is a significant loss of large cells in the basal nucleus of Meynert in the substantia innominata. Which of the following neurotransmitters is associated with these large cells?

- ○ (A) Glutamate
- ○ (B) Dopamine
- ○ (C) Acetylcholine
- ○ (D) GABA
- ○ (E) Vasoactive intestinal polypeptide

14. A 57-year-old man presents with dementia and choreiform movements, both of which have worsened over the past several years according to his family. The man's physician discovers that the man's father and two uncles died of a similar disease. MRI of this patient would most likely reveal loss of which of the following structures?

- ○ (A) Lenticular nucleus
- ○ (B) Head of the caudate nucleus
- ○ (C) Hippocampus
- ○ (D) Globus pallidus
- ○ (E) Dorsomedial nucleus of the thalamus

15. Diseases of the basal nuclei are, in general, neurodegenerative diseases that result in death of the cell body and/or degeneration of their processes. In which of the following basal nuclei diseases does glutamate excitotoxicity play a primary role?

- ○ (A) Hepatolenticular degeneration
- ○ (B) Parkinson disease
- ○ (C) Sydenham chorea
- ○ (D) Tardive dyskinesia
- ○ (E) Huntington disease

16. The net result of corticostriatal excitation of striatal neurons is best described by which of the following sequences through the direct pathway?

- ○ (A) Disinhibition of thalamocortical neurons with resultant increase in activity of cerebral cortical neurons
- ○ (B) Disinhibition of thalamocortical neurons and inhibition of cortical neurons
- ○ (C) Disinhibition of thalamocortical neurons with no change in the firing characteristics of cortical neurons

○ (D) Inhibition of thalamocortical neurons with resultant decrease in the firing patterns of cortical neurons

○ (E) Inhibition of thalamocortical neurons with resultant increase in the firing rate of cortical neurons

17. Which of the following is the neurotransmitter substance most specifically associated with subthalamic neurons that project to the medial segment of the globus pallidus?

○ (A) Acetylcholine
○ (B) GABA
○ (C) Glutamate
○ (D) Dopamine
○ (E) Glycine

Questions 18 through 21 are based on the following patient:

A 69-year-old man initially had a resting tremor in his right hand, but the left hand soon showed this motor deficit. As the disease progressed, the man developed difficulty in initiating voluntary movements and, once initiated, they were reduced in velocity and amplitude. He has a stooped, hunched posture and a shuffling gait; he walks with short steps and more or less slides his feet over the floor.

18. Which of the following best describes this man's inability to initiate a voluntary movement?

○ (A) Bradykinesia
○ (B) Akinesia
○ (C) Athetosis
○ (D) Hypometria
○ (E) Titubation

19. Once initiated, this patient's voluntary movements are reduced in velocity and amplitude and he may have difficulty stopping the movement once it is started. Which of the following best describes this characteristic movement disorder?

○ (A) Bradykinesia
○ (B) Akinesia
○ (C) Athetosis
○ (D) Hypometria
○ (E) Chorea

20. Which of the following most specifically describes the gait seen in this man?

○ (A) Inability to walk in tandem
○ (B) Festinating gait
○ (C) Titubation
○ (D) Hyperkinetic
○ (E) Athetoid

21. The symptoms experienced by this man are most likely related to cell loss in which of the following nuclei?

○ (A) Subthalamic nucleus
○ (B) Medial segment of the globus pallidus

○ (C) Substantia nigra, pars reticulata
○ (D) Basal nucleus of Meynert
○ (E) Substantia nigra, pars compacta

22. A 17-year-old boy is brought to the internist by his mother. Tests reveal elevated levels of amino acids in the urine (aminoaciduria) but no neurologic deficits. The physician learns from the mother that the boy's father was "treated" for a motor disorder. Which of the following is the most likely diagnosis in this boy?

○ (A) Parkinson disease
○ (B) Wilson disease
○ (C) Alcoholic cerebellar degeneration
○ (D) Sydenham chorea
○ (E) Huntington disease

23. The neurotransmitter associated with striatopallidal projections and with pallidothalamic projections is

○ (A) Dopamine
○ (B) Acetylcholine
○ (C) GABA
○ (D) Glutamate
○ (E) Histamine

24. A 71-year-old woman has a sudden onset of movement disorders while on a cruise. MRI a few days later reveals a hemorrhagic lesion in the area served by the lateral striate arteries. Which of the following outlined areas represents the most likely location of this lesion? (   )

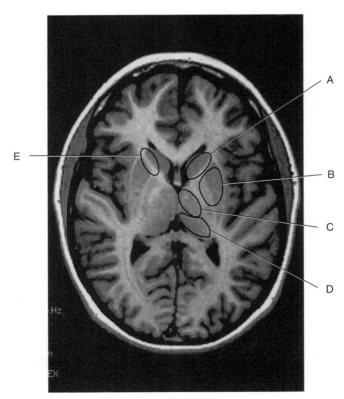

Figure 26–2

25. Which of the following structures contains neuron cell bodies whose axons collectively form the ansa lenticularis and lenticular fasciculus? ( )

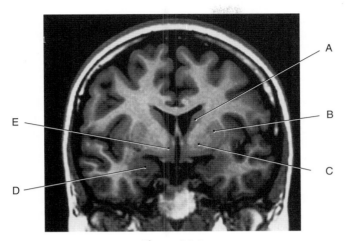

Figure 26–3

ANSWERS

1. **(D)** In this patient, the apparent enlargement in the ventricular space is caused by loss of brain parenchyma rather than an obstruction of CSF flow and resultant increase in pressure. MRI reveals a loss of the head of the caudate nucleus (from the lateral wall of the anterior horn of the lateral ventricle). This results in the anterior horns of the lateral ventricle appearing much larger than normal. Hydrocephalus ex vacuo may be present in patients with few or no neurologic deficits (general brain atrophy) or may be present in patients with loss of brain tissue resulting from a prior stroke or neurodegenerative process (with characteristic deficits).
Fn2e 419, also 106

2. **(E)** Parkinson disease, a loss of dopamine-containing cells in the substantia nigra/pars compacta, characteristically results in a resting tremor. The patient's fingers are loosely flexed and the fingers and hand have rhythmic movements while the patient is at rest. These tremors may decrease, or disappear entirely, when the patient performs a voluntary movement.
Fn2e 420–421

3. **(D)** Violent uncontrolled flinging movements of the extremities are called ballistic movements. When confined to one side of the body these are hemiballistic movements (or hemiballism). Ballistic movements are characteristically seen in patients with lesions in the subthalamic nucleus.
Fn2e 417

4. **(B)** Lesions of the subthalamic nucleus result in hemiballistic movements on the contralateral side. This is because the motor expression of the movements is through the corticospinal tract. In this patient a lesion in the left subthalamic nucleus, through its connections with the pallidum and dorsal thalamus, modifies inputs to the left motor cortex. The altered output from the left motor cortex (unpredictable, excitatory burst of activity) influences the right side of the body via the corticospinal tract.
Fn2e 416–417

5. **(C)** Hemiballistic movements appear suddenly and are usually the result of a vascular lesion in the subthalamic nucleus.
Fn2e 417

6. **(D)** GABAergic neurons located in the reticular part of the substantia nigra are indistinguishable from those in the medial segments of the pallidum. These cells project to the tectum (as nigrotectal fibers) and to the thalamus (as nigrothalamic fibers). These GABAergic nigral neurons tonically inhibit their target cells.
Fn2e 411

7. **(E)** Sydenham chorea is a childhood disease that may appear after an infection with group A β-hemolytic streptococci. The symptoms may appear weeks or even months after the infection and may include disturbances of movement, weakness, hypotonia, and difficulty attending to tasks. Children with Sydenham chorea usually recover completely.
Fn2e 421

8. **(A)** Pallidothalamic fibers originating from cells of the medial segment of the globus pallidus are GABAergic and, consequently, have an inhibitory influence on their target cells. Under the influence of inhibitory pallidothalamic fibers, the activity of thalamocortical neurons is decreased and there may be a corresponding decrease in the activity of cells of the motor cortex.
Fn2e 411, 413, 414

9. **(E)** Asterixis, or wing-beating tremor (flapping tremor), is characteristically seen in patients with hepatolenticular degeneration. The upper extremities are thrown up and down, and the tremor may be at the wrist or of the entire extremity. The fingers may spread and the hand may dorsiflex at the wrist. The extremity tends to move in an up-and-down arc.
Fn2e 421

10. **(B)** Loss of neurons in the putamen, the resultant gliosis, and appearance of small cavities are the main histopathologic features of hepatolenticular degeneration. Similar changes may also be seen in the cerebral cortex, especially of the frontal lobe.
Fn2e 421

11. **(E)** Hepatolenticular degeneration is an inherited disorder of copper metabolism. The metal accumulates in the liver, brain, and cornea. The accumulation in the liver results in necrotic nodules and progressive liver damage. Copper may also damage the tubules of the kidney, resulting in aminoaciduria. Treatment consists of removing copper from the body.
Fn2e 421

12. **(A)** The combination of motor deficits experienced by this patient, kidney and liver dysfunction, and the

occurrence of a yellow-green ring in the cornea are characteristic of hepatolenticular degeneration (Wilson disease). Treatment consists of administering medications to reduce the toxic levels of copper and to prevent its further accumulation.
Fn2e 421

13. **(C)** The large cells within the basal nucleus of Meynert contain acetylcholine. These large cells are lost in Alzheimer disease.
Fn2e 409

14. **(B)** This patient suffers from a disease inherited from his father, a disease characterized by progressively severe motor disturbances and dementia. This is Huntington disease. One characteristic of this disease is a loss of striatal neurons, most noticeable as a distinct loss of the head of the caudate nucleus.
Fn2e 419–420

15. **(E)** Corticostriatal projections release glutamate at their synapses on striatal neurons. Normally this results in excitation of the postsynaptic membrane of the striatal cell. For largely unknown reasons, the glutamate is not cleared quickly from the N-methyl-D-aspartate receptor site. The persistence of glutamate opens many calcium channels. The resulting influx of calcium leads to a sequence of events that results in cell death.
Fn2e 419–420

16. **(A)** Corticostriatal projections are glutaminergic and excite striatopallidal cells. These inhibitory (GABAergic) striatopallidal neurons, in turn, inhibit the pallidothalamic neurons that project to the thalamus. The result is that these thalamocortical neurons are removed from their usual inhibitory (GABAergic) influence by the pallidothalamic projection; the thalamocortical neurons are disinhibited. In this scenario, the thalamocortical neurons are more active, resulting in more activity in cortical neurons.
Fn2e 413–414

17. **(C)** Subthalamopallidal fibers use the excitatory neurotransmitter glutamate. Normally, these projections are kept largely in check by the inhibitory (GABAergic) pallidosubthalamic projection. However, disease processes that upset this balance may result in motor disturbances. The cerebral cortex also sends an excitatory input to the subthalamic nucleus.
Fn2e 410–411

18. **(B)** Inability, or significant difficulty, in initiating a voluntary movement is akinesia. Experimental studies in animals have shown that some neurons of the basal nuclei are involved in planning and initiating movement. When circuits through the basal nuclei are disrupted, akinesia, among other motor disturbances, results. Akinesia is one of the cardinal symptoms of disorders of the basal nuclei.
Fn2e 415, 420–421

19. **(A)** Bradykinesia is characterized by movements that are initiated slowly and are reduced in velocity and amplitude compared to normal. The decreased motor activity in bradykinesia is caused primarily by activity of antagonist muscles, rather than weakness of the muscles attempting the movement. Like akinesia, bradykinesia is one of the cardinal symptoms in patients with disease of the basal nuclei.
Fn2e 415, 420–421

20. **(B)** In addition to the stooped posture, this patient has a characteristic shuffling gait. He moves in short, choppy steps that may become more rapid as he progresses. He acts like his feet are stuck to the floor. This is called a festinating gait.
Fn2e 420–421

21. **(E)** The symptoms in this patient relate to loss of dopamine-containing cells in the substantia nigra and pars compacta and of their nigrostriatial terminals in the neostriatum. This loss of nigral neurons, and the characteristic motor disturbances, are seen in patients with Parkinson disease.
Fn2e 420–421

22. **(B)** Inherited motor disorders related to the basal nuclei are Huntington disease and Wilson disease. In the latter, the accumulation of copper in the liver results in cell damage and elevated amino acid levels in the urine. Liver damage may precede the onset of neurologic symptoms by several years.
Fn2e 421

23. **(C)** The predominate neurotransmitter of cells in the neostriatum and globus pallidus is γ-aminobutyric acid (GABA). The action of striatopallidal fibers and pallidal efferent fibers is to inhibit the cells on which their axons terminate.
Fn2e 412–413

24. **(B)** The lateral striate arteries (also commonly called the lenticulostriate arteries) are branches of the M_1 segment of the middle cerebral artery. These small penetrating vessels serve much of the superior portions of the putamen and globus pallidus. The inferior parts of these nuclei receive a significant blood supply from the anterior choroidal artery.
Fn2e 243, 245, 406–407

25. **(C)** The ansa lenticularis and lenticular fasciculus contain pallidothalamic fibers. These inhibitory fibers originate from neurons in the medial (internal) segment of the globus pallidus, course through these bundles, and terminate primarily in the ventral lateral nucleus of the thalamus. These are the main efferent pathways of the basal nuclei.
Fn2e 411–413

CHAPTER 27

The Cerebellum

1. A 39-year-old woman presents to the neurologist with the complaint that she "has trouble walking." The examination reveals an ataxic gait. There is no loss of muscle strength. Sensations from the face and body are normal. MRI reveals a tumor in the anterior lobe of the cerebellum. Which of the following lobules collectively form the anterior cerebellar lobe?

○ (A) Lobules I–III
○ (B) Lobules III–V
○ (C) Lobules I–V
○ (D) Lobules VI–VIII
○ (E) Lobules VI–IX

2. A 21-year-old woman complains to her family physician of frequent, and sometimes severe, headaches that are refractory to nonprescription medications. Suspecting a brain tumor, the physician orders MRI, which reveals an arteriovenous malformation in the anterior lobe. The venous side of this malformation appears to be a large channel entering the straight sinus. Which of the following represents the most likely source of arterial blood to this malformation?

○ (A) Posterior inferior cerebellar artery
○ (B) Anterior inferior cerebellar artery
○ (C) Superior cerebellar artery
○ (D) Posterior cerebral artery
○ (E) Anterior choroidal artery

3. A newborn presents with multiple developmental defects. MRI reveals defects within the cerebellum, including absence of the posterolateral fissure. In the normal infant this fissure separates which of the following parts of the cerebellum from each other?

○ (A) Anterior lobe from posterior lobe
○ (B) Anterior lobe vermis from paravermal area
○ (C) Posterior lobe vermis from paravermal area
○ (D) Flocculus from nodulus
○ (E) Flocculonodular lobe from posterior lobe

4. The MRI of a 57-year-old man with chronic alcoholism reveals a decrease in size of the anterior lobe of the cerebellum. The individual folia are smaller than normal, and the fissures between folia and lobules are larger than normal. This change in size of the cerebellar cortex is partially related to loss of cortical neurons.

Which of the following represents the efferent neuron of the cerebellar cortex?

○ (A) Granule cell
○ (B) Purkinje cell
○ (C) Superior stellate cell
○ (D) Basket cell
○ (E) Golgi cell

5. Which of the following cells of the cerebellar cortex exert an excitatory influence on other cells and processes on which they make synaptic contacts?

○ (A) Purkinje cell
○ (B) Golgi cell
○ (C) Basket cell
○ (D) Superior stellate cell
○ (E) Granule cell

Questions 6 through 8 are based on the following patient:

A 77-year-old man arrives at the dental clinic of a large medical center for routine dental care. The dentist notices that this man has difficulty with some motor tasks and refers him to a neurologist. The neurologic examination reveals that the man is unable to perform rapid alternating movements on the right side and has a tremor that worsens as he tries to touch his nose with his right index finger starting from arm's length. CT reveals a hemorrhagic lesion in the anterior lobe of the cerebellum involving cortex and nuclei.

6. Which of the following most specifically describes this patient's inability to perform a rapid alternating movement?

○ (A) Titubation
○ (B) Truncal ataxia
○ (C) Dysarthria
○ (D) Dysdiadochokinesia
○ (E) Hypometria

7. At the neurologist's request, the man extends his arm and then tries to touch his nose with his right index finger.

169

As his finger approaches his nose a tremor becomes so intense that he is unable to touch his nose. Which of the following most correctly describes this tremor?

- ○ (A)   Static tremor
- ○ (B)   Resting tremor
- ○ (C)   Intention tremor
- ○ (D)   Titubation
- ○ (E)   Hypermetria

8.   The lesion in this patient most likely originates from a hemorrhage of which of the following vessels?

- ○ (A)   Left superior cerebellar artery
- ○ (B)   Right superior cerebellar artery
- ○ (C)   Left anterior inferior cerebellar artery
- ○ (D)   Right anterior inferior cerebellar artery
- ○ (E)   Right quadrigeminal artery

9.   A 74-year-old woman presents to the emergency department with an unsteady wide-based gait and an inability to walk heel-to-toe (walk in tandem). CT reveals a lesion in the cerebellum. Which of the following represents the most likely location of this lesion?

- ○ (A)   Hemisphere (lateral zone) plus dentate nucleus
- ○ (B)   Cortex of the anterior lobe
- ○ (C)   Nodulus plus fastigial nucleus
- ○ (D)   Brachium conjunctivum
- ○ (E)   Cortex of the posterior lobe

10.   Which of the following structures is composed primarily of cerebellar efferent fibers, that is, of fibers leaving the cerebellum?

- ○ (A)   Restiform body
- ○ (B)   Juxtarestiform body
- ○ (C)   Brachium pontis
- ○ (D)   Brachium conjunctivum
- ○ (E)   Posterior spinocerebellar tract

Questions 11 through 14 are related to the following patient:

A 59-year-old morbidly obese man with uncontrolled hypertension is brought to the emergency department after becoming nauseated. The examination reveals that the man has diplopia (double vision) on attempted gaze to the right, the right eye is largely immobile, and the pupil on this side is dilated. In addition, this patient has ataxia on the left side of his body and a slight tremor, also on the left. The tremor is most evident in the upper extremity. Suspecting a stroke, the physician orders CT, which reveals a hemorrhagic lesion involving cerebellar efferent fibers as well as adjacent structures.

11.   Which of the following is most likely the best localizing sign in this patient?

- ○ (A)   Left-sided tremor
- ○ (B)   Left-sided ataxia
- ○ (C)   Diplopia in right eye
- ○ (D)   Dilated right pupil
- ○ (E)   Largely immobile right eye

12.   Recognizing that ataxia is a sign of a lesion of the cerebellum or of its efferent pathways, which of the following represents the most likely location of this lesion?

- ○ (A)   Superior cerebellar peduncle (brachium conjunctivum) on the left
- ○ (B)   Superior cerebellar peduncle (brachium conjunctivum) on the right
- ○ (C)   Cerebellothalamic (dentatothalamic) fibers on the right
- ○ (D)   Cerebellothalamic (dentatothalamic) fibers on the left
- ○ (E)   Ventral lateral nucleus of the thalamus on the left

13.   Realizing the likely position of this lesion as being in the midbrain, damage to which of the following structures would most likely explain the tremor in this patient?

- ○ (A)   Corticospinal fibers on the right
- ○ (B)   Red nucleus on the left
- ○ (C)   Decussation of the superior cerebellar peduncle
- ○ (D)   Red nucleus on the right
- ○ (E)   Pretectal nuclei on the right

14.   Which of the following represents the combination of deficits seen in this patient?

- ○ (A)   Weber syndrome
- ○ (B)   Claude syndrome
- ○ (C)   Benedikt syndrome
- ○ (D)   Wallenberg syndrome
- ○ (E)   Foville syndrome

15.   A 63-year-old woman presents to the emergency department with motor disturbances. The evaluation, which includes MRI, reveals a large tumor in lateral portions of the cerebellum on the left. Which of the following is most specifically descriptive of the overall motor deficits experienced by this patient?

- ○ (A)   Spasticity, spastic paralysis
- ○ (B)   Flaccid paralysis
- ○ (C)   Increased muscle tone with hyperreflexia
- ○ (D)   Resting tremor
- ○ (E)   Dyssynergy, decomposition of movement

16.   A male newborn presents with developmental defects. MRI reveals malformations of the cerebellum that most certainly include cells of the cortex. In the normal infant, excitation of granule cells by mossy fibers will most likely result in which of the following sequence of events?

- ○ (A)   Excitation of Purkinje cells, which excites cerebellar nuclear cells
- ○ (B)   Excitation of Purkinje cells, which inhibits cerebellar nuclear cells
- ○ (C)   Inhibition of Purkinje cells, which allows cerebellar nuclear outflow to proceed unchanged
- ○ (D)   Inhibition of Basket cells, which excites Purkinje cells
- ○ (E)   Excitation of stellate cells, which excites Purkinje cells

17. Which of the following is the exclusive source of climbing fibers to the cerebellar cortex?

○ (A) Inferior olivary neurons projecting to the ipsilateral cerebellum
○ (B) Lateral reticular nucleus neurons projecting to the ipsilateral cerebellum
○ (C) Pontine neurons projecting to the contralateral cerebellum
○ (D) Inferior olivary neurons projecting to the contralateral cerebellum
○ (E) Vestibular nuclei neurons projecting to the contralateral cerebellum

18. A 9-year-old girl is brought to the pediatrician for motor disturbances that are getting progressively worse. The examination reveals truncal ataxia, titubation, and nystagmus. MRI reveals a tumor. Which of the following is the most likely location of this lesion?

○ (A) Anterior lobe cortex
○ (B) Anterior lobe cortex plus cerebellar nuclei
○ (C) Posterior lobe hemisphere plus the dentate nucleus
○ (D) Nodulus and fastigial nucleus
○ (F) Flocculus only

Questions 19 through 21 are based on the following patient:

A 68-year-old woman presents to her family physician with persistent headache and motor disturbances. The history reveals that the headaches are refractory to over-the-counter medications and the motor problems have been getting worse over the past 9 months. Cranial nerve function is normal. This patient is unable to perform rapid alternating movements, cannot touch her index finger to her nose because of tremor, and has a slurred, garbled pattern of speech. In addition, she has difficulty accurately pointing to a moving target, such as when the physician moves his index finger from right to left in front of the woman. Excepting the slurred speech, all motor deficits are on the patient's right side. MRI reveals a large tumor within the parenchyma of the cerebellum.

19. The slurred, garbled speech in this patient is the result of dyssynergy of the nucleus of vocalization. Which of the following most specifically describes this pattern of speech?

○ (A) Dysmetria
○ (B) Dysarthria
○ (C) Dyslexia
○ (D) Apraxia
○ (E) Dysphagia

20. Which of the following most specifically describes the inability of this patient to point accurately to a moving or stationary target?

○ (A) Static tremor
○ (B) Resting tremor
○ (C) Hypometria/Hypermetria

○ (D) Alexia
○ (E) Impaired check (rebound phenomenon)

21. Based on the deficits experienced by this patient, which of the following represents the most likely location of the tumor in this woman?

○ (A) Midline of the anterior vermis plus fastigial nucleus
○ (B) Hemisphere on the left plus dentate and parts of the interposed nuclei
○ (C) Midline of the posterior vermis plus the fastigial nucleus and nodulus
○ (D) Hemisphere on the right plus dentate and parts of the interposed nuclei
○ (E) Fastigial nuclei bilaterally

22. Which of the following represents the most likely source of histaminergic fibers to the cerebellar cortex?

○ (A) Pontine nuclei
○ (B) Hypothalamus
○ (C) Raphe nuclei
○ (D) Olivary nuclei
○ (E) Reticular nuclei

23. A 29-year-old man presents to the internist's office with motor disturbances. The initial examination reveals signs and symptoms consistent with a lesion in the cerebellum. Cerebellar efferent fibers do not project directly to lower motor neurons. Consequently, the motor expression of a cerebellar lesion/dysfunction is predominately through which of the following pathways?

○ (A) Vestibulospinal fibers
○ (B) Reticulospinal fibers
○ (C) Spinocerebellar fibers
○ (D) Corticospinal fibers
○ (E) Hypothalamospinal fibers

24. Which of the following cerebellar nuclei projects bilaterally to brainstem nuclei that, in turn, exert influence on spinal motor neurons innervating axial (postural) muscles?

○ (A) Fastigial
○ (B) Globose
○ (C) Emboliform
○ (D) Dentate
○ (E) Lateral

25. A 4-year-old girl is brought to the pediatric neurologist by her mother, who says that her daughter is lethargic and frequently throws up. Suspecting a tumor, the physician orders MRI, which reveals a large tumor in the fourth ventricle that appears to originate from the choroid plexus. Which of the following most likely represents the blood supply to this part of the choroid plexus as well as to the tumor?

○ (A) Posterior inferior cerebellar artery
○ (B) Anterior inferior cerebellar artery
○ (C) Posterior spinal artery
○ (D) Long circumferential branches of the basilar artery
○ (E) Superior cerebellar artery

26. An 87-year-old woman is brought to her family physician by her son. The woman complains of headache. MRI reveals a tumor in the middle cerebellar peduncle. Which of the following labeled areas represents the most likely location of this tumor? (   )

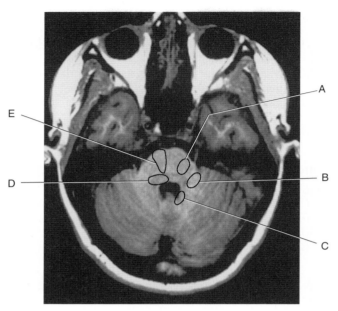

Figure 27–1

27. A 31-year-old woman with uncontrolled hypertension presents to her family physician with headache and intermittent nausea. Cranial nerve function is normal, and she has no overt motor signs or symptoms. MRI reveals the lesion shown here.

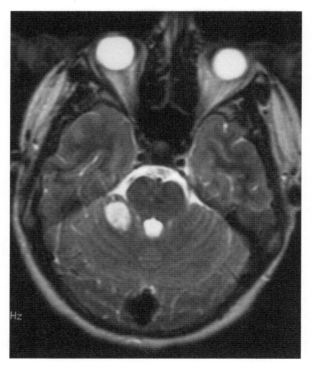

Figure 27–2

Which of the following most accurately describes the location of this lesion?

○ (A) Anterior lobe of cerebellum on patient's right
○ (B) Posterior lobe of cerebellum on patient's right
○ (C) Anterior lobe of cerebellum on patient's left
○ (D) Middle cerebellar peduncle on patient's left
○ (E) Posterior lobe of cerebellum on patient's left

28. A 49-year-old man is brought to the emergency department by his wife. He is lethargic, is nauseated, and has difficulty following instructions. The wife states that he became ill in the morning and has gotten progressively worse all day long. The physician orders CT, which reveals a large hemorrhage into the cerebellar hemisphere causing herniation of the cerebellar tonsil into the foramen magnum. Which of the following labeled structures represents the tonsil of the cerebellum? (   )

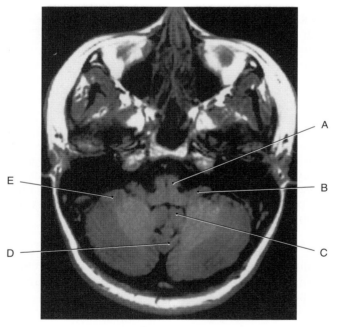

Figure 27–3

29. A 61-year-old morbidly obese man with diabetes presents to the emergency department after an episode of dizziness and nausea. Cranial nerve function is normal, but the man has general dysmetria. CT reveals a hemorrhagic lesion in the area of the cerebellum outlined below. See Figure 27–4.

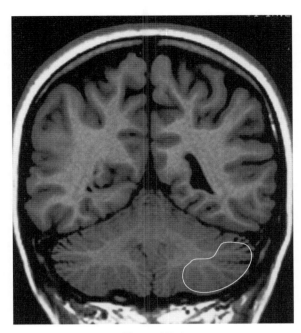

Figure 27–4

Which of the following vessels is the primary source of blood supply to this area of the cerebellum?

- ○ (A) Anterior inferior cerebellar artery
- ○ (B) Posterior inferior cerebellar artery
- ○ (C) Medial branch of the superior cerebellar artery
- ○ (D) Lateral branch of the superior cerebellar artery
- ○ (E) Branches of P$_4$

30. Lobules of the cerebellum are designated by Roman numerals. Vermis lobule by the numeral (i.e., III) and hemisphere portion of the same lobule by the same numeral preceded by an H (i.e., HIII). Which of the following lobules collectively comprise the posterior lobe?

- ○ (A) I (HI) to V (HV)
- ○ (B) III (HIII) to VII (HVII)
- ○ (C) V (HV) to IX (HIX)
- ○ (D) VI (HVI) to IX (HIX)
- ○ (E) X (HX)

31. Excitation of stellate cells or basket cells by the parallel fibers of granule cells will, through their synaptic contacts on Purkinje cells, have which of the following effects on neurons of the cerebellar nuclei?

- ○ (A) Excitation only
- ○ (B) Inhibition only
- ○ (C) Excitation and inhibition based on the receptor
- ○ (D) Disinhibition
- ○ (E) Excitation followed by inhibition through the same circuits

32. Which of the following cerebellar nuclei are functionally related to the paravermal zone of the cerebellar cortex?

- ○ (A) Globose and emboliform
- ○ (B) Globose only
- ○ (C) Emboliform only
- ○ (D) Dentate
- ○ (E) Fastigial

ANSWERS

1. **(C)** The anterior lobe is located between the anterior medullary velum and the primary fissure and consists of lobules I through V (from rostral to caudal). Only lobules II through V have hemisphere portions in the anterior lobe; the hemisphere portions are designated by the prefix "H" (HII through HV).
FN2e 424–425

2. **(C)** The anterior lobe is served by the superior cerebellar artery. This vessel is usually composed of a medial branch serving the more medial portions of the anterior lobe (and the rest of the superior cerebellar surface) and a lateral branch serving more lateral areas. In addition, penetrating branches of these arteries provide the blood supply to most of the cerebellar nuclei.
FN2e 427–428

3. **(E)** The posterolateral fissure is the first to appear in the developing cerebellum. This fissure appears in the caudal area of the cerebellar plate and passes from the midline laterally to separate the flocculonodular lobe from the posterior lobe when fully formed.
FN2e 174–175, 424–425

4. **(B)** The Purkinje cell is the only neuron in the cerebellar cortex whose axons exit the cortex as cerebellar cortical efferent fibers. The majority of Purkinje cell axons either end in the cerebellar nuclei (as cerebellar corticonuclear fibers) or in the vestibular nuclei (as cerebellar corticovestibular fibers). The action of Purkinje cells is inhibitory to their targets.
FN2e 428–430

5. **(E)** The granule cell is the only neuron in the cerebellar cortex that is excitatory to its targets; these cells are glutaminergic. All other neurons of the cerebellar cortex, including the Purkinje cell, which is the efferent neuron of the cortex, are inhibitory to their targets. The predominant neurotransmitter associated with these inhibitory neurons is γ-aminobutyric acid (GABA).
FN2e 428–430

6. **(D)** The inability to perform rapid alternating movements (dysdiadochokinesia) is usually tested by asking the patient to rapidly pronate and supinate his/her hand against the thigh. A patient with a cerebellar lesion will be unable to perform this task either rapidly or smoothly.
FN2e 441–442

7. **(C)** One of the standard tests for a patient with a cerebellar lesion is to ask him/her to touch the index finger to the nose. As the finger approaches the nose the tremor becomes worse; the patient is never really able to

touch the nose. An easy way to remember this relationship is that as the patient "intends" to do a precise movement the tremor becomes progressively worse ("intention" tremor). This may also be called a kinetic tremor because it becomes worse during movement.
FN2e 441

8. **(B)** The deficits experienced by this patient are on his right side. In brief, efferent fibers from the cerebellar nuclei project to the contralateral thalamus, which projects to the ipsilateral motor cortex, which projects to the contralateral spinal cord. Consequently, a lesion within the right side of the cerebellum, as in the infarct in this patient, results in deficits on the right (same) side of the body.
FN2e 427–428, 439–441

9. **(C)** Lesions of midline cerebellar structures such as the nodules and fastigial nucleus result in unsteady gait (truncal ataxia), a wide-based stance, and the patient may be unable to walk in tandem. In general, lesions of the medial portion of the cerebellum result in tremor, ataxia, and gait disturbances that affect the axial portion of the body. The patient may appear intoxicated when he/she walks. Dyssynergia related to the more distal musculature is largely absent in patients with medial lesions.
FN2e 435–436

10. **(D)** The brachium conjunctivum (superior cerebellar peduncle) is composed of axons that originate mainly from cells of the dentate, emboliform, and globose nuclei. These fibers leave the cerebellum (most cross in the decussation of the superior cerebellar peduncle) and distribute to a variety of centers in the neuraxis concerned with motor function. Lesions of the brachium conjunctivum prior to its decussation result in motor deficits on the same side.
FN2e 438–440

11. **(E)** The largely immobile right eye is the best localizing sign as it points to involvement of the nucleus or root of the oculomotor nerve. Diplopia may result from lesions of the oculomotor as well as of the abducens and/or trochlear nerves. While a dilated pupil may be seen in an oculomotor nerve/nucleus lesion, this condition may also be seen resultant to lesions in the orbit that involve, for example, the ciliary ganglion or the short ciliary nerves. Ataxia and tremor may result from lesions at several locations in the neuraxis.
FN2e 216, 395–396, 438

12. **(C)** The localizing sign in this patient places the lesion in the immediate location of the oculomotor nerve. Because the ocular motor deficit is on the right side, the lesion is on the right side (lower motor neurons or their axons are involved). Located immediately (and laterally) adjacent to the oculomotor fibers are cerebellothalamic fibers that originated in the left cerebellum, crossed in the decussation of the superior cerebellar peduncle, and are ascending on the right side as cerebellothalamic fibers. These will terminate primarily in the ventral lateral nucleus of the thalamus.
FN2e 438–440

13. **(D)** This lesion is on the right involving the fibers of the oculomotor nerve and cerebellothalamic fibers. The red nucleus is located immediately medial to the cerebellothalamic fiber bundle, and fibers of the oculomotor nerve pass through medial portions of this nucleus. Axons arising from neurons in the red nucleus cross the midline in the anterior (ventral) tegmental decussation. Those fibers that descend to the spinal cord (as the rubrospinal tract) terminate primarily in the cervical plexus and influence motor neurons innervating upper extremity musculature. The right red nucleus projects to the left spinal cord.
FN2e 380–381, 438–440

14. **(B)** Collectively, the deficits seen in this patient (tremors and ataxia on the left, oculomotor losses on the right) are characteristic of the Claude syndrome. The Weber syndrome is an alternating hemiplegia (corticospinal loss on one side, oculomotor losses on the opposite side), and the Benedikt syndrome is basically Claude plus Weber. The Wallenberg and Foville syndromes are lateral medullary and lateral pontine syndromes, respectively.
FN2e 395–397, 435–438

15. **(E)** The general sign of cerebellar disturbances is a deterioration of coordinated smooth movements into the individual components of the movement. This general decomposition of a coordinated movement is called dyssynergy. Within this general framework of cerebellar dysfunction, a variety of specific motor problems are recognized, such as intention tremor, impaired check, or dysdiadochokinesia.
FN2e 441

16. **(B)** Granule cells are the only excitatory neurons in the cerebellar cortex. When activated by cerebellar afferent fibers ending as mossy fibers, the granule cells form excitatory synapses on Purkinje cells (via parallel fibers). The Purkinje cell is an inhibitory neuron. Consequently, when activated by the granule cell the action of the Purkinje cell is to inhibit the cerebellar nuclear cells on which its axons terminate.
FN2e 443–435

17. **(D)** The nuclei of the inferior olivary complex (dorsal accessory, medial accessory, and principal olivary nuclei) send their axons to the cerebellum via the restiform body. These olivocerebellar projections are exclusively to the cerebellar cortex on the contralateral side, where they end as climbing fibers on Purkinje cell dendrites. Climbing fiber terminals are excitatory to the dendritic tree of a Purkinje cell.
FN2e 430–432

18. **(D)** Medially located lesions, such as those involving the nodules, posterior vermis, and fastigial nuclei, may result in motor disturbances of axial musculature. The function of more distal musculature, such as that controlling the forearm and hand, is largely normal. More laterally located lesions will result in motor dysfunction of more distal musculature.
FN2e 435–436, 441

19. **(B)** The slurred speech of a patient with a cerebellar lesion is caused by a general state of incoordination of the muscles of vocalization. In this patient the muscles

that function to create sound are not paralyzed and the patient has not lost the ability to formulate speech.
FN2e 441

20. **(C)** In general, dysmetria is the inability of the patient to control the speed, distance, and accuracy of a movement. Within this category of movement disorder, hypometria is undershooting the intended target and hypermetria is overshooting the intended target. Dysmetria, hypometria, and hypermetria are characteristic of cerebellar disease.
FN2e 441

21. **(D)** Unilateral lesions within the cerebellum result in motor deficits on the same side of the body. This is because the (altered) efferent signals from the cerebellar nuclei course to the ventral lateral (VL) thalamic nucleus on the contralateral side. The VL projects to the overlying somatomotor cortex, which, in turn, projects to the spinal cord on the contralateral side, this being the same side of the body as the origin of cerebellar efferent information. When the altered cerebellar signals arrive at the somatomotor cortex, via the VL, there are correspondingly altered signals in the corticospinal tract on attempted voluntary movement.
FN2e 438–441

22. **(B)** Histamine-containing cells of the hypothalamus project to the cerebellar cortex, where they appear to end in all layers of the cortex. Monamine- and peptide-containing fibers in the cerebellum may decrease the spontaneous discharge rates of Purkinje cells or alter the response of this cell type to mossy fiber or climbing fiber activation.
FN2e 432

23. **(D)** The cerebellar nuclei influence the contralateral ventral lateral (VL) nucleus of the thalamus, which projects to the somatomotor cortex on the same side. The motor cortex influences the contralateral fibers. A cerebellar lesion results in abnormal signals to the VL, which results in altered thalamocortical signals to the motor cortex. The inability to perform a smooth coordinated movement is seen when the patient attempts a voluntary movement either on his/her own or at the request of the examining physician.
FN2e 440–441

24. **(A)** The fastigial (medial cerebellar) nucleus receives a somatotopically organized projection from the overlying cerebellar cortex. In turn, this nucleus projects bilaterally to the vestibular and reticular nuclei; these fastigial efferents are excitatory. The vestibular and reticular nuclei contribute vestibulospinal and reticulospinal fibers to the spinal cord. The action of these fibers is predominately excitatory to spinal motor neurons innervating paravertebral (axial) and proximal limb extensor muscles.
FN2e 435–437

25. **(A)** The posterior inferior cerebellar artery (PICA) is usually the last major branch of the vertebral artery before it joins its counterpart to form the basilar artery. PICA arches around the medulla, giving rise to branches that serve the posterolateral medulla, and then forms a sharp turn in the dorsal cerebellomedullary cistern (cisterna magna). As the PICA arches through the cisterna magna it lies against the tela choroidea of the posterior portion of the fourth ventricle, giving rise to branches that penetrate the tela to serve the choroid plexus within the fourth ventricle.
FN2e 99–100, 427–428

26. **(B)** The exit of the trigeminal nerve (clearly seen on this MRI) from the lateral aspect of the pons specifies the interface between the basilar pons and the middle cerebellar peduncle. While pontocerebellar fibers are continuous through this area, the basilar pons is anterior (ventral) to the trigeminal exit and the middle cerebellar peduncle is posterior (dorsal) to the exit.
FN2e 424, 426

27. **(A)** This lesion is in the lateral aspect of the anterior lobe on the patient's right. The basilar pons is rounded, and there is no indication that the plane of the image is through the middle cerebellar peduncle. The fourth ventricle is modest in size and, therefore, consistent with a plane through more rostral portions of the pons, cerebellum, and fourth ventricle. In addition, the delicate lines characteristic of the folia of the anterior lobe are seen in this image. These folia/lines pass from the cerebellar margin to, and across, the midline into the opposite hemisphere of the anterior lobe.
FN2e 425–426

28. **(C)** The cerebellar tonsils are distinct oval-shaped clusters of folia located in the caudoventral portion of the cerebellum posterior (dorsal) to the medulla and adjacent to each other at the midline. An event that causes an increase in pressure in the posterior fossa, such as hemorrhage into the cerebellar hemisphere, may result in the tonsils being pushed down through the foramen magnum (tonsillar herniation). The resultant pressure on the medulla may compromise the patient's ability to breath or affect heart rate. This is due to pressure on respiratory and cardiovascular centers of the medulla.
FN2e 425–426

29. **(A)** The inferior aspects of the cerebellum are served by the posterior and anterior inferior cerebellar arteries. The former (PICA) serves the medial portion of the inferior cerebellar surface while the AICA serves the lateral portions of the inferior surface and adjacent parts of the middle cerebellar peduncle. Penetrating branches of the AICA also serve a small caudal part of the dentate nucleus.
FN2e 427–428

30. **(D)** The posterior lobe of the cerebellum consists of lobules VI through IX and their corresponding hemisphere portions (HVI through HIX). The anterior lobe consists of lobules I through V (and HII through HV; there is no hemisphere to lobule I), and the flocculonodular lobe consists of the nodules (X) and the floccules (HX).
FN2e 424–425

31. **(D)** Cerebellar nuclear neurons receive inhibitory (GABAergic) input from Purkinje cells. When a parallel fiber excites a stellate or basket cell, the action of these inhibitory (also GABAergic) interneurons of the cerebellar cortex is to inhibit the Purkinje cell. In this respect

the inhibitory influence of the Purkinje cell over neurons of the cerebellar nuclei is removed; the cerebellar nuclear cells are disinhibited.

FN2e 433–434

32.   **(A)** The globose and emboliform nuclei receive input from a variety of sources as collaterals of cerebel-lar afferent fibers traveling to the overlying cortex of the paravermal zone. These nuclei also receive cerebellar corticonuclear fibers from the paravermal cortex and project, via the superior cerebellar peduncle, to brainstem and thalamic targets primarily on the contralateral side.

FN2e 425–427, 438

CHAPTER 28

Visual Motor Systems

1. A 41-year-old woman is brought to the emergency department after falling down a narrow flight of stairs. The patient's report of "seeing double" just before the fall prompted a neurologic examination. This examination shows that the patient is unable to look down with her right eye after first looking inward (to the left). This deficit is consistent with a lesion involving which of the following structures?

○ (A) The right abducens nerve
○ (B) The right inferior rectus muscle
○ (C) The right lateral rectus muscle
○ (D) The right trochlear nucleus
○ (E) The right trochlear nerve

Questions 2 and 3 are based on the following patient:

During a neurological examination, a 23-year-old man successfully looks quickly back and forth between the doctor's upraised hands. He is also able to look back and forth between the doctor's nose and the doctor's finger placed 3 inches from the patient's nose. He accurately follows the doctor's fingertip, when it is moved slowly back and forth in front of him. When a strip of paper with alternating black and white stripes is moved slowly from left to right in front of him, the patient's eyes move back and forth. However, his eyes remain motionless when the paper is moved in the opposite direction (slowly from right to left).

2. The deficit seen in this patient falls into which of the following classes of eye movements?

○ (A) Saccadic
○ (B) Vergence
○ (C) Vestibular
○ (D) Optokinetic
○ (E) Smooth pursuit

3. In the case of this patient, which of the following CNS structures might be involved in a lesion?

○ (A) The right abducens nucleus
○ (B) One of the accessory optic nuclei
○ (C) The right superior vestibular nucleus
○ (D) The right pontine reticular region
○ (E) The left abducens nucleus

Questions 4 and 5 are based on the following patient:

A 63-year-old woman is brought to the emergency department after losing consciousness. After she regains consciousness the neurologic examination reveals drooping of the left eyelid and an inability to look to the right, up, or down with the left eye. The pupil in the left eye is larger than that of the right eye. The woman has a paralysis of muscles on the right lower face. In addition, her right arm and leg are paralyzed but sensation is normal over the face and body.

4. Which of the following represents the most likely location of the lesion in this patient?

○ (A) An anterior and medial midbrain lesion on the right
○ (B) A lesion that compresses the midbrain from above
○ (C) An anterior and medial midbrain lesion on the left
○ (D) A lesion of the medial pons on the left
○ (E) A lesion of the lateral midbrain on the left

5. Which of the following is the most likely cause of the deficits experienced by this patient?

○ (A) A tumor of the pineal compressing the midbrain
○ (B) An occlusion of the paramedian arteries of the pons
○ (C) An occlusion of the penetrating arteries derived from the P_1 portion of the posterior cerebral artery
○ (D) An aneurysm of the superior cerebellar artery
○ (E) An occlusion of the quadrigeminal artery

6. A 69-year-old man complains to his family physician of occasional "double vision." The physician finds that when the patient looks left, the left eye abducts and the right eye adducts, but neither eye moves past primary position when looking to the right. This loss of conjugate gaze to the right is present for smooth pursuit movements, as well (e.g., the eyes will not follow a rightward moving target past mid position). Convergent movements are normal in both eyes. A lesion in which of the following structures best explains the symptoms experienced by this patient?

○ (A) The right abducens nucleus
○ (B) The left abducens nucleus
○ (C) The right abducens nerve
○ (D) The right abducens and oculomotor nerves in the cavernous sinus
○ (E) The right medial longitudinal fasciculus (MLF)

7.   A 32-year-old woman presents with the complaint of double vision. Her eyes appear normal when looking straight ahead. However, when she looks to the right, only her right eye moves, and when she looks to the left, only her left eye moves. Medial rectus function in both eyes appears normal when viewing a near target. These findings are most consistent with a lesion in which of the following structures?

○ (A) A bilateral lesion in the oculomotor nucleus
○ (B) A bilateral lesion in the abducens nucleus
○ (C) A lesion in the posterior commissure
○ (D) A lesion in the commissure of the superior colliculus
○ (E) A midline lesion involving both medial longitudinal fasciculi (MLF)

8.   A 70-year-old chain smoker presents to the emergency department with signs of a brainstem stroke, including hemiparesis on the left side. However, these symptoms resolved, leaving only slight weakness and lessened sensation on the left. The following visual motor symptoms persist. The patient accurately looks at targets to the left, but he is unable to accurately move the eyes to targets on the right. However, he is able to follow a target moved slowly from the right field into the left field and vice versa. Perimetry testing reveals normal visual fields. Caloric testing is normal. Which of the following represents the most likely location of the lesion that results in the symptoms experienced by this patient?

○ (A) The right abducens nucleus
○ (B) The right pontine reticular formation
○ (C) The left superior colliculus
○ (D) The left pontine reticular formation
○ (E) The right frontal eye field (area 8)

9.   A 42-year-old man is referred to the neurologist because he is experiencing intermittent headaches. He indicates that analgesics and various migraine medications prescribed by his general practitioner initially helped but now fail. He also complains of visual difficulties. The visual examination reveals that he can look at and track targets on both his left and right side. However, when targets are presented above his normal resting position, the eye movements toward the target are furtive and drift back toward normal position. Both eyes are involved. Which of the following is the most likely cause of the deficits experienced by this patient?

○ (A) A tumor located in the interpeduncular fossa
○ (B) A vascular lesion in the right paramedian reticular formation
○ (C) A subdural hemorrhage in the area of the intraparietal sulcus

○ (D) Blockage of the posterior inferior cerebellar artery feeding the visual vermis
○ (E) A pinealoma compressing the posterior commissure

10.   As part of a general neurologic examination of a 31-year-old man, the physician notes that the patient's left eyelid droops slightly and the pupils are uneven, with the left being smaller than the right. These findings are most consistent with which of the following?

○ (A) Adie syndrome
○ (B) Argyll Robertson pupil
○ (C) Blepharospasm
○ (D) Horner syndrome
○ (E) Weber syndrome

11.   A 79-year-old man presents with a complaint of episodes in which his eyelids close and he has to prop them open with his fingers to see. On the occasion of one of these episodes, one eye is held open and a cotton swab is placed against the corner of the eye. This provokes a normal corneal reflex in both eyes. Observation of the patient in this condition shows that while the upper lids are fully down, the lower lids are not raised to touch them. A lesion in which of the following structures would most likely explain the deficits experienced by this patient?

○ (A) In the facial nerves
○ (B) In the caudal central subdivision of the oculomotor nucleus
○ (C) In the facial motor nuclei
○ (D) In the face representations of supplemental motor cortex
○ (E) In the spinal trigeminal nuclei

12.   A 42-year-old man presents to his family physician and complains that "my face looks funny and food keeps escaping from my mouth when I eat." Examination shows the left side of his face is flaccid. Touching a cotton swab to the cornea of either the right or the left eye results in a forceful blink on the right but only limited movement of the left upper eyelid. The eyelids move up and down normally in conjunction with vertical eye movements. No other motor symptoms are observed. Which of the following represents the most likely diagnosis in this case?

○ (A) Pseudobulbar palsy
○ (B) Blepharospasm
○ (C) A stroke involving the face representation in right motor cortex
○ (D) Bell palsy
○ (E) A stroke involving the left trigeminal sensory nuclei

13.   A 23-year-old unconscious man is brought to the emergency department from the site of an automobile collision. The left pupil is much larger than the right. When a light is shown in the right eye, the right pupil constricts but the left remains dilated. When a light is shown in the left eye, the same effects are observed: right pupillary constriction and no response on the left. Based on these findings which of the following would be the next most appropriate step?

○ (A) Immediate surgery
○ (B) Perform a spinal tap
○ (C) Stabilize the neck and watch for further symptoms
○ (D) Test visual fields
○ (E) Obtain CT of the head

14. Pupillary reflexes are tested on a 49-year-old woman during a routine neurologic examination. When the light is shown in the left eye, both pupils constrict. They also constrict when the light is shown in the right eye. However, when the light is moved back and forth between the right and left eyes, it is clear that the response from illuminating the right eye is only half as effective as leftward illumination. A lesion in which of the following structures would most likely produce these signs?

○ (A) Right oculomotor nerve
○ (B) Right optic nerve
○ (C) Right optic tract
○ (D) Right olivary pretectal nucleus
○ (E) Right Edinger-Westphal nucleus

15. An 82-year-old man complains of severe visual loss, including an inability to read. The neurologic examination reveals that the eyes appear to be constantly darting about in a random, albeit conjugate, manner. Saccades to targets can be made, but fixation at the new target is fleeting. Vestibular slow and quick phases appear normal, although saccades also appear, impinging on the normal movements. A lesion in which of the following structures would most likely explain these signs and symptoms?

○ (A) The nucleus prepositus hypoglossi
○ (B) The pontine raphe
○ (C) The vestibulocerebellum
○ (D) The paramedian pontine reticular formation (PPRF)
○ (E) The superior colliculus

16. A 58-year-old smoker with uncontrolled hypertension presents to the emergency department with dizziness and nausea. Initial observation shows the presence of nystagmus. A neurologic examination reveals that he has some loss of pain and temperature sensation on the right side of his face. Caloric testing reveals a general loss of vestibular input on the right side. There is also hearing loss on this side. The patient can direct his eyes to targets on both the right and left. However, he is unable to follow a target moving slowly from left to the right. A lesion in which of the following would most likely explain this last finding?

○ (A) The right abducens nucleus
○ (B) An accessory optic system nucleus on the right
○ (C) The right paramedian pontine reticular formation
○ (D) The right vestibular nuclear complex
○ (E) The left supraoculomotor area

17. During a rightward saccade, motor neurons in the right abducens nucleus display a pulse and step of activity that brings the right eye to the appropriate position. Which of the following nuclei provide the input that is responsible for the step in activity?

○ (A) The right rostral paramedian pontine reticular formation
○ (B) The right interstitial nucleus of Cajal
○ (C) The left caudal paramedian pontine reticular formation
○ (D) The right lateral vestibular nucleus (Deiters)
○ (E) The right nucleus prepositus hypoglossi

18. During a rightward saccade, the motor neurons in the left abducens nucleus fall silent. Which of the following structures provide the input that is responsible for their temporary cessation of activity?

○ (A) The left rostral paramedian pontine reticular formation (PPRF)
○ (B) The left interstitial nucleus of Cajal
○ (C) The right caudal paramedian pontine reticular formation (PPRF)
○ (D) The right lateral vestibular nucleus (Deiters)
○ (E) The left caudal paramedian pontine reticular formation (PPRF)

19. During an upward saccade, the superior rectus motor neurons in the oculomotor nucleus show a pulse and step of neural activity. Which of the following represent the most likely source of this pulse of activity?

○ (A) The medial vestibular nucleus
○ (B) The rostral interstitial nucleus of the medial longitudinal fasciculus
○ (C) The interstitial nucleus of Cajal
○ (D) The nucleus prepositus hypoglossi
○ (E) The omnipause region of the raphe nuclei

20. The axons found in the left predorsal bundle originate, at the level of the pons, from which of the following?

○ (A) The intermediate gray layer of the right superior colliculus
○ (B) The intermediate gray layer of the left superior colliculus
○ (C) The superficial gray layer of the right superior colliculus
○ (D) The superficial gray layer of the left superior colliculus
○ (E) The stratum opticum of the left superior colliculus

ANSWERS

1. **(E)** The secondary actions of the superior oblique muscle are depression and abduction. They are tested because the primary action, intorsion, is difficult to observe. The presence of the intact rectus muscles will compensate for the oblique in abduction, but in the adducted state only the superior oblique is in a position

to strongly depress the eye. (The inferior rectus works best when the eye is adducted.) The described deficit could be due to weakness either in the right superior oblique muscle or in the right nerve that supplies it. The trochlear nerves decussate in the midbrain, so a deficit in the right eye would be caused by a lesion in the left trochlear nucleus, not the right.
FN2e 446–447

2.   **(D)** The first test checks for saccades. The second test checks vergence movements. The third test evaluates smooth pursuit. It is only the fourth test that the patient fails. It tests the optokinetic system. The optokinetic system allows the eyes to compensate for the individual's movements in space, which normally cause full-field movements of the visual scene across the retina. The normal response to such movements is a slow compensatory movement in the direction the scene shifts, followed by a quick recentering movement. These slow and fast movements alternate as optokinetic nystagmus (OKN). OKN is named for the direction of the fast phases, so this patient would be described as lacking leftward OKN, with an intact rightward OKN.
FN2e 446, 458–459

3.   **(B)** The accessory optic nuclei receive retinal inputs from ganglion cells that note parallel movements across their field. Thus, a defect in one of these nuclei could produce loss of optokinetic movements. A lesion in either abducens nucleus would produce deficits in all classes of movements for a particular direction. The pontine reticular region controls saccades, not the slow following phases of OKN. The vestibular nuclei play a role in evoking slow optokinetic movements, but a lesion there would also affect smooth pursuit, which appeared normal.
FN2e 458–459

4.   **(C)** The symptoms described are those of a crossed paralysis (deficit). The paralysis of the hand and leg by themselves could be caused by an ipsilateral high cervical lesion of the corticospinal tract. However, the paralysis of the lower face points to a contralateral lesion involving corticonuclear (corticobulbar) fibers above the motor decussation. The presence of ptosis (drooping lid), the inability to move the eye medially or upwards, and the mydriasis (dilated pupil) are the best localizing signs. They suggest involvement of the ipsilateral oculomotor nerve or nucleus. The oculomotor nerve runs adjacent to the corticospinal and corticonuclear (corticobulbar) fibers in the medial midbrain.
FN2e 450

5.   **(C)** It is the branches of the first segment of the posterior cerebral artery (P$_1$ segment) that supply the medial anterior midbrain.
FN2e 197

6.   **(A)** A lesion in the right abducens nucleus would paralyze the ipsilateral abducens muscle, eliminating abduction in the right eye. This lesion would also eliminate the abducens internuclear neurons resident in this nucleus. They activate the contralateral medial rectus motor neurons during conjugate gaze changes. Inputs for convergence access the medial rectus motor neurons directly, so the medial rectus muscle would still adduct for near targets. A lesion in the nerve would spare the internuclear neurons, and so not affect the actions of the contralateral medial rectus muscle.
FN2e 452

7.   **(E)** These symptoms characterize bilateral internuclear ophthalmoplegia (BINO). They are produced by lesions involving both medial longitudinal fasciculi in the region between the abducens and oculomotor nucleus. This lesion eliminates the axons of abducens internuclear neurons that project to medial rectus motor neurons in support of conjugate horizontal gaze. Although not described here, deficits in the vestibular reflexes would also be present because of loss of ascending vestibular nucleus axons in the MLF.
FN2e 452

8.   **(B)** The fact that smooth pursuit and vestibular reflexes are spared indicates that the lesion cannot involve motor neurons. It appears to be confined to the saccadic system. Usually, the superior colliculus and frontal eye fields are each able to compensate for loss of the other, and lesions in these regions would not account for the initial symptoms. The saccade deficits would be best explained by rupture of a vessel supplying the right pontine reticular formation, which controls rightward saccades through its projections to the right abducens nucleus. The symptoms in the body would relate to a transient interruption of blood supply to the adjacent medial lemniscus and corticospinal fibers.
FN2e 454–456

9.   **(E)** The symptoms described are those of a vertical gaze palsy. Axons that connect the two interstitial nuclei of Cajal with each other and with the oculomotor nuclei pass through the posterior commissure. Loss of the activity supplied by this vertical integrator would produce vertical saccades that could not hold the vertical target position and would instead move back toward resting position.
FN2e 455

10.   **(D)** In Horner syndrome there is a loss of sympathetic input to the head. The cardinal features are ptosis, a drooping lid resulting from inactivation of the superior tarsal muscle; miosis, a constricted pupil caused by the loss of the dilator pupillae's antagonism of the constrictor pupillae muscle's activity; and anhidrosis, from loss of activity in sweat glands.
FN2e 452–453

11.   **(B)** The symptoms are not consistent with blepharospasm in which there are bilateral contractions of the orbicularis oculi muscle, because the lower lid is not raised, and the eyelids are not squeezed shut. This eliminates A, C, and D. The presence of a blink reflex rules out E. The caudal central subdivision projects bilaterally to the levator palpebrae superioris muscle, which is tonically active to hold the upper lid up. If these motor neurons become inactive, both upper lids close. This syndrome is sometimes termed apraxia of lid opening.
FN2e 460–462

12. **(D)** The self description and the observed physical symptoms are consistent with malfunction of the facial nerve on the left side. Bell palsy, which is believed to usually be a sequelae of a herpetic infection of the facial nerve, produces a temporary loss of facial nerve function. The presence of a blink reflex in response to corneal stimulation on either side rules out involvement of the trigeminal sensory nuclei. The limited movement of the left upper eyelid with corneal stimulation is caused by the normal inhibition of the levator palpebrae muscle that occurs when the orbicularis oculi muscle closes the eye for a blink. The eyelid still moves up and down with vertical eye movements because these are regulated by the caudal central subdivision of the oculomotor nucleus and its target, the levator palpebrae muscle.
FN2e 462

13. **(E)** This pattern of pupillary response—no consensual response from right illumination and no direct response from left illumination—points to intact afferent limbs of the pupillary light reflex but loss of the efferent limb on the left. The presence of a fixed (unresponsive) dilated pupil in a trauma victim points to the possibility of uncal herniation, in which a space-occupying lesion (hemorrhage) presses down on the brain until the uncus and adjacent parts of the parahippocampal gyrus compress the third nerve. The superficially located preganglionic fibers appear to be particularly sensitive to compression. Because this is often followed by further compression of the brainstem, with lethal effect, it is essential to identify the extent of the lesion and to ascertain if there is blood in the brain and/or subarachnoid space. This must be done before any treatment and is most easily accomplished by CT and MRI.
FN2e 10–12, 460

14. **(B)** These responses suggest a relative afferent pupillary defect, which occurs when the optic nerve is compromised. The difference in sensitivity to light indicates that the afferent limb is involved, whereas the equivalent direct and consensual responses of the two pupils rules out the efferent limb (responses A and E). Because half the fibers cross in the optic chiasm and because of the presence of a partial crossing of olivary projections to the Edinger-Westphal nucleus, lesions in this part of the reflex pathway (responses C and D) produce equivalent losses of reflex activity on both sides that are more difficult to discern.
FN2e 459–461

15. **(B)** The pontine raphe contains omnipause neurons. These neurons inhibit the excitatory burst neurons (EBNs) in the paramedian pontine reticular formation (PPRF) during periods of foveation (fixation). Without this inhibition, the EBNs trigger spurious saccades, making fixation difficult and limiting the ability to acquire information by foveation.
FN2e 454–455

16. **(D)** The vestibular nuclei contain premotor neurons responsible for the slow movements in smooth pursuit and optokinetic nystagmus, as well as for vestibular compensatory movements. The lesion described is a variation of lateral medullary syndrome, which in this case involved the right vestibular and cochlear nuclei as well as portions of the spinal trigeminal nucleus.
FN2e 171, 456–457

17. **(E)** The step in activity, which holds the eye at the new target, is supplied by the ipsilateral nucleus prepositus hypoglossi. This nucleus receives a pulsatile signal from the excitatory burst neurons (EBNs) in the rostral paramedian pontine reticular formation and converts it (neural integration) into the appropriate tonic activity (step) for a horizontal saccade.
FN2e 453–455

18. **(C)** The inhibitory burst neurons (IBNs) located in the caudal paramedian pontine reticular formation are responsible for inhibiting the contralateral abducens motor neurons to allow conjugate eye movements. Remember, with gaze to the right, the medial rectus muscle of the left eye will contract while the lateral rectus muscle of the left eye will relax. The reverse is true for muscles on the right side when gaze is to the left.
FN2e 453–455

19. **(B)** The rostral interstitial nucleus of the medial longitudinal fasciculus (riMLF), located medially in the fields of Forel at the midbrain-diencephalon junction, contains burst neurons that provide the pulse in activity to superior rectus motor neurons during upward saccades. Because this signal is also provided to the interstitial nucleus of Cajal, which converts it into the tonic step in activity needed to maintain fixation, loss of riMLF seriously affects both components of activity needed for a vertical saccade.
FN2e 454–455

20. **(A)** The predorsal bundle contains axons whose cells of origin lie primarily in the contralateral intermediate gray layer. Therefore, the right colliculus controls saccadic movements to targets on the left. The superficial gray layer cells also project to the ipsilateral thalamus.
FN2e 256

CHAPTER 29

Visceral Motor Pathways

1. A 26-year-old medical student experiences acute "stage fright" as she begins an oral presentation to a large group of students and faculty. Which of the following is most likely to be among the physiologic manifestations of her anxiety?

- ○ (A) Decreased heart rate
- ○ (B) Excessive salivation
- ○ (C) Decreased sweating
- ○ (D) Increased blood flow to the abdominal viscera
- ○ (E) Decreased blood flow to the skin

2. A 27-year-old woman suffered a severe spinal cord injury at the C7 spinal cord level as a result of a sledding accident. After 2 months, she experiences autonomic dysreflexia; that is, noxious stimuli to the trunk and lower extremities evoke piloerection, sweating, hypertension, and urinary retention. Which of the following represent the most likely cause of these responses?

- ○ (A) Exaggerated parasympathetic reflexes
- ○ (B) Suppressed parasympathetic reflexes
- ○ (C) Exaggerated sympathetic reflexes
- ○ (D) Suppressed sympathetic reflexes
- ○ (E) Exaggerated crossed extensor reflexes

3. After surgery to treat an occluded left common carotid artery, a 71-year-old man exhibits, on the left side, flushing of the face, a slight ptosis, and a constricted pupil that does not dilate in dim light. These observations suggest that an unintentional consequence of the surgery was injury to which of the following?

- ○ (A) Cervical sympathetic trunk
- ○ (B) Vagus nerve
- ○ (C) Glossopharyngeal nerve
- ○ (D) Ventral roots of spinal nerves C6 to C8
- ○ (E) Facial nerve

Questions 4 and 5 are based on the following patient:

A 48-year-old man presents to his internist with severe epigastric pain. The evaluation, which includes a barium study and aspiration of stomach contents via a nasogastric tube, clearly suggests a gastric ulcer. Bilateral vagotomy is performed to relieve symptoms arising from gastric ulcerations.

4. In addition to reduced gastric acid secretion, which of the following consequences of interrupted vagus nerve function may be seen in this patient?

- ○ (A) Bradycardia
- ○ (B) Inability to attain penile erection
- ○ (C) Loss of vascular tone in the upper and lower extremities
- ○ (D) Reduced blood flow to the small intestine
- ○ (E) Loss of sweating in the trunk, but normal sweating in the extremities

5. The long-term effects of vagotomy on motility of the patient's small intestine are relatively mild. Which of the following is a fact that explains this finding?

- ○ (A) The intrinsic innervation of the gut can function autonomously to generate waves of smooth muscle contraction in response to the presence of chyme in the gut lumen.
- ○ (B) The central and peripheral pathways of the sympathetic nervous system, which are intact, provide the major excitatory input that promotes peristalsis.
- ○ (C) Intestinal motility is chiefly a function of striated muscle fibers, which are innervated by alpha motor neurons with cell bodies in the anterior horn of the lower thoracic spinal cord.
- ○ (D) The parasympathetic innervation of the small intestine is conveyed by pelvic nerves that originate from the sacral spinal cord.

6. A 22-year-old man who is a patient in a dental clinic insists that he is experiencing no pain or anxiety as the dentist uses a drill to prepare a carious tooth for restoration. However, his pupils are dilated despite the bright illumination of his face. Which of the following most likely explains this phenomenon?

- ○ (A) He is being stoic (experiencing more pain than he admits).
- ○ (B) He is, as he claims, relaxed and without severe pain.
- ○ (C) He has a bilateral Horner syndrome.
- ○ (D) He has an injury of the trigeminal nerve on the side of the carious tooth.
- ○ (E) He has an injury to sympathetic input to his eyes.

7. A pathologist who is examining sections of a skin biopsy specimen from a 47-year-old woman who exhibits symptoms of autonomic dysfunction wishes to determine whether blood vessels of the dermis have an intact sympathetic innervation. One way to demonstrate such nerve fibers is through the use of immunostaining. Which of the following represents the best choice of antibodies for this type of immunostaining?

- ○ (A) Acetylcholine
- ○ (B) Neuropeptide Y
- ○ (C) Vasoactive intestinal peptide
- ○ (D) Epinephrine
- ○ (E) Dopamine

8. Movement by an individual from a reclining to upright position normally evokes the baroreceptor reflex. Among the responses that occur is increased vascular tone (vasoconstriction) of blood vessels that supply which of the following?

- ○ (A) Brain
- ○ (B) Skin
- ○ (C) Heart
- ○ (D) Skeletal muscles
- ○ (E) Bone

9. Which of the following is characteristic of the vasopressor center of the brainstem?

- ○ (A) It is located in the rostral dorsolateral pons.
- ○ (B) It is the dorsal motor vagal nucleus.
- ○ (C) It is regulated by inhibitory input from the nucleus solitarius.
- ○ (D) It functions mainly through excitatory projections to the dorsal vagal motor nucleus.
- ○ (E) It functions through spinal projections to the principal olivary nuclei.

10. Which of the following is the origin of inhibitory nerve fibers that innervate the detrusor muscle of the bladder?

- ○ (A) Inferior mesenteric ganglion
- ○ (B) Anterior horn of the spinal cord at S3 and S4
- ○ (C) Intermediolateral cell column at L1 and L2
- ○ (D) Dorsal motor vagal nucleus
- ○ (E) Wall of the bladder

ANSWERS

1. **(E)** The extreme anxiety that many people experience before speaking to a group often evokes a group of symptoms that reflect a global increase in sympathetic outflow. These are likely to include increased heart rate, decreased blood flow to the abdominal viscera along with decreased peristalsis of the gastrointestinal tract, a dry mouth, and cold, wet skin as a result of decreased blood flow in the skin and increased sweating.
FN2e 472

2. **(C)** Severe spinal cord injuries at cervical levels disrupt the descending pathways that mediate regulation of sympathetic preganglionic neurons by higher centers such as the hypothalamus, solitary nucleus, and reticular formation. A result of the loss in descending control is, after a period of spinal shock, exaggerated segmental sympathetic reflexes.
FN2e 476

3. **(A)** It is likely that injury of the cervical sympathetic trunk occurred in association with the surgery. This would disrupt the preganglionic nerve fibers that terminate in the superior cervical ganglion, with a consequent loss of sympathetic tone to blood vessels of the face, the smooth muscle of the superior tarsal muscle, the pupillary dilator, and the sweat glands of the face.
FN2e 470, 472

4. **(D)** Digestive functions are promoted by parasympathetic outflow, so loss of vagus nerve function will likely result in diminished motility and secretion in the gastrointestinal tract from the esophagus to the left colic flexure where sacral parasympathetics take over. The decreased motility and secretion is less pronounced than might be expected for reasons discussed in the next question. Any effect of vagotomy on heart rate would be toward tachycardia because of the unopposed action of sympathetic tone. Sweating and vascular tone in the extremities would be unaffected by vagotomy because these functions are regulated only by the sympathetic division of the autonomic system. Penile erection is mainly under parasympathetic control, but this is conveyed by the sacral parasympathetic outflow, not the vagus.
FN2e 466, 474

5. **(A)** Parasympathetic innervation of the small intestine would be interrupted by bilateral vagotomy. However, the large population of neurons within the wall of the gastrointestinal tract (enteric nervous system) is organized into complex circuits that can mediate basic functions, such as peristalsis and secretion, in response to ingested material in the lumen. This can occur independently of regulation by parasympathetic and sympathetic input. Although the sympathetic pathways to the gut would be intact after vagotomy, activation of this pathway results in decreased motility, secretion, and blood flow in the gut.
FN2e 475

6. **(A)** Dilation of the pupils, despite bright illumination, suggests that the sympathetic system is activated, probably in response to intense anxiety or pain. Accompanying symptoms might include sweating and pallor. Interruption of the sympathetic outflow to the head and face would result in the Horner syndrome, which includes constriction, not dilation, of the pupil. Injury of the trigeminal nerve might result in loss of sensation to the teeth, but unless this is an irritative lesion (as in trigeminal neuralgia), increased sympathetic outflow is unlikely to be evoked.
FN2e 472

7. **(B)** Neuropeptide Y would be the best choice because it serves as a neurotransmitter or modulator that

is released by many sympathetic postganglionic fibers, including those that innervate blood vessels of the skin. Generally, sympathetic ganglion neurons use norepinephrine rather than epinephrine as a transmitter. In contrast, epinephrine is synthesized and released by most of the endocrine cells (modified sympathetic ganglion neurons) of the adrenal medulla.

FN2e 473

8. **(D)** The baroreceptor reflex counteracts the tendency of blood to pool in the vessels of the lower extremities and trunk owing to gravitational forces when an individual assumes an upright position. If this gravitational effect is unchecked, the most serious effect is a sudden decrease in blood flow to the brain. The reflex results in increased heart rate and selective vasoconstriction of vessels supplying skeletal muscle and abdominal viscera. Vascular tone is not increased in the brain, heart, or skin.

FN2e 476–477

9. **(C)** The vasopressor center is not a well-defined nucleus but rather a network of neurons located in the rostral ventrolateral medulla. Inhibitory input from the solitary nucleus is a key component of the pathways that mediate the baroreceptor and chemoreceptor reflexes. For example, a drop in pressure in the aortic and carotid sinuses results in reduced inhibition of the vasopressor center by the projection from the solitary nucleus. Output from the vasopressor center affects cardiovascular function by way of its projections to preganglionic sympathetic neurons in the spinal cord.

FN2e 476–477

10. **(A)** The smooth muscle of the bladder wall (detrusor muscle) is innervated by both sympathetic and parasympathetic neurons. Postganglionic neurons with cell bodies in the inferior mesenteric ganglion provide the sympathetic input, by way of the hypogastric plexus. During periods of urine storage, this sympathetic innervation inhibits the smooth muscle directly and, in addition, indirectly by inhibiting the local parasympathetic neurons that provide the excitatory innervation of the detrusor.

FN2e 477

CHAPTER 30

The Hypothalamus

1. An 80-year-old woman complains that for the past 6 months she has been bothered by frequent urination and the need to drink a lot of water. She states "I think I must be going crazy. I have to get up so often during the night that I hardly get any sleep." Blood glucose levels in this patient are within normal limits; however, MRI reveals a small lesion within her hypothalamus. Assuming that this lesion is the cause of the patient's condition, which hypothalamic nucleus is most likely involved?

- (A) Arcuate nucleus
- (B) Suprachiasmatic nucleus
- (C) Supraoptic nucleus
- (D) Ventromedial nucleus
- (E) Medial mammillary nucleus

2. A 40-year-old woman presents with hypertension and an abnormal appearance that includes truncal obesity, violet-colored stretch marks, a moonlike face, and a dorsal cervical hump. Furthermore, an excessive amount of adrenal cortisol is present in the patient's blood. Based on these observations, the patient most likely has

- (A) acromegaly
- (B) hypothyroidism
- (C) hyperprolactinemia
- (D) Cushing disease
- (E) Graves disease

3. A 40-year-old man presents with a headache that has persisted for the past 2 months. The examination reveals bitemporal hemianopsia, but somatomotor and somatosensory functions are normal. Blood tests indicate that hormone levels are within normal limits. MRI reveals a large pituitary tumor, 2.5 cm in diameter, that is impinging on the optic chiasm. What type of tumor is this likely to be?

- (A) Nonsecreting macroadenoma
- (B) Rhabdomyoma
- (C) Nonsecreting microadenoma
- (D) Astrocytoma
- (E) Prolactinoma

4. A 10-year-old boy is brought to a family physician by his parents. The parents state that he has no appetite and has not eaten normally since he was involved in a motor vehicle collision 3 months earlier. The examination reveals an emaciated and lethargic boy. Cranial nerve function and somatomotor and somatosensory functions are normal. Reflexes are normal. MRI reveals a small lesion within the hypothalamus. Which of the following labeled hypothalamic areas is most likely involved in the lesion? (   )

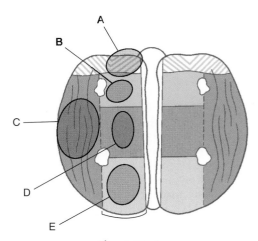

Figure 30–1

5. A 30-year-old man presents to his family physician with the complaint that he has been having trouble remembering things. The examination reveals an otherwise healthy man with normal cranial nerve function and a normal somatomotor and somatosensory examination. His wife explains that his memory problems began when he fell off his bicycle and hit his head about 6 months ago. Although he has no trouble remembering things that happened before the biking accident, his memory for more recent events seems fuzzy. She states, "When I tell

him something, it's like it goes in one ear and comes out the other." MRI reveals a small lesion within the hypothalamus. Which of the following labeled hypothalamic nuclei is most likely involved in the lesion? (   )

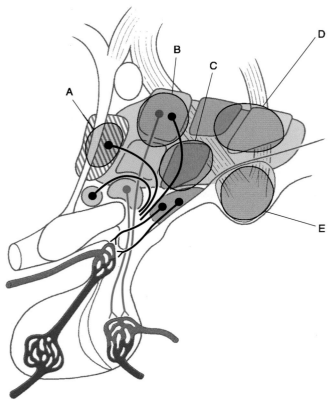

Figure 30–2

6.   A 6-year-old girl is brought to the pediatric neurologist by her mother, who states that the daughter "has not been herself" since she fell from her gym set. The examination reveals a well-developed and well-nourished girl. There is cutaneous vasodilation on the left side of her body. She is hypothermic (96.9°F). Her mother says that the girl seems more passive and does not eat as much as she used to. MRI is scheduled to identify any potential intracranial lesions. A lesion at which of the following sites could explain the symptoms in this patient?

○ (A) Anterior lobe of the pituitary
○ (B) Caudolateral hypothalamus
○ (C) Preoptic area of the hypothalamus
○ (D) Rostromedial hypothalamus
○ (E) Posterior lobe of the pituitary

7.   The posterior (dorsal) boundary between the hypothalamus and the dorsal thalamus is represented by which of the following?

○ (A) Lamina terminalis
○ (B) Hypothalamic sulcus
○ (C) Column of the fornix

○ (D) Massa intermedia
○ (E) Substantia innominata

8.   A 49-year-old alcoholic man is diagnosed with diabetes insipidus. Based on this information, the patient would most likely experience which of the following?

○ (A) Polyphagia
○ (B) Polydipsia
○ (C) Polyodontia
○ (D) Polycythemia
○ (E) Polyneuralgia

9.   A 49-year-old man is brought to the emergency department by the police. The examination reveals an unkept, intoxicated, and emaciated man. He remembers where he was born and grew up, but he does not seem to remember where he has been for the past several years, other than "living on the street." In addition to a good diet (and no alcohol), administration of which of the following would most likely improve this patient's general mental function?

○ (A) L-Dopa
○ (B) Vitamin C
○ (C) Vitamin E
○ (D) Neostigmine
○ (E) Thiamine

10.   Which of the following is the large, but diffusely arranged, fiber bundle that traverses the lateral hypothalamic area and interconnects the septal area, lateral hypothalmus, and midbrain?

○ (A) Anterolateral system
○ (B) Stria terminalis
○ (C) Medial forebrain bundle
○ (D) Internal capsule
○ (E) Stria medullaris thalami

11.   A 29-year-old anorexic woman is brought to her family physician by her husband. He states that she will not eat, drinks excessive amounts of alcohol, and was terminated at her job as a computer programmer because she could not remember how to write new programs. The examination reveals an emaciated, lethargic woman who is unable to recall recent details in her life. To fill in the details she makes up facts that seem unrelated to her actual life experiences. This patient most likely has which of the following?

○ (A) Wallenberg syndrome
○ (B) Korsakoff syndrome
○ (C) Klüver-Bucy syndrome
○ (D) Cushing disease
○ (E) Brown-Séquard syndrome

12.   A 14-year-old boy is brought to his family physician by his parents. The boy is 6-feet tall, weighs 170 pounds, and is extremely weak although he appears muscular. His parents report that since he was a baby he has always been "big for his age." Tests reveal an excessive production of growth hormone. This boy is most likely suffering from which of the following?

- (A) Cushing disease
- (B) Acromegaly
- (C) Korsakoff syndrome
- (D) Gigantism
- (E) Prolactinoma

13. Which of the following nuclei receive direct input from the retina and mediate hormonal fluctuations that are related to cycles of light and darkness?

- (A) Supraoptic
- (B) Medial preoptic
- (C) Dorsomedial
- (D) Suprachiasmatic
- (E) Paraventricular

14. A 34-year-old woman presents to her internist complaining of frequent urination. The physical examination reveals a rotund patient with disproportionately large hands and feet, a large nose and thickened lips, and prominent supraorbital ridges. Further tests reveal that the woman is diabetic and has an excessive production of growth hormone. This woman is most likely suffering from which of the following?

- (A) Cushing syndrome
- (B) Korsakoff syndrome
- (C) Acromegaly
- (D) Gigantism
- (E) Pinealoma

15. A 17-year-old boy is brought to an endocrinologist for insatiable hunger. His mother explains that over the past several months her son has become anxious and agitated (he is normally very calm), and he has a low-grade fever all of the time (99.5°F to 100.2°F). The endocrinologist orders MRI, which reveals a small hypothalamic lesion. Damage to which of the following would most likely explain the clinical problems experienced by this patient?

- (A) Rostromedial hypothalamus
- (B) Mammillary nuclei
- (C) Caudolateral hypothalamus
- (D) Suprachiasmatic nucleus
- (E) Periventricular zone

16. Which of the following hypothalamic nuclei is described as being "sexually dimorphic," that is, generally larger in males than in females?

- (A) Lateral hypothalamic nucleus
- (B) Medial preoptic nucleus
- (C) Suprachiasmatic nucleus
- (D) Posterior hypothalamic nucleus
- (E) Paraventricular nucleus

17. A 31-year-old man visits his family physician. He explains that over the past year or so he seems to have lost interest in sex (decreased libido) and when interested he has a lot of trouble getting and maintaining an erection (impotence). Suspecting an organic problem, the

physician orders MRI, which reveals a large tumor of the pituitary gland extending through the diaphragma sella into the suprasellar cistern. This patient is most likely suffering from which of the following?

- (A) Excessive secretion of growth-stimulating hormone
- (B) Excessive secretion of follicle-stimulating hormone
- (C) Excessive oxytocin production
- (D) Hyperprolactinemia
- (E) Hyperparathyroidism

18. Through which of the following fiber bundles do axons of the paraventricular nucleus pass to reach the posterior lobe of the pituitary?

- (A) Postcommissural fornix
- (B) Tuberoinfundibular tract
- (C) Stria medullaris thalami
- (D) Medial forebrain bundle
- (E) Supraopticohypophysial tract

19. The mother of a 16-year-old girl brings her daughter to the gynecologist suspecting that her daughter is pregnant. The mother noticed that her daughter's bras were "wet," and, when questioned, the daughter admitted that she had fluid coming out of her breasts. The examination reveals a healthy, nonpregnant girl who the gynecologist indicates to the mother is still a virgin. Which of the following would most likely explain this condition in this girl?

- (A) Excessive growth hormone
- (B) Pinealoma
- (C) Prolactinoma
- (D) Overproduction of corticotropin
- (E) Overproduction of antidiuretic hormone (vasopressin)

20. A 79-year-old man is diagnosed with an aneurysm at the bifurcation (apex) of the basilar artery. During the surgery to clip this aneurysm some of the small perforating branches of P_1 are inadvertently occluded by the clip. Which of the following structures would be most adversely affected by this disruption of blood supply?

- (A) Pituitary (anterior and posterior lobes)
- (B) Preoptic area
- (C) Supraoptic and suprachiasmatic nuclei
- (D) Paraventricular nucleus
- (E) Mammillary and posterior nuclei

21. A 34-year-old woman visits her gynecologist and complains that her breasts are tender. She also notes that when she self-examined her breasts about a month ago she expressed a small amount of white fluid. The woman states that she had a hysterectomy at age 31. Suspecting a small brain lesion, the physician orders MRI, which reveals a tumor. Which of the following labeled areas represents the most likely location of this neoplasm? See Figure 30–3. (   )

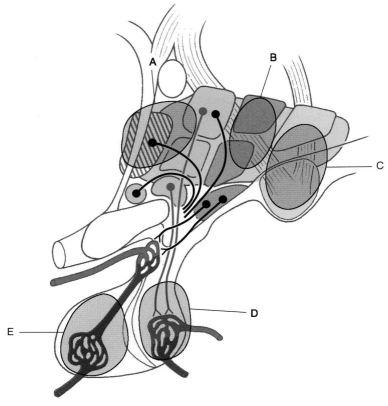

Figure 30–3

ANSWERS

1. **(C)** The supraoptic nucleus produces antidiuretic hormone (ADH) that is released into the blood from the posterior lobe of the pituitary. ADH causes the resorption of water from the collecting tubules of the kidney, thus returning water to the blood supply. Damage to the supraoptic nucleus can decrease the amount of circulating ADH. This diminishes the amount of water that is resorbed in the kidneys. Instead, the water exits the body via a copious output of urine. Consequently, the patient usually feels excessively thirsty all of the time and compensates by drinking large quantities of water. This condition is known as diabetes insipidus.
FN2e 488

2. **(D)** Cushing disease is a form of hyperadrenalism that is caused by an overproduction of corticotropin from the pituitary and secondarily by an excessive adrenal cortisol secretion. It is characterized by a variety of physical changes in appearance, including central truncal obesity, moonlike facies, and violaceous striae (violet-colored stretch marks). Hypertension is commonly present.
FN2e 490

3. **(A)** "Nonsecreting" tumors of the pituitary are so-named because they do not secrete hormones. As a result, they often go undetected until they are quite large and impinge on neighboring structures, such as the optic pathway. Accordingly, patients having one of these tumors often present with headaches and visual disturbances. Pituitary tumors are generally not malignant.
FN2e 489

4. **(C)** The lateral hypothalamic zone contains the lateral hypothalamic nucleus. Activation of this nucleus promotes feeding behavior. However, when the lateral hypothalamic nucleus is destroyed the patient will have a loss of appetite and a resultant loss of weight, producing an emaciated appearance.
FN2e 483

5. **(E)** Lesions of the mammillary nuclei lead to anterograde amnesia. People having anterograde amnesia have no difficulty remembering events that occurred before the lesion. However, memories for events occurring after the lesion are limited to a period of minutes. These people usually find it difficult to learn new skills.
FN2e 483

6. **(B)** The caudolateral hypothalamus normally functions to activate sympathetic activities (including cutaneous vasocontriction) and shivering. These influences cause an increase in body temperature. A lesion in the caudolateral hypothalamus results in the inhibition of sympathetic activities and a possible reduction in body temperature.
FN2e 491

7. **(B)** The hypothalamic sulcus is a shallow groove lying posterior (dorsal) to the hypothalamus. The hypo-

thalamic sulcus separates the hypothalamus from the dorsal thalamus.
FN2e 480–481

8. **(B)** Patients with diabetes insipidus have a decreased amount of antidiuretic hormone (ADH). The main clinical features of diabetes insipidus are polydipsia (increased amounts of water intake) followed by polyuria (excessive urination) and hyperosmolarity. This may be exacerbated by the consumption of alcohol.
FN2e 488

9. **(E)** Anterograde amnesia, a difficulty in recalling new events and turning these into long-term memory, is seen in patients with poor nutrition and thiamine deficiency. This is a particular problem in chronic alcoholism.
FN2e 483

10. **(C)** The medial forebrain bundle, composed of numerous axons, traverses the lateral zone of the hypothalamus. These axons interconnect the hypothalamus with structures lying both rostral and caudal to the hypothalamus.
FN2e 480, 486

11. **(B)** Korsakoff syndrome is characteristically seen in chronic alcoholics who are severely malnourished. These patients have difficulty remembering and learning new tasks (a loss of recent memory) and may attempt to compensate by confabulating events.
FN2e 483

12. **(D)** Growth hormone is produced by the adenohypophysis. An overproduction of growth hormone before the closure of the epiphyseal plates of long bones results in gigantism. The child will show growth patterns that consistently exceed what is expected for the chronologic age.
FN2e 489

13. **(D)** The suprachiasmatic nucleus lies in close proximity to the optic chiasm and receives direct input from the retina. It is thought that the suprachiasmatic nucleus responds to light-darkness cycles by influencing the release of hormones. Hormonal fluctuations that occur in response to the light-darkness cycle are known as circadian rhythms.
FN2e 483

14. **(C)** Excessive production of growth hormone after the epiphyseal plates have closed results in large, exaggerated facial features and unusually large hands and feet. These patients are not unusually tall and may have cardiac problems (such as cardiomegaly) and hypertension.
FN2e 489–490

15. **(A)** The rostromedial area of the hypothalamus functions in behavioral and physiologic states indicative of contentment and general well-being. These include an increase in parasympathetic activity, relaxed and passive behavior, a sense of satiety, and decreased body temperature. Lesions in this area of the hypothalamus result in deficits opposite of the expected function of those seen in the normal individual.
FN2e 491

16. **(B)** Neurons of the medial preoptic nucleus manufacture gonadotropin-releasing hormone (GnRH). GnRH is transported to the anterior lobe of the pituitary, where it causes the release of gonadotropins (luteinizing hormone and follicle-stimulating hormone). Because gonadotropin release is continuous in males and cyclical in females, the medial preoptic nucleus tends to be more active and consequently larger in males than the medial preoptic nucleus in females. Because of its gender-related variation in size, the medial preoptic nucleus is often described as being sexually dimorphic (i.e., having two forms as a function of gender).
FN2e 480

17. **(D)** Excessive production of prolactin in men may cause decreased sexual drive, impotence, and infertility. Hyperprolactinemia in males is usually the result of a pituitary tumor.
FN2e 490

18. **(E)** The hormones antidiuretic hormone and oxytocin are manufactured by the paraventricular and supraoptic nuclei. These hormones are transported via the supraopticohypophysial tract to the posterior lobe of the pituitary, where they are released into the bloodstream.
FN2e 487

19. **(C)** A tumor of the prolactin-producing cells of the anterior lobe of the pituitary (prolactinoma) results in hyperprolactinemia. In nonpregnant women or girls, this may result in milk production (galactorrhea) or amenorrhea (absence of menstrual periods).
FN2e 490–491

20. **(E)** Penetrating branches of P_1 traverse the interpeduncular fossa and enter the mammillary region of the hypothalamus to serve the mammillary and posterior nuclei. Although some of these vessels may enter the tuberal region, this area of the hypothalamus is served primarily by penetrating branches of the posterior communicating artery. Anterior hypothalamic areas are served primarily by penetrating branches of A_1 and penetrating branches of the anterior communicating artery.
FN2e 484

21. **(E)** This woman has hyperprolactinemia resulting from a tumor of the prolactin-secreting cells of the anterior lobe of the pituitary. Milk production in a nonpregnant female (her prior hysterectomy makes intrauterine pregnancy impossible) is one of the diagnostic features of this type of tumor.
FN2e 482, 490

CHAPTER 31

The Limbic System

Questions 1 through 3 are based on the following patient:

A 27-year-old man is brought to the emergency department from the site of an automobile collision. The initial examination reveals a stuporous man with extensive facial and scalp lacerations. Suspecting a brain injury, the physician orders CT. This reveals fractures in the facial skeleton and bilateral damage to the rostral 3 to 4 cm of the temporal lobes. The lacerations are repaired, and the patient is hospitalized and medicated to control brain swelling.

1. After recovering from the initial trauma, this man begins to compulsively explore his hospital room, aimlessly and repeatedly examining objects and places. Which of the following most specifically describes this condition?

- ○ (A) Hyperorality
- ○ (B) Hyperphasia
- ○ (C) Hyperphagia
- ○ (D) Visual agnosia
- ○ (E) Hypermetamorphosis

2. This patient also is compelled to examine objects, even inappropriate ones such as the plastic cap of a medicine bottle or a roll of film, by placing them in his mouth. Which of the following most precisely describes this condition?

- ○ (A) Hyperphagia
- ○ (B) Hyperorality
- ○ (C) Auditory agnosia
- ○ (D) Dementia
- ○ (E) Hypermetamorphosis

3. The behavioral aberrations seen in this patient, when correlated with the CT finding of bitemporal contusions, suggest that this man most likely has which of the following?

- ○ (A) Wernicke aphasia
- ○ (B) Wallenberg syndrome
- ○ (C) Korsakoff syndrome
- ○ (D) Klüver-Bucy syndrome
- ○ (E) Wernicke-Korsakoff syndrome

4. One important pathway through which the amygdaloid complex influences the hypothalamus is a fiber bundle that travels in close association with the tail and body of the caudate nucleus. This fiber bundle is the

- ○ (A) Stria medullaris thalami
- ○ (B) Amygdalofugal pathway
- ○ (C) Stria terminalis
- ○ (D) Medial forebrain bundle
- ○ (E) Mammillothalamic tract

5. The projections to the mammillary body from the hippocampal complex originate primarily from where?

- ○ (A) Ammon's horn
- ○ (B) Subiculum
- ○ (C) Dentate gyrus
- ○ (D) Hippocampus proper
- ○ (E) Indusium griseum

6. A 61-year-old woman is brought to the emergency department by her husband after developing lethargy and drooping of the lower side of the face on the right. Suspecting a vascular event, the physician orders CT, which reveals an ischemic infarction in the area of the hippocampal formation, part of the amygdaloid complex and adjacent anterior (ventral) parts of the internal capsule. This infarction most likely originated from occlusion of which of the following vessels?

- ○ (A) M_1
- ○ (B) Lateral posterior choroidal artery
- ○ (C) Posterior communicating artery
- ○ (D) A_1
- ○ (E) Anterior choroidal artery

7. The circuit of Papez is a pathway within the brain that is related, in part, to emotion and emotional responses. Which of the following schemes correctly depicts the complete Papez circuit?

○ (A) Mammillary body → cingulate gyrus → subiculum (hippocampal complex) → anterior nucleus of thalamus → cingulate gyrus
○ (B) Cingulate gyrus → subiculum (hippocampal complex) → mammillary body → anterior nucleus of thalamus → cingulate gyrus
○ (C) Cingulate gyrus → subiculum (hippocampal complex) → anterior nucleus of thalamus → cingulate gyrus → mammillary body
○ (D) Mammillary body → anterior nucleus of thalamus → subiculum (hippocampal complex) → amygdala → cingulate gyrus
○ (E) Cingulate gyrus → subiculum (hippocampal complex) → anterior nucleus of thalamus → amygdala → mammillary body

8. A 2-year-old girl has a history of near-drowning, having been submerged in a semi-frozen lake for 20 minutes. As a result of this experience, there are bilateral infarcts in the hippocampal complex. Which of the following behavioral disorders is this patient most likely to display?

○ (A) Aphasia
○ (B) A loss of immediate- and short-term memory
○ (C) Social crudeness
○ (D) A loss of long-term memory
○ (E) Hypersexuality

9. A 55-year-old alcoholic man presents with a long-standing memory deficit in which he has no recollection of events more than a few minutes old. Consequently, he appears confused. MRI reveals an obvious decrease in the size of the mammillary bodies, suggestive of a loss of neurons. The memory loss in this patient is known as what?

○ (A) Akinetic mutism
○ (B) Klüver-Bucy syndrome
○ (C) Alzheimer disease
○ (D) Sommer syndrome
○ (E) Korsakoff syndrome

10. A 26-year-old woman presents with a history of socially aberrant behavior. These include hypersexuality and hyperphagia (gluttony). In addition, the patient tends to examine objects within her environment by either tasting or smelling them. This patient has been referred to a neurologist for tests to identify a possible organic basis for these findings. MRI of this patient would most likely reveal lesions in which of the following structures?

○ (A) Mammillary bodies
○ (B) Hippocampus
○ (C) Amygdaloid complex
○ (D) Septal nuclei
○ (E) Prefrontal cortex

11. A 35-year-old man presents with a long-standing history of episodic fear and panic attacks. Sometimes during these panic attacks, the patient has displayed inappropriate and antisocial behavior. Through electroencephalographic studies, it is shown that there is episodic seizure activity occurring in a particular part of the brain. Assuming that the patient's history of aberrant behavior may have resulted from this abnormal increase in neuronal activity, what is the most likely site for the origin of the seizure activity?

○ (A) Nucleus accumbens
○ (B) Amygdala
○ (C) Septal nuclei
○ (D) Hippocampal complex
○ (E) Cingulate gyrus

12. A 75-year-old man, suspected of having Alzheimer disease, is referred to a neurologist. The primary symptom exhibited by this patient seems to be some loss of memory. The patient states "My memory seems to be shot. I sometimes find myself entering a part of the house, knowing that I must have gone there for some reason, but I can't remember what it was." Assuming that this patient's memory loss is due to the presence of neurofibrillary tangles and neuritic plaques, typically associated with Alzheimer disease, which of the following parts of the brain would most likely be involved?

○ (A) Subiculum
○ (B) Cingulate gyrus
○ (C) Amygdala
○ (D) Paracentral lobule
○ (E) Inferior parietal lobule

13. A 19-year-old man arrives in the emergency department from the site of an automobile collision. CT reveals a contusion injury to the uncus. In addition to the cortex of the uncus, which of the following parts of the limbic system is also most likely involved in this lesion?

○ (A) Prefrontal cortex
○ (B) Amygdaloid complex
○ (C) Hippocampal formation
○ (D) Cingulate gyrus
○ (E) Subcallosal area

Questions 14 and 15 are based on the following patient:

A 42-year-old homeless man is brought to the emergency department by the local authorities. The examination reveals an emaciated, unkempt, and intoxicated man. He has gaze palsies and generalized dysmetria. In response to specific questions he states that he used to be an automobile mechanic in Chicago, was married, and played college baseball. In response to questions about recent events he says he "can't remember" but says he "is a good friend of the mayor's wife and slept in the governor's house a few days ago."

14. In response to some questions this patient appears to be "making up" answers or stringing together unrelated or inappropriate facts. Which of the following most specifically identifies this type of response?

- ○ (A) Aphasia
- ○ (B) Aphonia
- ○ (C) Agnosia
- ○ (D) Confabulation
- ○ (E) Dysphagia

15. Taking all the deficits experienced by this man together, which of the following most likely represents his condition?

- ○ (A) Klüver-Bucy syndrome
- ○ (B) Wernicke aphasia
- ○ (C) Wernicke-Korsakoff syndrome
- ○ (D) Thalamic syndrome
- ○ (E) Parinaud syndrome

16. Which of the following fiber bundles represent the main efferent pathway of the subiculum and, to a lesser degree, the hippocampus?

- ○ (A) Stria terminalis
- ○ (B) Medial forebrain bundle
- ○ (C) Stria medullaris thalami
- ○ (D) Fornix
- ○ (E) Cingulum

ANSWERS

1. **(E)** The compulsion to explore the immediate environment is hypermetamorphosis. This patient may behave as if looking for something or some person and will repeatedly explore the same areas/objects. He/she will not know what he/she is looking for and may behave in a manic-depressive manner.
FN2e 501

2. **(B)** The compulsion of this patient to examine objects by placing them in his mouth is hyperorality. In addition to objects that should go into the mouth, such as food, a spoon, or a straw, the patient will place inappropriate items into his/her mouth, such as tree bark, nails, or a letter opener.
FN2e 501

3. **(D)** This patient experienced bilateral damage to the temporal lobes, including the uncus, amygdaloid complex, and rostral aspects of the hippocampal formation. An injury in this location may result in a constellation of deficits collectively called the Klüver-Bucy syndrome. This syndrome includes visual, auditory, and temporal agnosia; hyperphagia; hyperorality; hypersexuality; hypermetamorphosis; and amnesia, aphasia, or dementia. Such patients may also show placidity.
FN2e 501

4. **(C)** The stria terminalis is a relatively small bundle of axons that originate primarily from the corticomedial

nuclei of the amygdala. After a trajectory immediately adjacent to the caudate nucleus, the stria terminalis arches dorsally over the dorsal thalamus, to eventually lie in the groove separating the dorsal thalamus and the body of the caudate nucleus. The stria terminalis projects to a variety of hypothalamic nuclei.
FN2e 248, 501–502

5. **(B)** Fibers of the postcommissural fornix originate primarily from the subiculum of the hippocampal complex and not from the hippocampus proper (Ammon's horn). These fibers form the subiculum terminate in large part within the medial nucleus of the mammillary body.
FN2e 499

6. **(E)** The anterior choroidal artery originates from the internal carotid artery close to the origin of the posterior communicating artery. This artery courses in a caudolateral direction along the general route of the optic tract and along the medial aspect of the temporal lobe. In this position, branches of the anterior choroidal artery serve the optic tract, adjacent parts of the internal capsule and anterior (ventral) parts of the lenticular nucleus, the hippocampal formation, parts of the amygdaloid complex, and the choroid plexus in the temporal horn. The weakness of facial muscles is explained by the interruption of penetrating branches into the genu of the internal capsule.
FN2e 123–124, 496

7. **(B)** The complete circuit of Papez is usually described as beginning in the cortex of the cingulate gyrus. Axons from here then project directly or indirectly (via relays in the entorhinal cortex of the parahippocampal gyrus) to the subiculum of the hippocampal complex. Axons originating from the subiculum form the postcommissural bundle of the fornix and terminate in the medial nucleus of the mammillary body. The medial mammillary nucleus projects axons, via the mammillothalamic tract, to the anterior nucleus of the thalamus. The anterior nucleus of the thalamus then sends axons to the cingulate gyrus, thus completing the circuit.
FN2e 496, 499

8. **(B)** The primary function of the hippocampal formation is the processing of memory. Specifically, the hippocampal formation functions to convert immediate and short-term memories into long-term memories. People with lesions of the hippocampal formation have no trouble remembering events that occurred before their brain lesion. However, after the brain lesion, memories are limited to events occurring within the past few minutes and long-term memories cannot be formed.
FN2e 499, 500

9. **(E)** The Korsakoff syndrome is a condition related to thiamine deficiency and often occurs in individuals having chronic alcoholism due to poor diet. Neuronal degeneration is often seen in the mammillary bodies and sometimes in the dorsomedial nucleus of the thalamus and the hippocampal formation. The Korsakoff syndrome includes a failure of the conversion of short-term

memory into long-term memory. These patients improve with proper diet and supplemental thiamine.
FN2e 499, 500

10. **(C)** Bilateral lesions of the amygdaloid complex cause behavioral changes that are known as the Klüver-Bucy syndrome. Some of the deficits characterized by this syndrome include hypersexuality, hyperphagia, and hyperorality.
FN2e 501

11. **(B)** The amygdala contains an abundance of aversion centers. Seizure-induced activation of these aversion centers may elicit feelings of tremendous fear. A subject experiencing this fear may reflexively display violent, self-protective behavior.
FN2e 504

12. **(A)** Specific types of neural pathologic processes characterize Alzheimer disease, including neurofibrillary tangles and neuritic plaques. Early in the course of this disease, these processes are typically present within the subiculum and entorhinal cortices, where they adversely affect the processing of memory.
FN2e 500

13. **(B)** The amygdaloid complex lies immediately internal to the cortex of the uncus. Although not a part of the limbic "lobe," the amygdaloid complex is an important component of the limbic "system."
FN2e 494–496

14. **(D)** The stringing together of incorrect or patently unrelated facts in a reasonably fluent response is confabulation. In this patient's response, he slept somewhere, but not in the governor's home, and he may have a friend, but it is not likely to be the mayor's wife.
FN2e 500

15. **(C)** The Wernicke-Korsakoff syndrome includes memory deficits, confabulations, and motor deficits associated with degenerative changes in the cerebellum resulting from excessive alcohol consumption. Chronic alcoholics may present with this syndrome because of their poor diet accompanied by the toxic effects of alcohol on the brain.
FN2e 500

16. **(D)** The fornix originates from neurons located in the subiculum and the hippocampus. These axons form the fimbria of the hippocampus and then the various parts of the fornix (crus, body, and column; there is also a fibria on the crus of the fornix). They finally diverge into pre- and postcommissural portions at the level of the anterior commissure. The hippocampal commissure are those fornix fibers that cross the midline immediately inferior to the splenium of the corpus callosum.
FN2e 248, 497–499

CHAPTER 32

The Cerebral Cortex

1. A 61-year-old woman has a severe headache, confusion, and difficulty understanding the physician. When asked to write her name and address on a tablet, she is unable to write words that are recognizable even through she is not weak or paralyzed. Which of the following would best describe this inability to write legibly?

- ○ (A) Aphonia
- ○ (B) Agraphia
- ○ (C) Alexia
- ○ (D) Agnosia
- ○ (E) Ageusia

2. During a brain cutting, the neuropathologist observes what appears to be a delicate line in the cerebral cortex bordering on the calcarine sulcus in a 63-year-old man who died of a brain tumor. Which of the following would most likely explain this observation?

- ○ (A) Stria terminalis
- ○ (B) Molecular layer
- ○ (C) Inner band of Baillarger
- ○ (D) Striae medullares
- ○ (E) Stria of Gennari

3. An 17-year-old boy is brought to the emergency department after an automobile collision. The neurologic examination reveals severe damage to the spinal cord at C4-C5. Which of the following layers of the cerebral cortex contain the large pyramid- shaped neurons whose axons (as corticospinal fibers) are damaged in this patient?

- ○ (A) Layer I
- ○ (B) Layer II
- ○ (C) Layer III
- ○ (D) Layer IV
- ○ (E) Layer V
- ○ (F) Layer VI

Questions 4 to 6 are related to the following patient:

A 54-year-old hypertensive man is brought to the emergency department by his family. He appears confused and initially seems uncooperative. A careful neurologic examination reveals that he has difficulty reading and understanding instructions from the attending physician. When he speaks, the sentences are a tangle of unrelated, inappropriate, or apparently made-up words. The patient appears to be unaware of the fact that, when he speaks, he makes no sense.

4. Based on the information gathered during the neurologic examination, this patient is most likely suffering from which of the following?

- ○ (A) Broca aphasia
- ○ (B) Brown-Séquard syndrome
- ○ (C) Parinaud syndrome
- ○ (D) Benedikt syndrome
- ○ (E) Wernicke aphasia

5. The CT of this patient reveals a hemorrhagic lesion in the cerebral cortex. Which of the following represents the most likely location of this lesion?

- ○ (A) Inferior frontal gyrus
- ○ (B) Superior parietal lobule
- ○ (C) Inferior parietal lobule
- ○ (D) Precentral gyrus
- ○ (E) Cingulate gyrus

6. The CT reveals a hemorrhagic infarction in the territory of the middle cerebral artery. Based on the deficits experienced by this patient, which of the following M_4 branches are most likely compromised?

- ○ (A) Orbitofrontal and polar temporal
- ○ (B) Parietal, angular, and posterior temporal

○ (C) Anterior temporal
○ (D) Central and precentral
○ (E) Central, parietal, and precentral

7. Which of the following layers of the cerebral cortex contain neuron cell bodies whose axons project, as corticocortical fibers, to the ipsilateral and the contralateral cerebral cortex?

○ (A) Layers I and II
○ (B) Layers III and V
○ (C) Layers V and VI
○ (D) Layers III and VI
○ (E) Layers II and IV

8. A 72-year-old man is brought to his physician's office by his wife. Her major concern is, beginning several days ago, her husband talked, but he made "absolutely no sense at all." The physician asks the man where he lives and the patient replies, "I green tree at brick and the cat live wire tangle." Which of the following would most correctly describe this pattern of speech?

○ (A) Aphonic
○ (B) Alexic
○ (C) Paraphasic
○ (D) Aphrodisic
○ (E) Apraxic

9. A small tumor is removed from the cerebral cortex of a 12-year-old girl. When this tumor is examined, the neuropathologist identifies many large pyramidal cells and, with a special stain, some large basket cells whose processes extend into all layers of the cortex. Considering these two types of cells together would suggest that this lesion involved which of the following layers of the cerebral cortex?

○ (A) Layer I
○ (B) Layers I and II
○ (C) Layer III
○ (D) Layer IV
○ (E) Layer V

10. The MRI of a 57-year-old, right-handed woman reveals a lesion in the lateral aspect of the left hemisphere involving the inferior frontal gyrus, lateral portions of the pre- and postcentral gyri, the inferior parietal lobule, and portions of the adjacent superior temporal gyrus. Which of the following is the most prominent deficit in this patient?

○ (A) Blindness in the left eye
○ (B) Language comprehension and use
○ (C) Right-sided paralysis of the lower extremity
○ (D) Paralysis of all eye movement
○ (E) Aphonia

Questions 11 and 12 are based on the following patient:

A 61-year-old man is brought to the emergency department after a fainting spell at work. He is aphasic, his tongue deviates to the right when protruded, and he has an obvious weakness of the right upper extremity. CT reveals blood within some gyri of the cortex and in the sulci between these hemorrhagic gyri. Several days after this event the muscle weakness persists and the patient answers most questions with single short words such as "yes," "thanks," and "eat." His speech is slow, and words are poorly enunciated.

11. Based on the combined deficits seen in this patient, which of the following is the likely location of this lesion?

○ (A) Right frontal lobe
○ (B) Left frontal lobe
○ (C) Right parietal lobe
○ (D) Left parietal lobe
○ (E) Left cingulate gyrus

12. Which of the following most correctly designates the language deficits experienced by this patient?

○ (A) Nonfluent aphasia
○ (B) Aphonia
○ (C) Fluent aphasia
○ (D) Agraphia
○ (E) Areflexia

13. A 67-year-old woman suffered a cerebral infarction 3 weeks ago. She frequently forgets to put her left arm into the sleeve of her robe or blouse, always leaves food on the left side of her plate, and frequently bumps into things on her left side. She has no language disorders or paralysis of speech. Which of the following represents the most likely site of cerebral cortical damage in this patient?

○ (A) Motor cortex in the right hemisphere
○ (B) Parietal association cortex in the left hemisphere
○ (C) Parietal association cortex in the right hemisphere
○ (D) Inferior temporal cortex in the left hemisphere
○ (E) Inferior temporal cortex in the right hemisphere

Questions 14 and 15 are based on the following patient:

A 28-year-old man is brought to the emergency department. The paramedics explain that the man was shot in the head during the robbery of a convenience store. The man survives, but CT reveals significant damage in the regions of the brain shown in Figure 32–1.

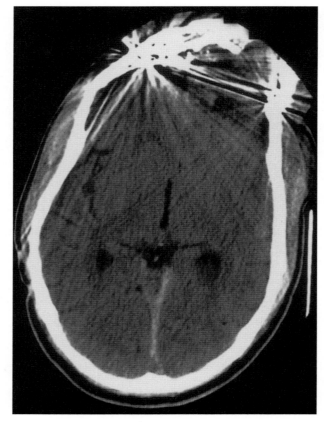

Figure 32-1

(C) Left superior temporal, supramarginal, and angular gyri
(D) Right inferior frontal gyrus
(E) Right superior temporal, supramarginal, and angular gyri

17.   A 67-year-old man suffered a stroke several months ago. He is asked by an occupational therapist to assemble a small block construction. The patient has a model to copy, but even his best effort (shown below) is not successful.

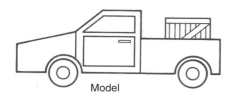

Model

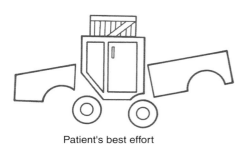

Patient's best effort

Figure 32-2

Which of the following other symptoms is this patient also most likely to have?

(A) Confusion in recognizing familiar faces
(B) Inability to draw an accurate floor plan of his home
(C) Difficulty in reading fine print
(D) Paralysis of the right upper and lower extremities
(E) Difficulty in comprehending spoken language

14.   Which of the following is most likely to be observed in this patient as he recovers?

(A) Bilateral blindness
(B) Broca aphasia
(C) Wernicke aphasia
(D) High degree of distractibility and an inability to plan and carry out any complicated activity
(E) Loss of long-term memory

15.   Which of the following signs or symptoms would also most likely be observed in this man?

(A) Bilateral loss of pain and temperature sensation
(B) Visual hallucinations
(C) Inability to recognize faces of close friends
(D) Increased level of stubbornness
(E) Wernicke aphasia

16.   A 57-year-old man suffered a cerebral infarction 3 days ago. When the neurology resident walks into his hospital room and asks how he is doing, the man smiles and says, "The house was dried for sun went gone to bread but don't in the spring?" Damage in which of the following brain areas would most likely result in this characteristic sign?

(A) Bilateral prefrontal lobe
(B) Left inferior frontal gyrus

Questions 18 through 20 are based on the following patient:

A 52-year-old right-handed executive is brought in to the emergency department after suffering a severe headache and falling to the floor in the middle of a business meeting. He is conscious, but in emotional distress. When asked to describe what happened, he obviously understands the question but is only able to say, with considerable effort, "Fall down." His speech is labored and he uses very few words, but he is able to give generally appropriate answers.

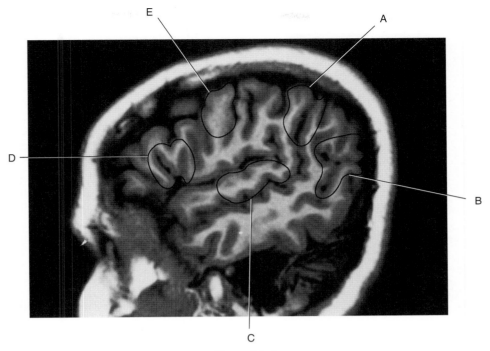

Figure 32–3

18. Which of the outlined areas above, each representing the site of a potential lesion in the left hemisphere, is the most likely location of the infarction in this patient? (   )

19. Which of the following signs would also most likely be observed in this man?

○ (A) Left homonymous hemianopia
○ (B) Weakness in the left face and upper extremity
○ (C) Weakness in the right face and upper extremity
○ (D) Loss of pain and temperature sensation in the left face and upper extremity
○ (E) Loss of pain and temperature sensation in the right face and upper extremity

20. Which of the following vessels represents the most likely source of blood supply to the infarcted area of the cortex in this man?

○ (A) Anterior cerebral artery, A_2 division
○ (B) Middle cerebral artery, M_2 division
○ (C) Middle cerebral artery, M_4 division
○ (D) Posterior cerebral artery, P_3 division
○ (E) Lenticulostriate arteries

21. Which of the following neuron types represent the predominant output neuron of the cerebral cortex?

○ (A) Spiny stellate cell
○ (B) Basket cell
○ (C) Chandelier cell
○ (D) Pyramidal cell
○ (E) Spiny stellate cell

22. Which of the following Brodmann number(s) is associated with the primary auditory cortex?

○ (A) 3, 1, 2
○ (B) 4
○ (C) 7
○ (D) 17
○ (E) 41

23. A 52-year-old man complains to his physician of persistent headache. MRI reveals a convexity meningioma impinging on the prefrontal association cortex. Which of the following thalamic nuclei projects primarily to this association cortex?

○ (A) Anterior
○ (B) Ventral lateral
○ (C) Dorsomedial
○ (D) Ventral posterolateral
○ (E) Pulvinar

Questions 24 and 25 are based on the following patient:

A 64-year-old man had a hemorrhage into his brain 2 months ago. He is now living at home and visiting an occupational therapist twice a week. His coordination is good and he can hold a pencil, write legibly, and copy simple drawings. However, he is unable to draw an accurate floor plan of his apartment. He gets the rooms in the wrong places and some walls are missing. When he draws the numbers on a clock face, all the numbers end up in the right half of the clock face.

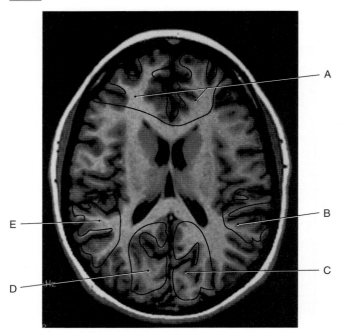

Figure 32–4

24. Which of the outlined cortical regions at left, each representing the site of a possible lesion, is the most likely location of cortical damage in this patient? See Figure 32–4. (   )

25. Which of the following arteries is the most likely vessel from which the hemorrhage occurred in this patient?

○ (A) Anterior cerebral artery, A_2 division
○ (B) Middle cerebral artery, M_2 division
○ (C) Middle cerebral artery, M_4 division
○ (D) Posterior cerebral artery, P_3 division
○ (E) Lenticulostriate arteries

26. Which of the following labeled areas of the cerebral cortex is composed of heterotypical granular cortex? See Figure 32–5. (   )

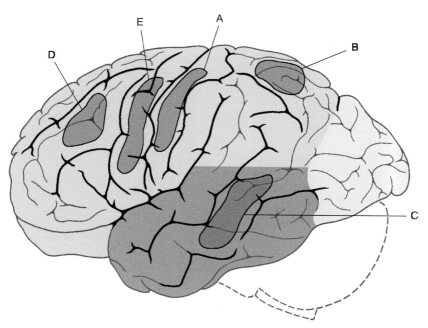

Figure 32–5

27. Which of the following labeled areas of the cerebral cortex contains an especially prominent layer V characteristically containing large pyramidal cells? See Figure 32–6. (   )

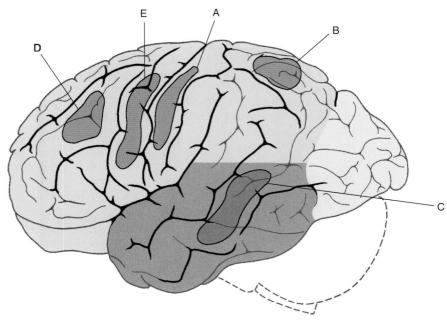

Figure 32–6

ANSWERS

1. **(B)** Agraphia is seen in patients with lesions in the area of the inferior parietal lobule (Wernicke aphasia). This results from an inability of the cortex to process input and to create the sequence of motor events necessary to write an intelligible sentence. The inability to write is not caused by muscle weakness.
FN2e 517

2. **(E)** The primary visual cortex bordering on the edges of the calcarine sulcus contains a distinct horizontally oriented (parallel to the surface of the cortex) lamina of fibers in layer IV. This lamina of fibers is the stria of Gennari (also called the outer band of Baillarger), and it is characteristic of the primary visual cortex.
FN2e 507

3. **(E)** Corticospinal fibers originate from pyramid-shaped cells located in layer V of the cerebral cortex. These fibers originate primarily from motor areas but may also arise from areas of the parietal lobe.
FN2e 389, 508–509

4. **(E)** The combination of deficits experienced by this patient clearly suggests a lesion in the area of the inferior parietal lobule of the dominant (usually the left) hemisphere. This combination of deficits is characteristic of a patient with Wernicke (fluent or receptive) aphasia.
FN2e 516–517

5. **(C)** The hemorrhage in the cerebral cortex in this patient is located in the area of the angular and supra-marginal gyri; collectively, these form the inferior parietal lobule.
FN2e 238–239, 516–517

6. **(B)** The blood vessels that serve the inferior parietal lobule are M₄ branches. These are the parietal and angular branches of the middle cerebral artery, and it is most likely that posterior temporal branches would also serve the general area of the angular gyrus.
FN2e 126, 516–517

7. **(D)** Corticocortical fibers may project from one cortical area to another on the ipsilateral side (association fibers) or to some portion of the contralateral side via the corpus callosum (callosal fibers). These fibers originate mainly from layers III and VI, although some cortico-cortical fibers also arise in layer V.
FN2e 508–509

8. **(C)** This patient has the ability to speak. The words may actually be clear and melodic, but the resultant sentences are a tangle that make no sense. This is paraphasic speech. It is seen in patients with Wernicke aphasia.
FN2e 517

9. **(E)** While pyramidal cells are found in several layers of the cerebral cortex, basket cells are located almost exclusively in layers III and V. The combination of large pyramidal cells and basket cells specifies layer V of the cerebral cortex.
FN2e 509

10. **(B)** This patient has a lesion that involves both the Broca area, as well as the Wernicke area, in the dominant hemisphere. This patient will exhibit global aphasia, reflecting the extensive cortical areas involved, and will have profound language deficits.
FN2e 518

11. **(B)** The weakness of the right upper extremity, as well as the aphasia, indicates a lesion in the left

frontal lobe (the dominant hemisphere). It involves the inferior frontal gyrus and the adjacent portion of the precentral gyrus, the latter representing part of the motor cortex.
FN2e 516–518

12. **(A)** The inability of this patient to speak at the initial examination and his difficulty in speaking at a subsequent examination are characteristic of a patient with a lesion of the inferior frontal gyrus in the dominant hemisphere. This is nonfluent aphasia, also called expressive aphasia or Broca aphasia.
FN2e 516

13. **(C)** Contralateral neglect and contralateral inattention are characteristic symptoms of right posterior parietal lobe damage. The patient basically "ignores" the left side of the body or things in the left side of his/her environment.
FN2e 518

14. **(D)** Injury to the prefrontal cortex produces a set of symptoms that include difficulty in carrying out a complex, multi-step activity, such as giving a dinner party. Patients with prefrontal damage tend to be distracted from an activity by any slight competing stimulus.
FN2e 518–520

15. **(D)** Even though a person with prefrontal lobe damage is easily distracted sometimes, he or she is not receptive to suggestions from others and may be extremely obstinate in sticking to a course of action, even when there are obvious problems with the plan.
FN2e 518–520

16. **(E)** The paraphasic speech (sometimes called "word salad") exhibited by this patient is typical of Wernicke aphasia. The affected area is called the Wernicke area. This area of cerebral cortex includes the angular and supramarginal gyri (the inferior parietal lobule) and immediately adjacent parts of the superior temporal gyrus.
FN2e 516–519

17. **(B)** Constructional apraxia (difficulty in building a block structure) is a common symptom of damage in the right posterior parietal lobe. A related symptom involves difficulty in depicting spatial relationships in a drawing or a map.
FN2e 518–519

18. **(D)** The patient exhibits classic signs of Broca

aphasia. The Broca area includes the pars orbitalis and pars triangularis of the inferior frontal gyrus.
FN2e 516–518

19. **(C)** The Broca area is adjacent to the face and hand representation of the precentral gyrus. Infarction, tumor, or trauma that affects the Broca area is likely to also affect the face and hand areas of the primary motor cortex.
FN2e 389–391, 516–518

20. **(C)** Branches of the M_4 division supply the Broca area. The specific branches of M_4 that serve the Broca area are usually the orbitofrontal and precentral arteries.
FN2e 242–243, 390, 514–515

21. **(D)** Virtually all output signals from the cerebral cortex to other areas of the cerebral cortex, the basal ganglia, the brainstem, and the spinal cord are carried by axons that arise from pyramidal cells.
FN2e 508–510

22. **(E)** Primary auditory cortex is located in the transverse gyri of Heschl, designated as area 41 in the commonly used classification system of Brodmann. The medial geniculate nucleus is the primary source of input of the primary auditory cortex.
FN2e 336–337, 512, 514

23. **(C)** The dorsomedial nucleus is the primary source of thalamocortical input to prefrontal association cortex.
FN2e 223–227, 513–514

24. **(E)** These symptoms are associated with damage in parietal association cortex in the nondominant (right) hemisphere. In about 95% of the general population the left hemisphere is the dominant hemisphere.
FN2e 518–519

25. **(C)** Branches of the M_4 division supply parietal association cortex. The postcentral, parietal, and angular arteries are the M_4 branches that serve this part of the lateral aspect of the hemisphere.
FN2e 126, 242, 390, 514–515

26. **(A)** Heterotypical agranular cortex has a thicker than average layer IV. This is a feature characteristic of primary sensory areas of the cortex including the postcentral gyrus.
FN2e 510–511

27. **(E)** Of the cortical areas indicated, the precentral gyrus (primary motor cortex) has the thickest layer V.
FN2e 510–511

CHAPTER 33

The Neurologic Examination

1. A neurologist performs an examination on a 17-year-old boy in preparation for joining a sports team. During this neurologic examination, which of the following cranial nerves (CN) may not be tested?

- ○ (A) Olfactory, CN I
- ○ (B) Oculomotor, CN III
- ○ (C) Abducens, CN VI
- ○ (D) Vagus, CN X
- ○ (E) Spinal accessory, CN XI

2. During a routine neurologic examination of a 51-year-old man, the physician detects dysarthria. Testing of which of the following cranial nerves (CNs) might be instructive regarding the location of the lesion that results in this deficit?

- ○ (A) CNs III, IV, and VI
- ○ (B) CNs V and XI only
- ○ (C) CN VII only
- ○ (D) CNs VII, IX, X, and XII
- ○ (E) CNs IX and XII only

3. In the course of a routine physical examination of a 22-year-old man, the physician touches a wisp of cotton to the man's cornea. In response, the man blinks. The afferent and efferent limbs of this reflex are formed, respectively, by peripheral branches of which of the following cranial nerves (CNs)?

- ○ (A) CNs III and V
- ○ (B) CNs V and VII
- ○ (C) CNs V and VI
- ○ (D) CN V for both limbs
- ○ (E) CNs VII and XII

4. A 16-year-old girl is having a physical examination as part of her application to join a sports team. When the physician looks at the girl's face she is slightly "cross-eyed"; the right eye is rotated slightly inward. This would suggest a weakness of which of the following muscles of the eye?

- ○ (A) Tarsal
- ○ (B) Left medial rectus
- ○ (C) Right medial rectus
- ○ (D) Right superior oblique
- ○ (E) Right lateral rectus

5. A 49-year-old man is brought to the emergency department from the site of an automobile collision. During the neurologic examination, the physician notes that muscle strength is "1/5" in the lower extremities. This would most likely indicate which of the following?

- ○ (A) Complete muscle paralysis
- ○ (B) Minimal contractions; palpation reveals muscle contraction but no movement
- ○ (C) Muscle contracts but patient is unable to lift lower extremity
- ○ (D) Patient can lift lower extremity
- ○ (E) Patient can overcome resistance of physician

6. A 16-year-old boy is brought to the emergency department from the site of a motorcycle crash. The motor examination reveals a profound weakness in both lower extremities. Which of the following most specifically describes this boy's condition?

- ○ (A) Quadriplegia
- ○ (B) Hemiplegia
- ○ (C) Paraplegia
- ○ (D) Monoplegia
- ○ (E) Alternating hemiplegia

7. During the routine neurologic examination of a 31-year-old woman, the physician asks the woman to slide her right heel down her left shin beginning at the knee. The woman is able to initiate the movement and she has the muscle strength to complete the movement. However, she is unable to keep the heel precisely aligned with the shin during the movement. This abnormal movement is most likely a consequence of dysfunction of which of the following structures?

- ○ (A) Corticospinal tract
- ○ (B) Basal nuclei
- ○ (C) Anterolateral system
- ○ (D) Reticulospinal tracts
- ○ (E) Cerebellum

8. A 68-year-old man is not able to perceive vibration when a tuning fork (128 Hz) is applied to the medial malleolus on his left leg. The integrity of which of the following structures is tested by this part of the neurologic examination?

- ○ (A) Corticospinal fibers
- ○ (B) Posterior columns
- ○ (C) Anterolateral system
- ○ (D) Reticulospinal and vestibulospinal fibers
- ○ (E) Raphespinal fibers

9. Which of the following is an abnormal reflex or sign in an adult with a lesion in the CNS but may be seen in a normal infant?

- ○ (A) Gag reflex
- ○ (B) Corneal reflex
- ○ (C) Bárány sign
- ○ (D) Babinski sign
- ○ (E) Romberg sign

10. A physician conducts a neurologic examination on a 49-year-old man who has headaches. The physician notices that the margins of the optic discs are blurred. The disc and associated blood vessels appear elevated, and there are small hemorrhages at and around the disc margins. Which of the following most specifically describes this condition in this man?

- ○ (A) Optic atrophy
- ○ (B) Papilledema
- ○ (C) Glaucoma
- ○ (D) Miosis
- ○ (E) Coloboma

11. During a routine neurologic examination of a 32-year-old woman, the physician notices that the woman's left eye will not abduct on attempted gaze to the left. In addition to the eye movement disorder, which of the following would this woman also most likely have?

- ○ (A) Glaucoma
- ○ (B) Ptosis
- ○ (C) Diplopia
- ○ (D) Papilledema
- ○ (E) Miosis

12. In the course of a routine neurologic examination of a 61-year-old woman, the physician notices the patient's tongue deviates to the left on attempted protrusion. Which of the following muscles is not functioning properly when the physician asks the woman to protrude her tongue?

- ○ (A) Left genioglossus
- ○ (B) Left styloglossus
- ○ (C) Left hyoglossus
- ○ (D) Right styloglossus
- ○ (E) Right genioglossus

13. The neurologic examination of a 17-year-old boy involved in a motorcycle crash reveals that he is unable to turn his head to the right against resistance. This finding would suggest damage to which of the following cranial nerves?

- ○ (A) Right accessory
- ○ (B) Left accessory
- ○ (C) Right vagus
- ○ (D) Right seventh
- ○ (E) Left seventh

14. In the example shown here the integrity of which muscle stretch reflex is being examined?

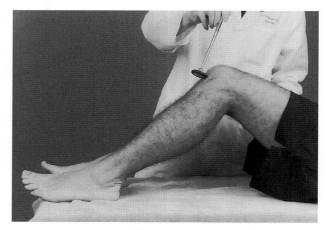

Figure 33–1

- ○ (A) Gastrocnemius
- ○ (B) Biceps femoris
- ○ (C) Tibialis anterior
- ○ (D) Quadriceps femoris
- ○ (E) Adductor magnus

15. The maneuver shown here is most likely a test for which of the following?

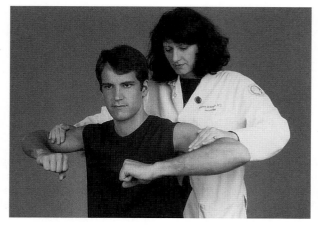

Figure 33–2

- ○ (A) Triceps muscles stretch reflex
- ○ (B) Muscle strength
- ○ (C) Limb proprioception
- ○ (D) Pain and thermal sense
- ○ (E) Asterixis

16. During the neurologic examination of a 22-year-old woman, the physician notices that the biceps muscle stretch reflex is barely discernible. Which of the following most specifically describes this observation?

- ○ (A) Hyperreflexia
- ○ (B) Areflexia
- ○ (C) Hyporeflexia
- ○ (D) Hypometria
- ○ (E) Hypermetria

17. During the neurologic examination of a 61-year-old man, the physician asks the man to slide his left heel down his right shin beginning just distal to the knee. The man is not able to initiate the movement, although muscle strength appears to be normal. Although slow to initiate, the finger-to-nose test is normal. The inability of the man to initiate the heel-to-shin movement is most likely a consequence of dysfunction of which of the following?

- ○ (A) Corticospinal tract
- ○ (B) Basal nuclei
- ○ (C) Anterolateral system
- ○ (D) Reticulospinal tracts
- ○ (E) Cerebellum

18. To test the gag reflex in a 72-year-old woman experiencing difficulty in swallowing, the physician would most likely do which of the following?

- ○ (A) Touch the hard palate with a tongue depressor
- ○ (B) Apply a noxious substance to the anterior two thirds of the tongue
- ○ (C) Touch the upper or lower lip, or the angle of the mouth, with a pin
- ○ (D) Touch the posterior pharyngeal wall with a tongue depressor
- ○ (E) Touch the inner surface of the cheek with a pin

19. During a routine neurologic examination, the physician asks a 21-year-old man to open his mouth and say "Ah." The man's uvula elevates slightly but stays on the midline. The integrity of which of the following is tested by this maneuver?

- ○ (A) Hypoglossal nerve
- ○ (B) Accessory nerve
- ○ (C) Vagus nerve
- ○ (D) Glossopharyngeal nerve
- ○ (E) Facial nerve

20. A 16-year-old girl is brought to the internist's office by her mother. The girl complains that her voice is hoarse, but the physical examination indicates that she does not have a sore, or infected throat, or any type of sinus condition. A lesion involving peripheral branches of which of the following cranial nerves (CN) would most likely explain this girl's hoarse voice?

- ○ (A) CN XII
- ○ (B) CN XI
- ○ (C) CN X
- ○ (D) CN IX
- ○ (E) CN VII

21. During the routine neurologic examination of a 22-year-old man, a test is conducted to compare bone and air conduction of sound. First, a 256-Hz tuning fork is applied to the mastoid process and, when sound is no longer perceived in that ear, the tuning fork is brought to the external auditory meatus of the same ear.

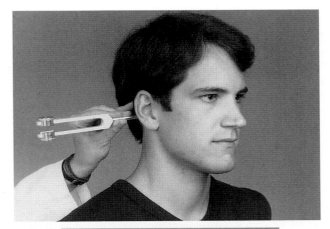

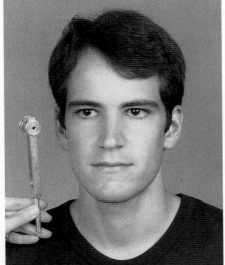

Figure 33–3

This procedure is known as what?

- ○ (A) Weber test
- ○ (B) Rorschach test
- ○ (C) Pap test
- ○ (D) Rinne test
- ○ (E) Bárány caloric test

22.   Sensory testing of the face, cornea, and oral cavity provides the greatest amount of information concerning the integrity of which of the following nerves?

- ○ (A)   Oculomotor
- ○ (B)   Facial
- ○ (C)   Glossopharyngeal
- ○ (D)   Vagus
- ○ (E)   Trigeminal

23.   Which of the following maneuvers will activate the afferent limb of the jaw jerk reflex?

- ○ (A)   Pin applied to lower lip
- ○ (B)   Gentle tap on chin
- ○ (C)   Gentle tap on frontalis muscle
- ○ (D)   Pin applied to tongue
- ○ (E)   Application of noxious substance to tongue

24.   During a routine neurologic examination of a 27-year-old woman, the physician discovers what is called a "blind spot" (also called a physiologic scotoma) in the visual field of this patient. Which of the following most specifically explains this observation?

- ○ (A)   A small scotoma resultant to a retinal detachment
- ○ (B)   Occlusion of the central retinal artery
- ○ (C)   A visual defect resulting from an increase in intracranial pressure transmitted along the subarachnoid space surrounding the optic nerve
- ○ (D)   A spot in the visual field corresponding to the optic disc where there are no rods, cones, or ganglion cells
- ○ (E)   A visual defect corresponding to a lesion of the crossing fibers of the optic chiasm

25.   Which of the following is most likely being tested in the examination of the 22-year-old man shown here?

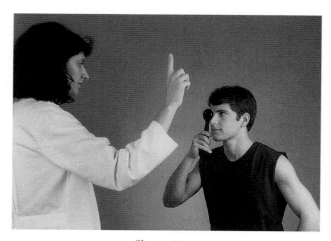

Figure 33–4

- ○ (A)   Pupillary light reflex
- ○ (B)   Eye movements
- ○ (C)   Visual fields by confrontation
- ○ (D)   Corneal reflex
- ○ (E)   Configuration of the optic disc

26.   During a neurologic examination of a 69-year-old man, the physician tests lateral gaze by moving his finger back and forth 15 to 20 inches in front of the man's eyes. When the physician moves his finger to the patient's left, he is testing the integrity of which of the following?

- ○ (A)   Left lateral rectus motor neurons (CN VII), right superior oblique motor neurons (CN IV)
- ○ (B)   Right lateral rectus motor neurons (CN VI), left medial rectus motor neurons (CN III)
- ○ (C)   Left lateral rectus motor neurons (CN VI), right inferior oblique motor neurons (CN III)
- ○ (D)   Right medial rectus motor neurons (CN III), left medial rectus motor neurons (CN III)
- ○ (E)   Left lateral rectus motor neurons (CN VI), right medial rectus motor neurons (CN III)

27.   During the neurologic examination of a 49-year-old man, the physician asks the man to slide his right heel down his left shin starting at the knee. Although palpation reveals obvious and immediate contractions of the muscles of the hip and thigh, the man is unable to elevate the lower extremity and to approximate the heel to the shin. The remainder of the examination reveals no tremor, nystagmus, or other abnormal movements. The inability to perform this movement is most likely a consequence of dysfunction of which of the following structures?

- ○ (A)   Corticospinal tract
- ○ (B)   Basal nuclei
- ○ (C)   Anterolateral system
- ○ (D)   Reticulospinal tracts
- ○ (E)   Cerebellum

ANSWERS

1.   **(A)** The olfactory nerve is not routinely tested during the neurologic examination. This is primarily because the function of this nerve is generally compromised by sinus disease or smoking in many individuals. A decrease in the patient's ability to perceive odors is not always indicative of a neurologic disorder.
FN2e 522

2.   **(D)** Dysarthria is a disorder of speech. It may result from a number of different causes, including lesions of cranial nerves or lesions within the brain. Lesions involving CN VII (muscles of facial expression), CNs IX and X (pharyngeal and laryngeal muscles), and CN XII (movements of the tongue) may cause dysarthria. Patients with lesions of the internal capsule may experience dysarthria from damage to corticonuclear (corticobulbar) fibers that traverse the internal capsule.
FN2e 522

3.   **(B)** The afferent limb of the corneal reflex travels via the ophthalmic division of the trigeminal nerve. The cell bodies of origin for these fibers are in the ipsilateral trigeminal ganglion. These primary sensory trigeminal

fibers terminate in the spinal trigeminal nucleus (pars caudalis). Collaterals of trigeminothalamic fibers terminate on motor neurons of the facial nucleus, this being the origin of the efferent limb of the reflex.
FN2e 213–215, 527

4. **(E)** Inward (medial) rotation of the right eye in this girl relates to weakness of the lateral rectus muscle and/or possible damage to the root of the abducens nerve on the right. The eye is rotated slightly medially owing to the unopposed action of the medial rectus muscle. If asked to look to the right, the girl's right eye would not abduct.
FN2e 212–213, 527

5. **(B)** The degree of muscle strength is graded 0 to 5: 0/5 is complete paralysis, 5/5 is normal muscle strength, and 3/5 is the ability to hold the limb against gravity. A 1/5 indicates that there are very minor muscle contractions that the physician can feel but there is no effective movement. The muscle contraction is palpable and may be visible but does not result in a productive movement.
FN2e 532

6. **(C)** A motor deficit of both lower extremities is paraplegia. This is usually accompanied by sensory deficits, such as a loss of pain and thermal sensations, and of proprioception, discriminative touch, and vibratory sense. Quadriplegia refers to deficits in both upper and both lower extremities, hemiplegia to upper and lower extremities on one side, and monoplegia to one extremity. Monoplegia is usually the result of a plexus lesion or proximal peripheral nerve lesion.
FN2e 533

7. **(E)** The heel-shin maneuver is an important part of the neurologic examination and may be used to test more than one system. In this situation, the woman is able to initiate the movement and has the muscle strength to perform the movement. Her inability to perform the movement, specifically the fact that her heel wobbles and is not able to be held on the shin, is limb ataxia. This is indicative of a lesion in the cerebellum that would involve cortex as well as more lateral portions of the cerebellar nuclei.
FN2e 441–442, 534–536

8. **(B)** Vibratory sense is conveyed by fibers in the posterior columns. For the lower extremities, these fibers have their cell bodies of origin in the ipsilateral posterior root ganglia and their central processes form the gracile fasciculus. An inability to perceive vibration may indicate a peripheral neuropathy or damage to fibers in the posterior columns.
FN2e 536–537

9. **(D)** The Babinski sign is dorsiflexion of the great toe in response to stroking along the lateral border of the sole of the foot. While indicative of some type of abnormal process in an adult, the Babinski sign can be elicited in a normal infant. This is most likely caused by incomplete myelination of the CNS in the very young.
FN2e 533

10. **(B)** Swelling of the optic disc, with venous engorgement and peripapillary hemorrhages, is called papilledema. The most common cause of papilledema is an increase in intracranial pressure.
FN2e 526

11. **(C)** A weakness of any of the extraocular muscles will result in varying degrees of diplopia (double vision). As a matter of fact, the primary complaint of the patient will be that he/she sees double when looking in the direction of paralyzed recti muscles. Paralysis of the oblique muscles results in double vision when looking in the direction opposite the paralyzed muscle. The patient may have other deficits, but diplopia will be the most obvious symptom.
FN2e 216–217, 526

12. **(A)** Deviation of the tongue to the left on attempted protrusion is caused by muscle weakness on that side. Protrusion of the tongue is mediated through the action of the genioglossus muscle. Consequently, if the left genioglossus muscle is weak or paralyzed, the action of the healthy right genioglossus muscle will pull the tongue to the left.
FN2e 396–398, 530

13. **(B)** The accessory nerve innervates the trapezius muscle and the sternocleidomastoid muscle. Injury to this nerve will result in drooping of the shoulder on the side of the lesion and an inability to rotate the head to the side opposite the lesion. In this boy, an inability to rotate the head to the right is indicative of damage to the left accessory nerve.
FN2e 203–206, 530

14. **(B)** Tapping the patellar tendon results in stretch of the muscle spindles in the quadriceps femoris muscle, which actually consists of four parts: the rectus femoris, vastus medialis, vastus intermedius, and vastus lateralis. In response to the patellar tendon tap, these muscles contract and the leg moves.
FN2e 533–534

15. **(B)** Elevating the arms against resistance is one component of the test for general muscle strength. Different muscle groups of the upper and lower extremities can be used (e.g., triceps, quadriceps).
FN2e 531–533

16. **(C)** A muscle stretch reflex that is significantly decreased in intensity or strength is hyporeflexia. Hyperreflexia refers to an excessively brisk reflex and areflexia to the absence of a reflex.
FN2e 533

17. **(B)** In this situation, muscle strength appears to be normal, indicating that the corticospinal tract is most likely functioning properly. The normal finger-to-nose test suggests that the cerebellum is not likely to be involved in the lesion. However, the fact that the man has significant difficulty initiating the movement (bradykinesia) indicates that the basal nuclei are involved in a lesion or in a neurodegenerative process.
FN2e 415–416, 530, 533

18. **(D)** Touching the posterior pharyngeal wall excites the afferent limb of the gag reflex. The efferent limb

travels on fibers of the glossopharyngeal nerve to the stylopharyngeus muscles.
FN2e 530

19. **(C)** The muscles of the uvula are innervated by branches of the vagus nerve (CN X). A lesion involving the vagus nerve results in a deviation of the uvula away from the side of the lesion, owing to the action of muscles on the healthy side.
FN2e 398, 530

20. **(C)** The vocalis muscle is innervated by the recurrent laryngeal branch of the vagus nerve. The motor neurons for these fibers are found in the ipsilateral nucleus ambiguus. Interruption of this pathway results in a hoarse, gravely voice.
FN2e 530

21. **(D)** The Rinne test compares bone conduction versus air conduction in the same ear. In the normal individual, the bone conduction of sound disappears first, but when the tuning fork is brought to the external auditory meatus, the patient perceives sound.
FN2e 529–530

22. **(E)** General sensation, such as pain and thermal sense, from the face, oral cavity, and cornea is transmitted over sensory branches of the trigeminal nerve. The cell bodies of origin for these primary sensory fibers are located in the ipsilateral trigeminal ganglion. The central processes of these pain and thermal sense fibers terminate primarily in the spinal trigeminal nucleus, pars caudalis.
FN2e 527

23. **(B)** A gentle tap on the chin activates the muscle spindles in the masseter muscles, which, in turn, excite motor neurons in the trigeminal motor nucleus, which innervate the masseter muscle. This is a cranial example of a muscle stretch reflex.
FN2e 527

24. **(D)** The "blind spot" is actually a physiologic scotoma (a naturally occurring scotoma) within the temporal visual field that corresponds to the position of the optic disc that is located in the nasal half of the retina. The blind spot is located at about 12 degrees lateral (temporal) to the center of the visual field; this center corresponds to the position of the fovea. Nothing is seen in the blind spot because it lacks rods, cones, and ganglion cells.
FN2e 524–525

25. **(C)** The physician is testing the patient's visual fields by confrontation. This is the easiest and most common method used to test visual fields at bedside or in the clinic. This is a fast and reliable way to test all quadrants of the visual fields.
FN2e 524–525

26. **(E)** Testing lateral gaze, by moving a finger back and forth in front of the patient, tests the abducens nerve (CN VI) and portions of the oculomotor nerve (CN III). Movement to the left tests the integrity of motor neurons in the nucleus of CN VI (or the abducens nerve) on the left side and the medial rectus motor neurons in the nucleus of CN III on the right side. Interneurons in the left abducens nucleus communicate with medial rectus motor neurons in the oculomotor nucleus on the right side via the medial longitudinal fasciculus.
FN2e 452–454, 526–527

27. **(A)** In this case, the man lacks the strength to elevate his leg from the bed or gurney and to place the heel on his shin. This represents a profound muscle weakness. This indicates involvement of corticospinal fibers. The absence of tremor, nystagmus, or any other abnormal movement suggests that the basal nuclei and cerebellum are not involved.
FN2e 391–395, 530–533